Essentials of Dental Caries

Essentials of Dental Caries

Edited by **Kaley Ann**

New Jersey

Published by Foster Academics,
61 Van Reypen Street,
Jersey City, NJ 07306, USA
www.fosteracademics.com

Essentials of Dental Caries
Edited by Kaley Ann

International Standard Book Number: 978-1-63242-186-9 (Hardback)

Contents

Preface

This book aims to highlight the current researches and provides a platform to further the scope of innovations in this area. This book is a product of the combined efforts of many researchers and scientists, after going through thorough studies and analysis from different parts of the world. The objective of this book is to provide the readers with the latest information of the field.

This book discusses latest developments regarding etiology, pathogenesis, diagnosis and treatment of caries. With such advancements, it will soon become possible to completely defeat dental caries. It comprises of basic information regarding dental caries - its control, treatment and prevention, dental caries in kids and other minor caries. This book will be a valuable and rich source of information for students, practitioners, dentists and professionals engaged in this domain of medical science.

I would like to express my sincere thanks to the authors for their dedicated efforts in the completion of this book. I acknowledge the efforts of the publisher for providing constant support. Lastly, I would like to thank my family for their support in all academic endeavors.

Editor

Part 1

Caries Control and Prevention

Microbial Dynamics and Caries:
The Role of Antimicrobials

Andréa C.B. Silva[1], Daniela C.C. Souza[2], Gislaine S. Portela[2],
Demetrius A.M. Araújo[3] and Fábio C. Sampaio[2]
[1]Center of Sciences, Technology and Health,
State University of Paraiba, Araruna, Paraiba,
[2]Health Science Center, Federal University of Paraiba, João Pessoa, Paraiba,
[3]Center of Biotechnology, Federal University of Paraiba, João Pessoa, Paraiba,
Brazil

1. Introduction

The advancement of technology through the application of molecular techniques for identification and analysis of complex bacterial communities have demonstrated the diversity of the oral microbiota and the presence of numerous strains not previously described. Dental plaque is formed by the initial adhesion of pioneer bacterial species to film acquired from enamel, followed by secondary co-aggregation of these bacteria to other microorganisms of different genera and species. This mature dental plaque has some characteristics of multicellular organisms, such as cooperation mechanisms to obtain nutrients, resistance to environmental and communication stresses in order to regulate their growth (Marsh and Martin, 2009).

The understanding of the dental plaque structure as a microbial biofilm sheds light on the clinical relevance of antimicrobials usage (Zanatta et al, 2007). Biofilms have a more tolerant phenotype to antimicrobial agents, stress and host defenses than planctonic cultures, making them difficult to control (Socransky and Haffajee, 2002). This means that the effectiveness of agents used to prevent dental caries, specifically those compounds targeted to combat cariogenic pathogens, should be evaluated in biofilms rather than in traditional liquid cultures (Tenover, 2006). According to Wade (2010), high concentrations of Chlorhexidine (CHX) nearly eliminate all cells, and this is not interesting for microbiota balance in the oral biofilm. Successful antimicrobial agents are able to maintain the oral biofilm at levels compatible with oral health but without disrupting the natural and beneficial properties of the resident oral microflora (Marsh, 2010).

In this chapter, the etiology of dental caries will be briefly introduced focusing on the role of biofilms for initiation and progression of this disease. It will be followed by a thorough review of literature taking into account recent and novel antimicrobial strategies for biofilm control. Recent advances in anti-plaque agents, including those chemoprophylactic, antimicrobial peptides (anti-quorum sensing approach) and probiotics/replacement therapy will be analyzed. Both the discovery of new and effective drugs to control pathogenic biofilms as well as new delivery systems for oral environment will be the future focus of this research field.

2. Dental biofilm: Dynamics of biofilm formation

General microbial biofilms are defined as communities of microbes associated with any surface (Costerton et al., 1994). In dentistry the surface can be any tooth tissue (enamel, dentin), dental material or any other surface located in the oral cavity. This microbial complex system, also known as 'dental plaque" is organized as bacterial biofilm community that consists of more than 700 different bacterial species (Aas et al., 2005). It is also important to point out that the diverse community of microorganisms found on the tooth surface as a biofilm is embedded in extracellular matrix of polymers (Marsh, 2004).

Bacterial species are thought to play important role in the maintenance of oral health and in the etiology of oral diseases in humans (Socransky et al., 2002). Oral biofilms develop naturally and the resident plaque microflora contributes to the host defenses by preventing colonization by exogenous species (Marsh, 2003). Mechanisms contributing to colonization resistance include more effective competition for nutrients and attachment sites, production of inhibitory factors and creation of unfavorable growth conditions by the resident microflora (Marsh, 2004).

The composition of oral biofilms varies on distinct anatomical surfaces due to the prevailing physical and biological properties of each site (Bowden et al., 1975; Theilade et al., 1982). An important factor involved in oral biofilm formation is the need for specific intermolecular interactions between bacteria and receptors to occur selectively on the enamel surface. In addition to intermolecular interactions, initial attachment of bacteria on a surface is also mediated by nutrient availability, hydrophobicity and hydrophilicity between cell surface and substratum, proteins specificity (Marsh and Bradshaw, 1995).

Between routine oral hygiene procedures, communities re-form on enamel by sequentially adding bacterial constituents in a predictable manner. All bacteria exhibit the ability to adhere to at least one other species of oral bacteria and usually to multiple species. An inherent characteristic of many species of oral bacteria is their ability to recognize and attach to genetically distinct bacterial cells. This phenomenon is termed co-aggregation and has been linked to biofilm formation and maturation of dental plaque (Kolenbrander & Palmer, 2004). Microbial co-aggregation is also thought to be a universal trait of all biofilm bacteria (Rickard et al., 2003) enabling rapid colonization of surfaces and protection from external conditions contributing to survivability, particularly from antimicrobials (Filoche et al., 2004).

The spatial distribution of bacteria is affect by microbial metabolism which produces gradients in biologically significant factors. Gradients develop in key parameters that affect microbial growth (nutrients, pH, O_2, etc.). This will lead to vertical and horizontal stratification of the biofilm plaque and produce a mosaic of micro-environments (Marsh, 2000). These gradients are not linear and such heterogeneity may explain how organisms with apparently contradictory requirements (e.g. in terms of atmosphere, nutrition) are able o co-exist in plaque, and how they are able to influence the activity of antimicrobial agents at different locations within the biofilm (Marsh, 2003).

Biofilm communities are complex and dynamic structures that accumulate through sequential and ordered colonization of multiple oral bacteria (Kolenbrander et al., 2002). The development of a biofilm like dental plaque can be divided arbitrarily into several distinct phases:

Adsorption of host and bacterial molecules to the tooth surface to form of a conditioning film (acquired pellicle). Pellicle forms immediately following eruption or cleaning (Al-Hashimi and Levine, 1989) and directly influences the pattern of initial microbial colonization (Marsh, 2004).

Passive transport of oral bacteria to the pellicle-coated tooth surface. A non-specific reversible phase involving physic-chemical interactions among salivary bacteria and acquire enamel pellicle creates a weak area of net attraction facilitating reversible adhesion. Subsequently, strong, short-range interactions between specific molecules on the bacterial cell surface (adhesins) and complementary receptors in the pellicle can result in irreversible attachment (Lamont & Jenkinson, 2000) and can explain microbial tropisms towards surfaces. Many oral bacteria possess more than one type of adhesion on their cell surface.

Co-aggregation (co-adhesion) of later colonizers to already attached early colonizers. This co-aggregation that also involves specific interbacterial adhesion-receptor interactions (often involving lectins) leads to increased biofilm diversity (Kolenbrander et al., 2000). Co-adhesion may also facilitate the functional organization of dental plaque (Bradshaw et al., 1998).

Multiplication of attached microorganisms to produce confluent growth: Cell division leads to confluent growth and eventually, a three-dimensional spatially and functionally organized mixed-culture biofilm. Dental plaque functions as a true microbial community in which properties are greater than the sum of the component species (Marsh, 2004).

Active bacteria detachment from surfaces: Bacteria can respond to environmental cues and detach from surfaces, enabling cells to colonize elsewhere.

It has been suggested that oral biofilm formation consisted of two process involving separate mechanisms (Gibbons and van Houte, 1973). The first process was associated with adsorption of cells to the pellicle and required specific adhesions on the cell surface. The second step involved a build-up of cells biding to each other in a process termed co-adhesion.

Bacterial accretion through co-adhesion drives the temporal development of plaque biofilms that is characterized by bacterial successions and occurs over a time frame of weeks. The early biofilm consisted of pioneer organisms deposition followed by multiplication in morphologically distinct palisading columns of cocci (Rosan and Lamont, 2000). Pioneer species are predominantly streptococci (*S. sanguis*, *S. oralis* and *S. mitis*) (Marsh and Bradshaw, 1995). Although the oral streptococci initially predominate in plaque and can constitute up to 80% of early plaque, another significant colonizing species is *Actinomyces naeslundii*, and some haemophili (Rosan and Lamont, 2000).

Single cells of mainly Gram-positive coccoid cells can be seen by microscopy on pellicle-coated surfaces, together with a few rod-shaped organisms, after few hours (2-4h) of plaque formation (Marsh and Bradshaw, 1995). The attached cells then divide rapidly to form microcolonies in the first instance, which coalesce to form a confluent film of varying thickness (Nyvad and Fejerskov, 1989).

After 1-2 days, Gram-positive rods and filaments can be observed extending outwards from microcolonies of mainly coccoid cells. After several days of development, morphological and cultural microflora diversity increases. The biofilm depth increases and its structure becomes more varied. If plaque is left to develop undisturbed on exposed enamel surfaces for 2-3 weeks, a climax community will establish and bacterial composition will become relatively constant overtime (Marsh and Bradshaw, 1995).

A very important key point on biofilm formation is the synthesis of extracellular polyssacharides from sucrose by adherent bacteria (Figure 1). These insoluble molecules are considered very important contributors in the structural integrity and pathogenic properties of biofilms.

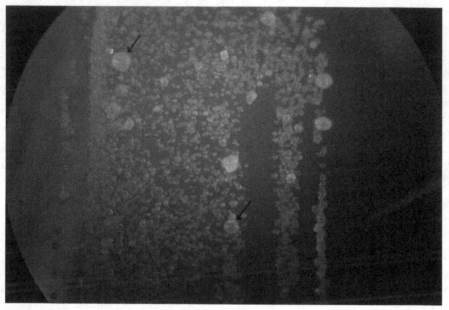

Fig. 1. Production of extracellular polymers of *S. mutans* UA159 under planktonic form of growth with sucrose enriched medium. Note arrows that indicate the presence of polymers. (40x)

Confocal laser scanning microscopy techniques has demonstrated that "dental plaque" has a similar architecture to biofilms from others sites. Dental plaque has open architecture, with channels traversing from the biofilm surface through to the enamel (Wood et al., 2000; Zaura-Arite et al., 2001). This structure will have important implications for penetration and distribution of molecules within plaque.

One of the most notable features of clinical relevance with respect to phenotype of micro-organisms growing on a surface is the increased resistance of biofilms to antimicrobial agents (Mah and O'Toole, 2001). Bacteria growing as a biofilm frequently express phenotypes that are different from those of planctonic bacteria and one possible consequence can be a reduced sensitivity to inhibitors. Most pre-clinical trials for testing oral antibacterial products used planctonic techniques where cells grow freely without any effect of biofilm structure. Therefore, most products that showed good in vitro results did not show similar effects under clinical evaluations (Guggenheim et al., 2004; Leibovitz et al., 2003; Marsh, 2004). The observation that genetic expressions of *S. mutans* are not the same for planctonic and biofilm forms of organization supports that most antimicrobials need biofilm techniques for reproducing more closely to the oral environment in *vivo* (Marsh, 2004).

A greater understanding of the significance of oral biofilms as a complex bacterial structure will have the potential to impact significantly on clinical practice (Marsh, 2004). Biofilms in nature are often difficult to investigate and experimental conditions are not completely defined. Therefore, a number of different laboratory-based experimental biofilm model systems have been developed (Palmer, 1999). These systems allow studies on biofilms under defined conditions. Such systems are necessary in order to perform well-controlled reproducible experiments (Tolker-Nielsen et al., 2000). Various multispecies models of biofilm testing procedures have been described and applied to problems of clinical relevance, most notably biofilm permeability and chemical control. These systems usually consist either of flow cells (Christersson et al., 1987; Larsen and Fiehn, 1995) or chemostats modified to allow for insertion and removal of colonizable surfaces (Bowden, 1999; Bradshaw et al., 1996; Herles et al., 1994), and these devices have contributed to our understanding of microbial adhesion and biofilm formation. In spite of the great development on oral biofilms studies, there is still a room for improvement. Thus, new insights will be presented in the near future on this topic.

3. Communication microbial biofilms: *Quorum sensing* mechanisms

In the dental biofilm bacteria do not exist as independent entities, but as a coordinated and metabolically integrated microbial community (Marsh & Bowden, 2000). This interaction provides enormous benefits to the participating organizations compared to the same bacteria grown in planctonic form, including: a wider range of habitat for growth, increased diversity, increased metabolic efficiency and greater resistance to environment, antimicrobial agents and host defenses (Shapiro, 1998; Marsh & Bowden, 2000).

The heterogeneity and high bacteria density within biofilms promote genotypic and phenotypic changes through releasing of self-inducers in the environment, leading to modification of gene expression (virulence genes of exoenzymes, exopolysaccharides) and at the same time, the acquisition of a important competitive advantage for survival and perpetuation in natural environments, highly competitive (eg, oral cavity, intestine), where hundreds of species coexist (Shei & Petersen, 2004). These virulence factors mediated by self-inductors were called "quorum sensing" (Fuqua et al., 1994).

The *quorum sensing* (QS) is a communication process among microorganisms mediated by population density. The main QS' regulation mechanism is given by production of auto-inducers released into the external environment, where they accumulate, and the interaction with its receptor, which may be intracellular or present in cell surface (Nealson et al, 1970; Hens et al., 2007). When its concentration reaches a certain threshold, it promotes the activation or repression of several genes causing cells to exhibit new phenotypes (Redfield, 2002).

The first indication that bacteria communicate through chemical signals came from studies of Nealson et al. (1970). They studied the bioluminescence regulation in the marine bacterium *Vibrio fischeri*, which has a symbiotic relationship with marine animals such as squid. In this regard, the host uses the light produced by the bacterium, to attract preys and partners or ward off predators, while the *V. fischeri* obtains necessary nutrients from its host (Nealson et al., 1970).

The luminescence is observed only when bacteria colonize the host's organs and by increasing the number of bacteria in the medium they are able to perceive cell density by detecting the auto-inducer concentration. Upon reaching a threshold concentration of self-induction, it is enough to trigger the process of gene transcription (Swem et al., 2009).

The self-inducers involved in this process may be of different chemical nature, in gram-negative organisms the signaling molecules are derived from N-acyl homoserine lactone (AHL) and its regulation occurs through homologous proteins LuxR and LuxI. The first protein acts as an enzyme (AHLsintetase) and second, when connecting to the AHL, forms the AHL-LuxR the complex, which is responsible for the activation and expression of numerous genes. In gram-positive, self-inducers usually correspond to small peptides (hepta and octapeptides). These peptides are usually secreted by carriers bound to ATP (ABC). Some interact with membrane-bound kinases sensors carrying a flag through the membrane; others are transported into the cell by oligopeptide permeases, which then interact with intracellular receptors (Swem et al., 2009; Rock Road, et al., 2010).

In QS systems via AHLs, the variation in the acyl chain (chain length, degree of oxidation and saturation) may confer some specificity to these communication systems. Thus, there seems to be some cross-talk among bacteria belonging to different genera. Part of this cross-talk may represent a way by which bacteria acquire information about the total population, allowing a response to competitors or prospective members (Williams, 2007). *E. coli* does not synthesize AHLs but express a homologous biosensor LUXR (SDIA). It is speculated that this system allows *E. coli* detecting communication signals of other gram-negative and exploiting such information for its own benefit (Ahmer, 2004).

The gram-negative bacterium, *Streptococcus mutans*, a major pathogen of dental caries, performs the quorum-sensing by releasing mediator peptides of gene expression. The signaling system involves at least six gene products encoded *comCDE, comAB and comX* (Cvitkovitch et al., 2003). The OMCC gene encodes a precursor peptide, which when cleaved and exported release a signal peptide, 21 amino acid or stimulating competence peptide (CSP). Through the quorum-sensing, it was found that the competence-stimulating peptide (CSP) was necessary for proper formation of *S. mutans* biofilm in addition to its virulence characteristics (Li et al., 2001).

The quorum sensing systems control a variety of microbial processes such as sporulation, virulence, biofilm formation, conjugation and production of extracellular enzymes (Miller & Bassler, 2001). Bacteria use QS to coordinate gene expression within species. Moreover, the same detection signals are used to inhibit or activate transcription programs between competing bacteria strains and other existing species in the same microenvironment (Bassler, 2002). Communication can still cross the borders of the kingdom, as QS effector molecules that can alter the eukaryotic transcription programs, found in epithelial cells and immune effector cells (Williams, 2007; Shin et al., 2005).

The discovery that *S. mutans* performs quorum-sensing of the system ideal in growing biofilms led us to investigate other features of this system in biofilm formation and biofilm physiology. The strategy for control of microorganisms by interfering in QS systems presents an important alternative for control of oral biofilms.

4. Antimicrobials: Mechanisms of action

Antimicrobials can be bactericidal (kill the microorganism directly) or bacteriostatic (prevent the microbe growth). In the case of bacteriostatic drugs, host defenses such as phagocytosis and antibody production usually destroy the microorganism. With the suspension of the second type of drug, bacteria can grow back. For bacteriostatic and bactericidal actions are apparent it is necessary to determine the MIC (Minimum Inhibitory Concentration) and MBC (minimum bactericidal concentration). As the therapeutic activity of antibiotics depends, among other factors, on their concentrations in body fluids, MICs and CBMs are essential determinations, since the establishment of the antibiotic regimen depends on them. The MIC and MBC are estimated in vitro, but used to determine bacteriostatic and bactericidal concentrations of antibiotics in body fluids (Maillard, 2002).

In Biofilms, MIC and MBC of antimicrobial agents usually must be greater than those required for plancttonic cells, due to its greater resistance to these drugs. In addition, optimal antimicrobials indicated for diseases that have bacteria organized in biofilms as etiological agent, must have good distribution in these structures. The main mechanisms of action of antimicrobials include: inhibition of cell wall synthesis, inhibition of protein synthesis, plasma membrane damage, inhibition of the synthesis of nucleic acids and inhibition of the synthesis of essential metabolites (Maillard, 2002).

Cell Wall Inhibition. The bacterium's cell wall consists of a network of macromolecules called peptidoglycan, which is found exclusively in bacteria's cell wall. Penicillin and other antibiotics prevent complete synthesis of peptidoglycan, consequently, the cell wall becomes fragile and cell undergoes lysis. As penicillin targets the synthesis process, only cells in active growth will be affected by this antibiotic. And as human cells do not have peptidoglycan, penicillin has low cytotoxicity to the host cell (Broadley et al. 1995).

Inhibition of Protein Synthesis. Protein synthesis is a characteristic common to all cells, both prokaryotes and eukaryotes, not presenting therefore a suitable target for selective toxicity. Eukaryotic cells have 80S ribosomes and prokaryotic cells have 70S ribosomes. The difference in the ribosome structure is responsible for selective toxicity to antibiotics that affect protein synthesis. However, the mitochondria (important cytoplasmic organelles) also has the 70S ribosomal unit similar to bacteria units. Antibiotics that act on the 70S ribosome may therefore have adverse effects on host cells. Among the antibiotics that interfere are the clorofenicol, erythromycin, streptomycin, and tetracycline (Nakamura & Tamaoki, 1968).

Damage to the plasma membrane. Certain antibiotics, especially polypeptide antibiotics, promote changes in the permeability of plasma membrane. These changes result in the loss of major metabolites of the microbial cell. For example, polymyxin B disrupts the plasma membrane by binding to membrane phospholipids (Lambert & Hammond, 1973). Likewise, planktonic cells, when exposed to higher concentrations of the chlorhexidine (CHX), suffer membrane rupture (Figure 2). This observation can be explained by the fact that CHX, which is positively charged, binds tightly to negatively charged bacteria membrane, causing its disruption (Gilbert & Moore, 2005).

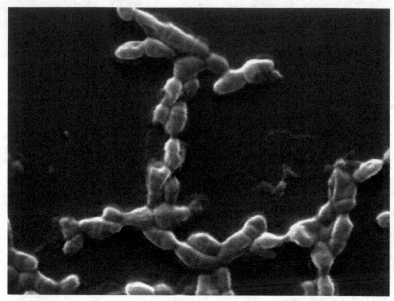

Fig. 2. Scanning electron micrograph of planktonic *S. mutans* UA159 cells exposed to chlorhexidine at 4.5 μg/ml. After 6h of CHX incubation, several wilted cells with spilled intracellular material could be observed (15 kV and 13.000x of magnification).

Inhibition of nucleic acids synthesis. Some antibiotics interfere with the processes of DNA transcription and replication of microorganisms. Some drugs with this mode of action have limited use due to interference with DNA and RNA of mammals. Others, such as rifampin and quinolones, are more widely used in chemotherapy by having a higher degree of selective toxicity (Silver, 1967).

Inhibition of Synthesis of Essential Metabolites. The enzymatic activity of a specific microorganism can be competitively inhibited by a substance (antimetabolites) that closely resembles enzyme's normal substrate (Russell and Hugo, 1994).

5. Recent advances in anti-plaque agents: Chemoprophylactic agents, antimicrobial peptides, anti-quorum sensing approach and probiotics/replacement therapy

Control of oral biofilms is essential for maintaining oral health and preventing dental caries, gingivitis and periodontitis. However, oral biofilms are not easily controlled by mechanical means and represent difficult targets for chemical control (Socransky, 2002). With the exception of chlorhexidine and fluoride, few of the existing oral prophylactic agents have significant effects (Petersen & Scheie, 1998; Wu & Savitt, 2002; Scheie, 2003). A likely explanation for this low efficiency is due to the fact that microorganisms organized in biofilms possess characteristics that differentiate them from planktonic cells, such as higher resistance to several antimicrobial agents; most studies so far use study models with planktonic cells, not reproducing the reality of the oral cavity. In addition, antimicrobials for oral use must have adequate diffusion in biofilms to be effective (Marsh, 2005).

Thus, many of these studies need to be revalidated, taking into account the oral environment. Recent approaches to the study of microbial gene expression and regulation in non-oral microorganisms have elucidated systems for transduction of stimuli in biofilms, such as two-component systems and quorum sensing (two-component and quorumsensing systems) that allow the coordinated gene expression in these structures. These studies based on understanding the regulation and expression in microbial biofilms can potentially benefit the development of new strategies for prevention and treatment of diseases caused by oral biofilms. Thus, the intervention should be directed at targets such as surface adhesion, colonization, co-adhesion, metabolism, growth, adaptation, maturation, climax community and detachment, and strategies must be based on surface modification, immunization, replacement therapy , interference with two-component systems and quorum sensing (Scheie, 2004).

These new drugs must be highly specific, have little ability to induce resistance in microorganisms and produce minimal effects on vital functions of human cells. In therapeutic approaches, the main target should be the mature and established biofilm. In this case, genes and proteins essential for viability of microorganisms represent the traditional targets for designing these antimicrobial drugs. Among these potential agents are included bacteriophages, inhibitors of the biosynthesis of fatty acids and antimicrobial peptides (Hancock, 1999, Payne et al. 2001; Sulakvelidze & Morris, 2001). In prophylactic approaches, the main targets are the pathogenic microorganisms directly involved in the formation of mono or multi-species biofilms. Promising targets for this purpose would be the two-component systems and quorum sensing, whose inference could be used to ensure the ecological balance in the biofilm, allowing the maintenance of health-related microbiota (Marsh, 2010). This approach would have a selective toxicity, since these systems are present in most microorganisms, but not in mammalian cells, which use other mechanisms of signal transduction.

Another important strategy is the modification of tooth surface or, more precisely, the film acquired from the enamel to prevent bacterial colonization and thus biofilm formation. The film acquired from enamel has binding sites for oral bacteria through specific and nonspecific binding mechanisms. An in vitro study showed that the combination of alkylphosphate and a nonionic surfactant changes the characteristics of tooth surface, making it less attractive for microorganisms. However, the clinical efficacy of these agents has been low, probably due to difficulties in obtaining the active components of these agents (Olsson, 1998).

Some properties of topical antimicrobial agents for oral use are essential to their success as high substantivity in the oral sites of biological action, low acute and chronic toxicity, and low permeability, being overall associated with their mechanism of action. Clinical activity of the antimicrobial agent depends on the drug formulation that must have a quick and efficient release vehicle. The supragingival plaque, film acquired from enamel and saliva may be primary sites of action for these agents, but the detailed understanding of these interactions is limited. These antimicrobials are retained by electrostatic bonds to carboxylic acids and phosphate and sulfate residues of proteins and glycoproteins in the oral mucosa, film acquired from enamel and plaque. The non-ionic antibacterials are retained by adsorption to lipophilic regions in these receptor sites. The ability of these antiplaque agents have to keep an optimal concentration in saliva over a long period, in addition to remaining in the bioactive form at the action sites, such as the teeth surfaces is extremely important and influence in the clinical effectiveness of these agents (Cummins & Creeth , 1992).

The analysis of retention characteristics and antimicrobial properties of clinically proven antiplaque agents suggest that they act multifunctionally and at multiple sites. Thus, they reduce growth and metabolism of bacteria in plaque, saliva and tooth surface, but also reduce the adhesion of potential settlers. Two generic routes to increase the antiplaque activity of these agents have received attention. Firstly the use of a combination of antimicrobial agents with similar but complementary activities uses only one route and mode of action. A second potential route is the use of a polymer that serves as auxiliary retention of only one antimicrobial used (Cummins, 1991b).

The total oral retention, salivary profile and agent concentrations on the plaque, film acquired from enamel and oral mucosa are not only indicators of biological activity in vivo, but they serve as potential indicators for this activity. This means that the increased release of a specific agent in vivo is not predictive of its increased clinical efficacy (Cummins, 1991b). The increased activity on the site or sites of biological action combined with agent's residence time in the oral cavity are the best predictors of agent's clinical activity (Creeth & Cummins, 1992).

Replacement therapy has been suggested as a strategy for replacement of pathogenic microorganisms modified to become less virulent. Some requirements for this type of approach are important, such as: the replaced organism must not cause disease by itself; it must persistently colonize and must possess a high degree of genetic stability. DNA technology has enabled to produce potential candidates for replacement therapy in the prevention of dental caries. Among these, there is the super-colonizing strain of *S. mutans*. This strain produces mutacin, which allows it to replace the wild-type strain efficiently. It lacks the enzyme lactate dehydrogenase and therefore is unable to produce lactate (Hillman et al., 2000). Other ureolitic recombinant strains have been constructed and are capable of hydrolyzing urea to ammonia, thereby offsetting the environment acidification (Clancy et al., 2000).

A possible future approach would be to use genetically modified microorganisms for releasing molecules that could interfere with pathways such as signal transduction of two-component and quorum sensing. However, it is important to emphasize that there is the possibility of a genetically modified strain subsequently undergoes transformation in oral biofilms and then becomes a pathogenic opportunistic strain (Scheie, 2004).

Immunization against oral diseases as dental caries and periodontal disease has been extensively studied in recent decades (Koga et al. 2002; Smith, 2002). The goal would be inhibiting or reducing the virulence of some microbial etiological agents. Several molecules involved in various stages of the pathogenesis of caries and periodontal disease could be susceptible to immune intervention and serve as targets for production of vaccines. Thus, it would be possible to eliminate microorganisms of the oral cavity with antibodies able to block adhesins or receptors involved in adhesion, or metabolically modify important functions or virulence. Efforts are being made for manufacturing active and passive vaccines, especially for tooth decay. In active immunization, an attenuated antigen induces a protective immune response when administered. In passive immunization, the ready antibody is administered (Sheie, 2004).

Studies on animals and humans using approaches with active and passive immunization have been successful, especially in passive immunization where there is impediment to recolonization of microorganisms related to dental caries (Koga et al. 2002; Smith, 2002) and also in periodontal disease (Booth et al., 1996). The vehicles for passive immunization, such as milk from immunized cows (Shimazaki et al., 2001) and transgenic plants (Ma et al., 1998), have been tested with promising results. Similarly, it was shown that recombinant chimeric microbial vectors that are non-virulent, but express antigens of S. mutans (Huang et al., 2001, Taubman et al., 2001) or P. gingivalis (Sharma et al., 2001) promoted protection against tooth decay and loss of alveolar bone in experimental animals.

One of the issues that still need to be solved is about which immune system should be stimulated, if the systemic immune system or that associated with mucosal. In the case of an anti-caries vaccine, it would be more interesting the oral administration and based on induction of the immune system associated with mucosa. A vaccine against periodontal disease should probably involve the systemic immune system and that associated with mucosa. A major problem is that approaches to immunization are usually directed against epitopes of isolate bacteria; however, both tooth decay and periodontal disease are diseases whose etiologic agent consists of a multispecies microbiota (Marsh, 1994). Moreover, since microorganisms have the ability to form biofilms and adapt to this environment, this can lead to changes in antigenicity which could affect the durability of protection induced by immunization.

An alternative approach are a new class of antibiotics called of antimicrobial peptides (AMP) that can be used against these microorganisms (White et al., 1995, Yount & Yeaman, 2004; Hancock & Sahl, 2006; Gardy et al., 2009); however, a poor understanding of the fundamental principles of the action mechanisms and structure-activity relationship of these drugs (Shai, 2002; Bechinger, 2009) has reduced the development of MPAs that can be used clinically.

The potential advantages of using antimicrobial peptides as antimicrobial drugs are significant (Hamill et al., 2008, Easton et al., 2009). They have a broad spectrum of activity against many strains of Gram positive and negative bacteria, including strains resistant to other drugs, and are also active against some fungi. Moreover, their interactions with bacterial components do not involve binding sites to specific proteins and thus do not induce resistance. The AMP bioavailability is reduced because they cannot be taken orally; however, topical applications and injections are available. Recently, AMP has been tested in clinical trials for various applications in oral candidiasis (Demegen Pharmaceuticals, 2010), infections associated with catheters (Melo et al., 2006) and infections in implant surfaces (Kazemzadeh-Narbat et al., 2010). These clinically tested AMPs are derived from natural peptides, this fact being responsible for its biggest drawback, which is the high production cost compared to other chemical antibiotics. For this reason, there is a critical need for development of new AMPs, powerful, small and with simple composition. The potential for the rational design of these drugs is often limited due to little knowledge about the details of its mechanism of action.

Since tooth decay is an infection, it would be logical to treat the disease with antibiotics or antimicrobials, such as antimicrobial peptides. However, most of these agents are not selective, have broad spectrum of action on the microorganisms such as chlorhexidine, iodopovidine, fluoride, penicillin or other antimicrobial/antibiotics. Importantly, the agents described above does not sterilize the oral cavity, since it is exposed to the external environment where there are many microbes, it is not a sterile space. Thus, the use of broad-spectrum agents for treating dental caries can suppress the infection, but will never eliminate it entirely (Luoma et al., 1978). In this context, due to the limitations of traditional strategies in the management of dental caries, a "probiotic" approach of the disease is necessary. The term "probiotic" used here means that mechanisms are used to selectively remove only the pathogen responsible for disease in an attempt to keep the oral ecosystem intact. Most efforts in this sense are derived from studies that have attempted to genetically modify strains of *Streptococcus mutans*, turning them into strains that in addition to not producing acids, still competing for the same ecological niche that wild strain of *S. mutans* (Hillman, 2002).

In theory and experimentally in laboratory animals, when this substitute organism is introduced, it completely shifts the wild *S. mutans* causing the disease. This action stops the decay process and also prevents the re-emergence of disease-causing organisms, eliminating the possibility of re-infection, since the "normal microbiota is complete." Another way to remove pathogens is developing specific antimicrobials for certain targets (Eckert et al., 2006). The basic principle is developing a cheap molecule that targets only the organism of interest, in this case *S. mutans*, *S sobrinus*, or other pathogens.

In the case of the oral cavity and tooth decay, this system is attractive from the perspective of eliminating all pathogens, thus preventing the re-growth of the original infection. There are also laboratory and clinical evidence demonstrating that when the biofilm's bacterial ecosystem is free of *S. mutans*, this bacterium finds it difficult to be reintroduced due to competitive inhibition with other microorganisms (Keene & Shklair, 1974; Shi, 2005). A criticism to probiotic approaches is that they target only one of the pathogens involved with the disease, being not directed at other pathogens that may be involved with the beginning of the process, as the case of dental caries.

6. The role of antimicrobials in the future

A better understanding of bacterial communities found in biofilms, such as its diversity and interactions among cells, provides opportunities for new methods to control biofilm formation (Wade, 2010). It has been shown that blocking communication mechanisms between cells in biofilms (quorum-sensing) can partially restore their susceptibility to antimicrobial agents (Bjarnsholt et al., 2005). Other benefits may include reduction of pathogenic microorganisms due to reduction in the virulence mechanism in the microorganism of interest. In the particular case of dental caries, blocking or reducing the activity of glycosyltransferase in *S. mutans* would be interesting, since these enzymes are implicated in the ability of this cariogenic bacterium.

In addition, probiotic approaches for oral use are being developed: such as the development of s *Lactobacillus paracasei* trains which maintain its co-aggregation activity with *S. mutans* even when dead (Lang et al., 2010), or *Lactobacillus reuteri* strains that are able to reduce the number of *S. mutans* in the mouth (Caglar et al., 2008) in order to decrease the incidence of tooth decay. Other bacterium normally found in the mouth, and important in this sense, is *Streptococcus salivarius*, which produces a bacteriocin that inhibits anaerobic Gram-negative bacteria and that in vivo was shown also to reduce the level of halitosis (Burton et al., 2006).

In conclusion, microbiota analysis methods independent of culture have allowed to understanding the diversity of the oral microbiota. So far, most studies have focused on the microbiota composition in the disease, but a better understanding of this microflora in health is required and also as probiotic organisms are capable of restoring and maintaining health in such environment. Thus, future studies are still needed, especially for analyzing the interactions between species and how to use this knowledge to develop new products for prevention and treatment of oral diseases.

7. References

Aas JA, Paster BJ, Stokes LN, Olsen I, Dewhirst FE. (2005). Defining the normal bacterial flora of the oral cavity. *J Clin Microbiol*, Vol. 43, n. 11, pp. 5721-32.

Ahmer BMM. (2004). Cell-to cell signaling on Escherichia coli and Salmonella enterica. *Mol Microbiol*, Vol. 52, p.933-945.

Al-Hashimi I, Levine MJ. (1989). Characterization of in vivo salivary-derived enamel pellicle. *Arch Oral Biol*, Vol. 34, n. 4, pp. 289-95.

Bassler BL. (2002). Small talk. Cell-to-cell communication in bacteria. *Cell*, Vol. 109, p. 421-424.

Bechinger B. (2009). Rationalizing the membrane interactions of cationic amphipathic antimicrobial peptides by their molecular shape. *Current Opinion in Colloid & Interface Science*, Vol. 14, pp. 349-355.

Bjarnsholt T, Jensen PO, Burmolle M, Hentzer M, Haagensen JA, Hougen HP, et al. (2005). *Pseudomonas aeruginosa* tolerance to tobramycin, hydrogen peroxide and polymorphonuclear leukocytes is quorum-sensing dependent. *Microbiology*; Vol. 151:(Pt 2), pp. 373–83.

Booth V, Ashley FP, Lehner T (1996). Passive immunization with monoclonal antibodies against *Porphyromonas gingivalis* in patients with periodontitis. *Infect Immun*, Vol. 64, pp. 422-427.

Bowden GH, Hardie JM, Slack GL. (1975). Microbial variations in approximal dental plaque. *Caries Res*, Vol. 9, n. 4, pp. 253-77.

Bowden GH. (1999). Controlled environment model for accumulation of biofilms of oral bacteria. *Methods Enzymol*, Vol. 310, pp. 216-24.

Bradshaw DJ, Marsh PD, Schilling KM, Cummins D. (1996). A modified chemostat system to study the ecology of oral biofilms. *J Appl Bacteriol*, Vol. 80, No. 2, pp. 124-30.

Bradshaw DJ, Marsh PD, Watson GK, Allison C. (1998). Role of Fusobacterium nucleatum and coaggregation in anaerobe survival in planktonic and biofilm oral microbial communities during aeration. *Infect Immun*, Vol. 66, No. 10, pp. 4729-32.

Broadley SJ, Jenkins PA, Furr JR, Russell AD. (1995). Potentiation of the effects of chlorhexidine diacetate and cetylpyridinium chloride on mycobacteria by ethambutol. *Journal of Medical Microbiology*, Vol. 43, pp. 458–460.

Burton JP, Chilcott CN, Moore CJ, Speiser G, Tagg JR. (2006). A preliminary study of the effect of probiotic *Streptococcus salivarius* K12 on oral malodour parameters. *Journal of Applied Microbiology*, Vol. 100, No. 4, pp. 754–64.

Caglar E, Kuscu OO, Cildir SK, Kuvvetli SS, Sandalli N. (2008). A probiotic lozenge administered medical device and its effect on salivary mutans streptococci and lactobacilli. *International Journal of Paediatric Dentistry*, Vol. 18. No. 1, pp. 35–9.

Christersson CE, Fornalik MS, Baier RE, Glantz PO. (1987). In vitro attachment of oral microorganisms to solid surfaces: evaluation of a controlled flow method. *Scand J Dent Res*, Vol. 95, No. 2, pp. 151-8.

Clancy KA, Pearson S, Bowen WH, Burne RA (2000). Characterization of recombinant, ureolytic *Streptococcus mutans* demonstrates an inverse relationship between dental plaque ureolytic capacity and cariogenicity. *Infect Immun*, Vol. 68, pp. 2621-2629.

Costerton JW, Lewandowski Z, DeBeer D, Caldwell D, Korber D, James G. (1994). Biofilms, the customized microniche. *J Bacteriol*, Vol. 176, No. 8, pp. 2137-42.

Cummins D (1991b). Zinc citrate/Triclosan: a new antiplaque system for the control of plaque and the prevention ofgingivitis: short term clinical and mode of action studies. *J Clin Periodontol*, Vol. 18, pp. 455-461.

Cummins D, Creeth JE. (1992). Delivery of Antiplaque Agents from Dentifrices, Gels, and Mouthwashes. *J Dent Res*, Vol. 71, No. 7, pp. 1439-1449.

Cvitkovitch DG et al. (2003). Quorum sensing and biofilm formation in streptococcal infections. *J Clin Investig*, Vol. 112, p.1626– 1632.

Demegen Pharmaceuticals. (2010). *Demegen Pharmaceticals Candidiasis Wedsite*.

Easton DM et al. (2009). Potential of immunomodulatory host defense peptides as novel anti-infectives. *Trends Biotechnol*, Vol. 27, pp. 582–590.

Eckert R, Qi F, Yarbrough k, He J, Anderson MH, Shi W. (2006). Adding selectivity to antimicrobial peptides: Rational design of a multi-domain peptide against Pseudomonas spp. *Antimicrobial Agents Chemother*, Vol. 50, No. 4, pp. 1480-1488.

Filoche SK, Zhu M, Wu CD. (2004). In situ biofilm formation by multi-species oral bacteria under flowing and anaerobic conditions. *J Dent Res*, Vol. 83, No. 10, pp. 802-6.

Fuqua WC et al. (1994). Quorum sensing in bacteria: the LuxR-LuxI family of cell density-responsive transcriptional regulators. *J Bacteriol, Vol.* 176, pp. 269-275.

Gardy JL et al. (2009). Enabling a systems biology approach to immunology: focus on innate immunity. *Trends Immunol*, Vol. 30, pp. 249–262.

Gibbons RJ, van Houte J. (1973). On the formation of dental plaques. *J Periodontol*, Vol. 44, No. 6, pp. 347-60.

Gilbert P, Moore LE. (2005). Cationic antiseptics: diversity of action under a common epithet. *J Appl Microbiol*, Vol. 99, pp. 703-715.

Guggenheim B, Guggenheim M, Gmur R, Giertsen E, Thurnheer T. (2004). Application of the Zurich biofilm model to problems of cariology. *Caries Res*, Vol. 38, No. 3, pp. 212-22.

Hamill P et al. (2008). Novel anti-infectives: is host defence the answer? *Curr Opin Biotechnol*, Vol. 19, pp. 628–636.

Hancock RE (1999). Host defence (cationic) peptides: what is their future clinical potential? *Drugs*, Vol. 57, pp. 469-473.

Hancock RE, Sahl HG. (2006). Antimicrobial and host-defense peptides as new anti-infective therapeutic strategies. *Nat Biotechnol*, Vol. 24, pp. 1551–1557.

Hense BA et al. (2007). Does efficiency sensing unify diffusion and quorum sensing? *Nat Rev Microbiol*, Vol. 5, pp. 230–39.

Herles S, Olsen S, Afflitto J, Gaffar A. (1994). Chemostat flow cell system: an in vitro model for the evaluation of antiplaque agents. *J Dent Res*, Vol. 73, No. 11, pp. 1748-55.

Hillman JD. (2002). Genetically modified *Streptococcus mutans* for the prevention of dental caries. *Antonie Van Leeuwenhoek*, Vol. 82, pp. 361-366.

Hillman JD, Brooks TA, Michalek SM, Harmon CC, Snoep JL, van Der Weijden CC (2000). Construction and characterization of an effector strain of *Streptococcus mutans* for replacement therapy of dental caries. *Infect Immun*, Vol. 68, pp. 543-549.

Huang Y, Hajishengallis G, Michalek SM (2001). Induction of protective immunity against *Streptococcus mutans* colonization after mucosal immunization with attenuated *Salmonella enterica* serovar typhimurium expressing an *S. mutans* adhesin under the control of in vivo-inducible nirB promoter. *Infect Immun*, Vol. 69, pp. 2154-2161.

Kazemzadeh-Narbat M et al. (2010). Antimicrobial peptides on calcium phosphate-coated titanium for the prevention of implant-associated infections. *Biomaterials*, Vol. 31, pp. 9519-9526.

Keene HJ, Shklair IL. (1974). Relationship of *Streptococcus mutans* carrier status to the development of carious lesions in initially caries free recruits. *J Dent Res*, Vol. 53, pp. 1295.

Koga T, Oho T, Shimazaki Y, Nakano Y (2002). Immunization against dental caries. *Vaccine*, Vol. 20, pp. 2027-2044.

Kolenbrander, PE, Andersen, RN, Kazmerak, KM, Palmer, RJ. (2000). Coaggregation and coadhesion in oral biofilms, In: *Community Structure and Co-Operation in Biofilms*, Allison, DG, Gilbert, P, Lappin- Scott, HM, Wilson, M, pp. 65–85, Society for General Microbiology Symposium 59, Cambridge University Press, Cambridge.

Kolenbrander, PE, Palmer, RJ. (2004). Human Oral Bacterial Biofilms, In: *Microbial Biofilms*, Ghannoum, M, O'Toole, G, pp. 85-117, American Society for Microbiology, Washington.

Kolenbrander PE, Andersen RN, Blehert DS, Egland PG, Foster JS, Palmer RJ, Jr. (2002). Communication among oral bacteria. *Microbiol Mol Biol Rev*, Vol. 66, No. 3, pp. 486-505.

Lambert PA, Hammond SM. (1973). Potassium fluxes. First indications of membrane damage in micro-organisms. *Biochemical and Biophysical Research Communications*, Vol. 54, pp. 796-799.

Lamont, RJ, Jenkinson HF. (2000). Adhesion as an ecological determinant in the oral cavity, In: *Oral Bacterial Ecology: The Molecular Basis*, Kuramitsu HK, Ellen RP, pp. 131–168, Horizon Scientific Press, Wymondham.

Lang C, Bottner M, Holz C, Veen M, Ryser M, Reindl A et al. (2010). Specific *Lactobacillus / Streptococcus mutans* coaggregation. *Journal of Dental Research*, Vol. 33, in press.

Larsen T, Fiehn NE (1995). Development of a flow method for susceptibility testing of oral biofilms in vitro. *APMIS*, Vol. 103, No. 5, pp. 339-44.

Leibovitz A, Dan M, Zinger J, Carmeli Y, Habot B, Segal R. (2003). Pseudomonas aeruginosa and the oropharyngeal ecosystem of tube-fed patients. *Emerg Infect Dis*, Vol. 9, No. 8, pp. 956-9.

Li YH et al. (2001). Natural genetic transformation of *Streptococcus mutans* growing in biofilms. *J Bacteriol*, Vol. 183, pp. 897–908.

Luoma H et al. (1978). A simultaneous reduction of caries and gingivitis in a group of schoolchildren receiving chlorhexidine-fluoride applications. Results after 2 years. *Caries Res*, Vol. 12, pp. 290-298.

Ma JK, Hikmat BY, Wycoff K, Vine ND, Chargelegue D, Yu L, *et al.* (1998). Characterization of a recombinant plant monoclonal secretory antibody and preventive immunotherapy in humans. *Nat Med*, Vol. 4, pp. 601-606.

Mah TF, O'Toole GA. (2001). Mechanisms of biofilm resistance to antimicrobial agents. *Trends Microbiol*, Vol. 9, No. 1, pp. 34-9.

Maillard J-Y. (2002). Bacterial target sites for biocide action. *Journal of Applied Microbiology*. Symposium Supplement, Vol. 92, 16S-27S.

Marsh PD (1994). Microbial ecology of dental plaque and its significance in health and disease. *Adv Dent Res, Vol.* 8, pp. 263-271.

Marsh, PD. (2000). Oral ecology and its impact on oral microbial diversity, In: *Oral Bacterial Ecology: The Molecular Basis*, Kuramitsu HK, Ellen RP, pp. 11-65, Horizon Scientific Press, Wymondham.

Marsh PD. (2003). Plaque as a biofilm: pharmacological principles of drug delivery and action in the sub- and supragingival environment. *Oral Dis*, Vol. 9, Suppl. 1, pp. 16-22.

Marsh PD. (2004). Dental plaque as a microbial biofilm. *Caries Res*, Vol. 38. No. 3, pp. 204-11.

Marsh PD. (2005). Dental plaque: biological significance of a biofilm and community life-style. *J Clin Periodontol*, Vol. 32, Suppl 6, pp. 7-15.

Marsh PD. (2010). Controlling the oral biofilm with antimicrobials. *Journal of Dentistry*, Vol. 38, S1; S11-S15.

Marsh PD, Bowden GHW. (2000). Microbial community interactions in biofilms. In: Allison DG et al. *Community Structure and Co-operation in Biofilms*. Society for General Microbiology Symposium Cambridge: Cambridge University Press, No. 59, pp. 167-198.

Marsh PD, Bradshaw DJ. (1995). Dental plaque as a biofilm. *J Ind Microbiol*, Vol. 15, No. 3, pp. 169-75.

Marsh PD, Martin MV. (2009). Oral Microbiology,5th edn. Edinburgh: Churchill Livingstone.

Melo MN, Dugourd D, Castanho MA. (2006). Omiganan pentahydrochloride in the front line of clinical applications of antimicrobial peptides. *Recent Pat Antiinfect Drug Discov*, Vol. 1, pp. 201-207.

Miller MB, Bassler BL. (2001). Quorum sensing in bacteria. *Annu rev microbiol*, Vol. 55, pp. 165-99.

Nakamura K, Tamaoki T. (1968). Reversible dissociation of *Escherichia coli* ribosomes by hydrogen peroxide. *Biochemica and Biophysica Acta*, Vol. 161, 368-376.

Nealson KH et al. (1970). Cellular control of the synthesis and activity of the bacterial luminescent system. *J Bacteriol*, Vol. 104, pp. 313-322.

Nyvad B, Fejerskov O. (1989). Structure of dental plaque and the plaque-enamel interface in human experimental caries. *Caries Res*, Vol. 23, No. 3, pp. 151-8.

Olsson J (1998). Inhibition of dental plaque by chemical surface modification. In: *Oral biofilms and plaque control*. Busscher HJ, Evans LV, editors. Amsterdam: Harwood Academic Publisher, pp. 295-309.

Palmer RJ, Jr. (1999). Microscopy flowcells: perfusion chambers for real-time study of biofilms. *Methods Enzymol*, Vol. 310, pp. 160-6.

Payne DJ, Warren PV, Holmes DJ, Ji Y, Lonsdale JT (2001). Bacterial fatty-acid biosynthesis: a genomics-driven target for antibacterial drug discovery. *Drug Discov Today*, Vol. 6, pp. 537-544.

Petersen FC, Scheie AAa (1998). Chemical plaque control: a comparison of oral health care products. In: Oral biofilms and plaque control. Busscher HJ, Evans LV, editors. Amsterdam: Harwood Academic Publisher, pp. 277-293.

Redfield RJ. (2002). Is quorum sensing a side effect of diffusion sensing? *Trends in Microbiology*, Vol. 10, No. 8, pp. 365-370.

Rickard AH, Gilbert P, High NJ, Kolenbrander PE, Handley PS. (2003). Bacterial coaggregation: an integral process in the development of multi-species biofilms. *Trends Microbiol*, Vol. 11, No. 2, pp. 94-100.

Rocha-Estrada J et al. (2010). The RNPP family of quorum-sensing proteins in Gram-positive bacteria. *Appl Microbiol Biotechnol*, Vol. 87, No. 3, pp. 913-923.

Rosan B, Lamont RJ. (2000). Dental plaque formation. *Microbes Infect*, Vol. 2, No. 13, pp. 1599-607.

Russell AD, Hugo WB. (1994). Antimicrobial activity and action of silver. *Progress in Medical Chemistry*, Vol. 31, pp. 351-371.

Shai Y. (2002). Mode of action of membrane active antimicrobial peptides. *Biopolymers*, Vol. 66, pp. 236-248.

Shapiro JA. (1998). Thinking about bacterial populations as multicellular organisms. *Annual Review of Microbiology*, Vol. 52, pp. 81-104.

Scheie AAa (2003). The role of antimicrobials. In: *Dental caries. The disease and its clinical management*. Fejerskov O, Kidd E, editors. Oxford: Blackwell Munksgaard, pp. 179-189.

Sharma A, Honma K, Evans RT, Hruby DE, Genco RJ (2001). Oral immunization with recombinant *Streptococcus gordonii* expressing *Porphyromonas gingivalis* FimA domains. *Infect Immun*, Vol. 69, pp. 2928-2934.

Sheie AA, Petersen FC. (2004). The biofilm concept: consequences for future prophylaxis of oral diseases? *Crit Rev Oral Biol Med*, Vol. 15, No. 1, pp. 4-12.

Shi W. (2005). Oral biofilm resistance to reinfection by *S. mutans*. In: Anderson M, ed. Selective removal of a specific microbe nearly precludes its reentry into the oral biofilm by competitive inhibition. Los Angeles.

Shimazaki Y, Mitoma M, Oho T, Nakano Y, Yamashita Y, Okano K, et al. (2001). Passive immunization with milk produced from an immunized cow prevents oral recolonization by *Streptococcus mutans*. *Clin Diagn Lab Immunol*, Vol. 8, pp. 1136-1139.

Shiner EK et al. (2005). Inter-kingdom signaling: deciphering the language of acyl homoserine lactones. *FEMS Microbiol Rev*, Vol. 29, pp. 935-947.

Silver SD. (1967). Acridine dye action at cellular and molecular levels. *Experimental Chemotherapy*, Vol. 4, pp. 505-511.

Smith DJ (2002). Dental caries vaccines: prospects and concerns. *Crit Rev Oral Biol Med*, Vol. 13, pp. 335-349.

Socransky S (2002). Dental biofilms: difficult therapeutic targets. *Periodontol 2000* 28:12-15.

Socransky SS, Haffajee AD. (2002). Dental biofilms: difficult therapeutic targets. *Periodontol 2000,*Vol. 28, pp. 12-55.

Socransky SS, Smith C, Haffajee AD. (2002). Subgingival microbial profiles in refractory periodontal disease. *J Clin Periodontol,* Vol. 29, No. 3, pp. 260-8.

Sulakvelidze A, Morris JG Jr (2001). Bacteriophages as therapeutic agents. *Ann Med,* Vol. 33, pp. 507-509.

Swem LR et al. (2009). A quorum-sensing antagonist targets both membrane-bound and cytoplasmic receptors and controls bacterial pathogenicity. *Mol Cell,* Vol. 35, No. 2, pp. 143-53.

Taubman MA, Holmberg CJ, Smith DJ (2001). Diepitopic construct of functionally and epitopically complementary peptides enhances immunogenicity, reactivity with glucosyltransferase, and protection from dental caries. *Infect Immun,* Vol. 69, pp. 4210-4216.

Tenover FC. (2006). Mechanisms of antimicrobial resistence in bacteria. *Am J Infect Control,* Vol. 34 (6 Suppl 1): 3S-10S discussion 64S-73S.

Theilade E, Fejerskov O, Karring T, Theilade J. (1982). Predominant cultivable microflora of human dental fissure plaque. *Infect Immun,* Vol. 36, No. 3, pp. 977-82.

Tolker-Nielsen T, Brinch UC, Ragas PC, Andersen JB, Jacobsen CS, Molin S. (2000). Development and dynamics of Pseudomonas sp. biofilms. *J Bacteriol,* Vol. 182, No. 22, pp. 6482-9.

Wade WG. (2010). New aspects and new concepts of maintaining "microbiological" health. *Journal of Dentistry,* 38, S1; S21-S25.

Wagner VE et al. (2007). Analysis of the hierarchy of quorum-sensing regulation in *Pseudomonas aeruginosa. Anal Bioanal Chem,* Vol. 387, pp. 469-479.

White SH, Wimley WC, Selsted ME. (1995). Structure, function, and membrane integration of defensins. *Cur Opinion Struc Biol,* Vol. 5, pp. 521-527.

Williams P. Quorum sensing, comunicação e reino cruzado de sinalização em todo o mundo bacteriano. *Microbiologia,* 2007.

Wood SR, Kirkham J, Marsh PD, Shore RC, Nattress B, Robinson C. (2000). Architecture of intact natural human plaque biofilms studied by confocal laser scanning microscopy. *J Dent Res,* Vol. 79, No. 1, pp. 21-7.

Wu C, Savitt E (2002). Evaluation of the safety and efficacy of overthecounter oral hygiene products for the reduction and control of dental plaque and gingivitis. *Periodontol 2000* 28:91-105.signatures in antimicrobial peptides. *Proc Natl Acad Sci,* Vol. 101, pp. 7363-7368.

Zanatta FB, Antoniazzi RP, Rösing CK. (2007). The effect of 0.12% chlorhexidine rinsing in previously plaque-free and plaque-covered surfaces. A randomized controlled clinical trial. *J Periodontol,* Vol. 78, n. 11, pp. 2127-2134.

Zaura-Arite E, van Marle J, ten Cate JM. (2001). Confocal microscopy study of undisturbed and chlorhexidine-treated dental biofilm. *J Dent Res,* Vol. 80, No. 5, pp. 1436-40.

2

Inhibitory Effects of the Phytochemicals Partially Hydrolyzed Alginate, Leaf Extracts of *Morus alba* and *Salacia* Extracts on Dental Caries

Tsuneyuki Oku, Michiru Hashiguchi and Sadako Nakamura
University of Nagasaki Siebold,
Japan

1. Introduction

Many studies on natural materials with anticariogenic effects have been carried out. Anticariogenic materials, such as polyphenols from oolong tea (Nakahara et al, 1993) and polyphenols from cacao (Ito et al, 2003), are known to be inhibitors of glucosyltransferases (GTases). These compounds have been used in foods to prevent or reduce dental caries. Sugar alcohols and oligosaccharides, which are not utilized as the substrate of GTase, are known as alternative sweeteners to sucrose (Kawanabe et al, 1992; Makinen et al, 1995; Ooshima et al, 1992; Van Loveren, 2004).

We investigated the potentiality of inhibitory effects of some phytochemicals on dental caries, because it is very interesting that phytochemical components inhibit the activity of not only GTase but also α-glucosidase. We have clarified that some phytochemicals such as partially decomposed alginate (Alg53), extractives from the leaves of *Morus alba* (ELM) and extractives from *Salacia chinensis* (ES) have inhibitory effects on disaccharidases such as maltase, sucrase and trehalase.

Alginate is a polyuronic saccharide that is isolated from the cell walls of a number of brown seaweed species around the world, and produced as an extracellular matrix by certain bacteria (Draget et al, 2003). It has a gelling ability, stabilizing properties and high viscosity. Alginate and its decomposed derivatives are widely used in foods, cosmetics and pharmaceutical industries (Ci et al, 1999; Johnson et al, 1997). Alginate hydrolysates exhibit many bioactivities, such as stimulating human keratinocytes, accelerating plant root growth and enhancing penicillin production from cultures of *Penicillium chrysogenum* (Ariyo et al, 1998; Kawada et al, 1997; Natsume et al, 1994). We have clarified that alginic acid with lowered molecule (mean molecular weight about 55,000) has suppressive effects on the elevation of blood glucose and insulin secretion (Oku et al, 1997) and improves defecation ant the fecal conditions (Oku et al, 1998).

Morus alba has traditionally been cultivated in China, Korea and Japan to use its leaves to feed silkworms. Recently, health benefits of *Morus alba* have been clarified and naturally occurring 1-deoxynojirimycin (DNJ) was isolated from its roots (Yagi et al, 1976). DNJ is glucose analogue with a secondary amine group instead of an oxygen atom in the pyranose ring of glucose. Then, DNJ has also been found in the leaves and fruits of *Morus alba* (Asano et al, 1994, 2001). Ever since, preventive effect of *Morus alba* on diabetes by α-glucosidase inhibitor has been extensively studied. Furthermore, *Morus alba* has been clarified multiple biological and physiological effects, as well as hypoglycemic, anti-oxidant and decrease in serum triacylglycerol (TG) level (Kojima et al, 2010). In a long term treatment study, intake of *Morus alba* does not cause harmful effects (Kimura et al, 2007).

The roots and stems of *Salacia* species plants have been used in the Ayurvedic system of Indian medicine to treat diabetes mellitus (DM) (Li et al, 2008). *Salacia* is a woody climbing plant belonging to the Celastrceae family that is found in limited regions of India and Sri Lanka. Currently, extracts of *Salacia* are consumed in commercial foods and food supplements in Japan for the treatment of diabetes and obesity. The water soluble portion of the methanolic extract inhibits α-glucosidase. Moreover, Beppu et al have reported that *Salacia reticulata* has improvement effect of fasting blood glucose and HbA1c levels in human including mild type 2 diabetics and has no toxicity (Beppu et al, 2006). The potential genotoxicity of *Salacia oblonga* extract was evaluated and it was determined not to be genotoxic (Flammang et al, 2006).

These phytochemicals, Alg53, ELM and ES competitively inhibit sucrase, maltase and trehalase of vesicles of the brush border membrane of rat intestine. The activity of GTase is inhibited by some polyphenols. We hypothesized that phytochemicals that inhibit α-glucosidases such as sucrase may also inhibit the synthesis of glucan from sucrose by GTase, because the latter is also a type of enzyme related to carbohydrate metabolism. Conversely, acarbose and DNJ are known to competitively inhibit sucrase and GTase, and suppress the postprandial elevation of blood levels of glucose and insulin (Newbrun et al, 1983). These chemicals are used as medicine for the treatment of DM.

We have investigated the anticariogenic effect of some phytochemicals using simple *in vitro* methods. The inhibitory effect of phytochemicals on the production of glucan from sucrose by GTase can be used for screening of the anticariogenic effects of natural materials. Surveys of natural materials with anticariogenic effects are important for reduction of the development of dental caries. Discovering new materials to prevent dental caries could expand the repertoire of the development of functional foods for oral health. These functional foods for oral health should be used in combination with different types of materials because the development of dental caries is related to multiple factors.

In this chapter, we introduce the procedures employed to evaluate the anticariogenic effects of phytochemicals. We also discuss the properties of three phytochemicals, Alg53, ELM and ES. Although many natural materials have been studied for anti-cariogenic effect, in our knowledge, this is the first and unique report that α-glucosidase inhibitor also inhibit GTase activity in natural materials. That is to say, Alg53, ELM and ES are expected as multiple functional food materials which have the effects of prevention to dental caries, diabetes and obesity. Moreover, if we search for natural materials that inhibit GTase, it might be a key point that certain materials have inhibition of α-glucosidase activity.

2. Evaluation of the anticariogenic effects of phytochemicals

Evaluation of the anticariogenic effects of phytochemicals is often tested on animals and eventually in humans. The *in vitro* experiments should be first done using a simple method.

Inhibitory Effects of the Phytochemicals Partially Hydrolyzed Alginate, Leaf Extracts of Morus alba and Salacia
Extracts on Dental Caries

23

Because the inducing factor of dental caries is complicate, some types of *in vitro* experiments have to be carried out and judged carefully to recognize characteristics of phytochemicals. Several typical methods are described below.

2.1 *In-vitro* experiments to evaluate anticariogenic effects

In vitro experiments to evaluate the anticariogenic effects of phytochemicals include observations of pH decline by acid production, inhibitory effects on glucan production by GTase from mutans streptococci and sucrose-dependent cell adhesion on smooth surfaces by mutans streptococci. In addition, antibacterial effect and the evaluation of plaque accumulation or enamel demineralization by using artificial mouth also have been investigated (Hinoide et al, 1984; Pigman et al, 1952). We have evaluated the anticariogenic effects of phytochemicals based on pH decline, glucan production by GTase and sucrose-dependent cell adhesion.

2.1.1 Evaluation of inhibitory effects on pH decline by acid production

Oral bacteria produce organic acids from sugars. If oral pH declines to approximately 5.5 due to organic acids produced, enamel demineralization of teeth begins. If organic acids produced from sugars by mutans streptococci are omitted or decreased and oral pH does not decline to 5.5, enamel demineralization is prevented by buffering action of saliva. Therefore, the degree of pH decline of the culture medium is measured during the incubation with oral bacteria (especially mutans streptococci) in the presence and absence of test substance with anticariogenic effects. Our procedure to measure pH decline is rapid and reliable. Cell suspension and phytochemical solution are added to 20 mM glucose solution in Stephan's buffer (pH 7.0) in a test tube (total volume, 1.0–2.0 mL), and incubated for 10–60 min at 37°C under anaerobic conditions after mixing. During incubation, the pH of the reaction medium is periodically measured with a portable pH meter (Hashiguchi-Ishiguro et al, 2009). Another method uses an incubation period of 24-48 h. But oral pH declines to about 4 immediately after the ingestion of sugars as glucose and sucrose (Lingström et al, 2000). Actually, the pH of reaction medium resulted in an immediate decline within 30 min in our study. In practical eating, if we intake sugars from meals or snacks, the food is masticated and swallowed within a few minutes and the pH in oral cavity declines. Therefore, the rapid and reliable method is suitable for *in vitro* assay.

2.1.2 Evaluation of inhibitory effects on glucan production by GTase

Water-insoluble and water-soluble α-linked glucans produced from sucrose due to the action of GTases adhere to the surfaces of teeth and promote the development of dental caries. GTase inhibitors disturb the production of these glucans and prevent the development of dental caries. The inhibitory effect of test substances on GTase has been evaluated by partially purified GTase from mutans streptococci, particularly *Streptococcus mutans* and *Streptococcus sobrinus*, which are considered to be the primary causative agents of dental caries in humans. Partially purified GTase can be conveniently used to evaluate the inhibitory effects of test substances on glucan production because it is stable and readily administered after preparation. If *S. mutans* and *S. sobrinus* are directly used to evaluate the inhibitory effects of test substances on glucan production, the assay is complicated and additional effort is required for the storage and administration of mutans streptococci. Hence, we are using a partially purified GTase from *S. mutans* and *S. sobrinus* to evaluate the inhibitory effects on glucan production. *S. sobrinus* GTase which synthesizes the water-insoluble glucan is released into the reaction medium during culture and that of *S. mutans* is localized mainly on the cell surface (Furuta et al, 1985). The properties and preparation method of GTase have been described (Baba et al, 1986; Furuta et al, 1985; Hamada et al, 1989).

An outline of our procedure to evaluate the inhibitory effect of phytochemicals on glucan production by GTase is given here. To measure the inhibition by phytochemicals for the synthesis of glucan from sucrose, 1 mL of 3% sucrose solution, 0.3 mL of GTase solution, 0.3 mL of test solution, and 1.4 mL of 0.1 M phosphate buffer are mixed and incubated at an angle of 20° for 24 h at 37°C. After the reaction is stopped in boiling water, the reaction mixture is centrifuged to separate water-insoluble and water-soluble glucans. The amount of total carbohydrate is measured using the phenol-sulfuric acid method (Dubois et al, 1956).

The phenol-sulfuric acid method is a popular and simple method for the determination of glucan produced by GTase (Koo et al, 2002). However, this method randomly determines the amount of whole carbohydrate in the sample without a clear difference between glucan production and the structure of phytochemicals in the reaction medium. Therefore, if the structure of test phytochemicals is similar to glucose polymer, alternative method is recommended to evaluate the inhibitory effect on glucan production. One method is the determination of radioactive carbon (^{14}C) transferred to glucan from ^{14}C-sucrose by GTase. Briefly, ^{14}C-sucrose is added to the reaction mixture mentioned above and incubated under identical conditions. After incubation, the amount of ^{14}C incorporated into glucan is measured by a liquid scintillation counter. This method requires specific facilities, but can specifically determine glucose incorporated to glucan fraction by GTase.

The preparation of GTase to evaluate inhibitory effects upon glucan production was carried out in our experiments. Briefly, to prepare partially purified GTase, after *S. sobrinus* 6715 was grown for 24 h at 37°C in 2 L of Brain Heart Infusion (Difco, Franklin Lakes, NJ, USA), the supernatant containing GTase was precipitated with 60% saturated $(NH_4)_2SO_4$ for 24 h at 4°C. Low-molecular weight (<30,000) proteins contained in the precipitate were removed using an ultrafiltration system (Millipore, Billerica, MA, USA). The crude GTase obtained was further purified by chromatography using a Bio-gel hydroxyapatite (BioRad, Hercules, CA, USA) column. GTase fractions eluted to 0.5 M with a linear gradient from 0.1 M to 0.6 M phosphate buffer (pH 6.8) were used for the assay of inhibitory effects of phytochemicals (Venkitaraman et al, 1995; Yanagida et al, 2000).

After *S. mutans* MT8148 was grown for 24 h at 37°C in 2 L of Brain Heart Infusion (Difco), the collected cells were suspended with 8 M urea to obtain the cell-extract solution. Low-molecular weight (<30,000) proteins contained in the solution were removed using an ultrafiltration system (Millipore). The resulting solution was used to evaluate the inhibitory effects on glucan production (Yanagida et al, 2000).

2.1.3 Evaluation of inhibitory effects on sucrose-dependent cell adhesion on smooth surfaces by mutans streptococci

When mutans streptococci are cultured in a medium containing sucrose, they strongly adhere on smooth surfaces. Dental biofilms are formed on teeth surface by interaction

Inhibitory Effects of the Phytochemicals Partially Hydrolyzed Alginate, Leaf Extracts of Morus alba and Salacia
Extracts on Dental Caries

25

between glucan and oral bacteria. Therefore, the measurement of sucrose-dependent cell adhesion is used to evaluate the formation of biofilms on teeth surface. If sucrose-dependent cell adhesion on the smooth surface is inhibited by phytochemicals, the test substance indicates the possibility to reveal anticariogenic effects.

This procedure has been described by Hamada and Torii (Hamada and Torii, 1978). After mutans streptococci (*S. sobrinus* or *S. mutans*) are grown in the medium, the collected cells are resuspended in the medium. The cell suspension (0.5 mL), sucrose solution (final concentration, 1%) and 0.3 mL of phytochemical solution are mixed in a new glass test tube, and incubated at angle 20° for 24 h at 37°C. After incubation, the reaction mixture containing nonadherent cell is gently removed by a Pasteur pipette. The glass test tube upon which mutans streptococci adhere to the surface is gently washed with distilled water at angle 20°. In the control, cell and glucan are not peeled by washing because of those are tightly adhere on test tube. Then, the cell and glucan are suspended in 1 N NaOH to measure absorbance at 550 nm.

We have tried to evaluate the inhibitory effect of phytochemicals using this method, described below (Hashiguchi-Ishiguro et al, 2011). The degree of inhibitory effects on cell adhesion correlated roughly with inhibition of glucan production by phytochemicals. Anticariogenic effects of extractives from red wine, apple polyphenols and propolis are evaluated using this method (Furiga et al, 2008; Hayacibara et al, 2005; Yanagida et al, 2000). In this method, the surface of glass test tube is used for smooth surface model of teeth. The glass test tube used in this method must be new one that has very smooth surface with no flaw. Human saliva-coated hydroxyapatite beads are used as teeth surface model in other method (Venkitaraman et al, 1995), because teeth consists mainly of hydroxyapatite. The model of latter method reflects the situation of oral environment. Koo et al have reported the details of the procedure (Koo et al, 2002, 2010).

2.2 *In-vivo* experiments to evaluate anticariogenic effects

If anticariogenic effects of phytochemicals are demonstrated by some *in vitro* experiments as described above, an *in vivo* experiment using experimental animals (e.g., rats) is carried out to confirm that the test material has anticariogenic effects in the systemic body. The animal experiment to evaluate anticariogenic effects consumes much expense and time. In other method, human plaque is also used the *in vivo* experiment. "Touch electrode method" and "plaque sampling method" are used for the purpose of measuring human plaque pH (Frostell, 1970; Stephan, 1940). Mühlemann et al develop " indwelling plaque pH telemetry method" (Graf H, et al 1966). In this section, we show an outline on animal experiment.

2.2.1 Animals and diets to evaluate anticariogenic effects

Fifteen-day-old specific pathogen-free Sprague–Dawley (SD) rats are suitable for caries studies. The first and second molars are coming through at this age. Mutans streptococci are inoculated to animals during this period. If inoculation lags behind, the prevalence of dental caries is reduced (Ooshima et al, 1994). The number of mutans streptococci that must be inoculated to definitely cause dental caries is very important. The breeding period after inoculation with mutans streptococci is about 55 days. Diet #2000 is a popular diet in animal experiments on caries (Keyes and Jordan, 1964) and contains 56% sucrose. If the percentage of sucrose is reduced, the prevalence of dental caries is also reduced. Phytochemicals are commonly added to the diet to evaluate anticariogenic effects. After breeding, the molar is removed and the degree of dental caries is scored. The details of the experimental protocol have been described (Ooshima et al, 1981; Tsunehiro et al, 1997). The typical procedure of caries scoring is the Keyes Caries Score (Keyes, 1958).

According to the established method, we have carried out animal experiments using phytochemicals that revealed anticariogenic effects *in vitro*. Young rats were fed with diet #2000 containing phytochemicals with anticariogenic effects for 60 days. However, our results were inconclusive. Therefore, we would like to describe some key points for the planning of animal experiments based on our experience.

2.2.2 Amount of mutans streptococci

If oral infection by mutans streptococci is not sufficient, dental caries is not induced in the experimental animal despite feeding with a caries-inducing diet. The amount of mutans streptococci adhered on teeth also influences the development of caries. Accordingly, the amount of mutans streptococci in the oral cavity should be measured periodically until the end of the experimental schedule. According to several studies, dental caries is definitely induced if the amount of mutans streptococci is $>10^5$ colony-forming units (CFU)/mL (Ooshima et al, 1993; Tsunehiro et al, 1997).

2.2.3 Amount of sucrose intake and texture of diets

Dental caries is positively correlated with the amount of sucrose intake (Sreebny, 1982). Therefore, the amount of diet that the animals ingest needs to be equal among feeding groups. Furthermore, the Vipeholm Dental Caries Study clarified that the texture of food containing sucrose influences the occurrence of dental caries (Gustafsson et al, 1954). In that study, subjects ate several foods (e.g., bread, chocolate, caramel) containing sucrose. The incidence of caries was higher in the group consuming "gooey" foods between meals than in the control group. Namely, the ingestion of sucrose that causes the adhesion to the teeth surface becomes a high risk of dental caries induction. Therefore, the texture and configuration of test materials containing phytochemicals added to the animal experimental diet are important to get significance. If the texture and taste of test substances are unique and likely to influence intake and adhesion, the method to reduce these factors should be implemented.

2.2.4 The indirect effect of anticariogenic substances on body except for tooth

The test substance might have multiple functions apart from anticariogenic effects. Test substances such as ELM, ES and Alg53, which have been used in our experiments, have inhibitory effect on α-glucosidase. Therefore, if experimental animals are given an α-glucosidase inhibitor and sucrose, the latter is not digested by intestinal disaccharidases and reaches the large intestine, where it is fermented by microbiota. These intestinal microbiota produce short-chain fatty acids, CO_2, NH_4 and H_2 (Oku, 2005). This action is similar to that of prebiotics such as non-digestible oligosaccharides and sugar alcohols ingested orally. These short-chain fatty acids are energy sources for the host and improve intestinal microflora. In this way, sucrose (the digestion of which in the small intestine is inhibited by

Inhibitory Effects of the Phytochemicals Partially Hydrolyzed Alginate, Leaf Extracts of Morus alba and Salacia
Extracts on Dental Caries

27

α-glucosidase) provides many beneficial effects. However, if a large amount of sucrose and α-glucosidase are ingested simultaneously, transient diarrhea is caused because of an increase in osmotic pressure in the large intestine. This mechanism is thought to identical to that of lactose intolerance.

When a diet containing ELM or ES is added to Diet #2000 and given to rats, most of the rats suffer osmotic diarrhea during the experimental period and growth is slightly suppressed. ELM and ES strongly inhibit sucrase activity. Hence, a lot of sucrose of Diet #2000 is transferred to the lower intestine and may cause osmotic diarrhea. Osmotic diarrhea may reduce the immune response, and disturb anticariogenic effect of phytochemicals in experimental animals. If experimental animals catch illness except for dental caries during the experiment, the risk of dental caries infection may increase. Therefore, the properties and functional effects of test substance apart from anticariogenic effects need to be examined, and the concentration and form of test substance added to diets should be investigated carefully before carrying out animal experiments.

3. Preparation and property of phytochemicals with anticariogenic effect

We have investigated the anticariogenic effects of phytochemicals such as ELM, ES and Alg53. Each of phytochemicals has unique properties and structure.

3.1 Extractive from the leaves of *Morus alba* (ELM)

Morus alba has been used for centuries in Japan as a tea infusion. *Morus alba* contains DNJ and some of its derivatives, which are well known as α-glucosidase inhibitors, as shown in Fig. 1 (Asano et al, 1994). D-glucose analogs such as voglibose, miglitol and acarbose, with nitrogen-in-rings, have been used for the treatment of DM (Drent et al, 2002; Raimbaud et al, 1992; Yasuda et al, 2003).

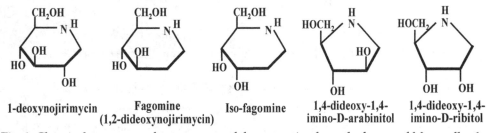

1-deoxynojirimycin   Fagomine   Iso-fagomine   1,4-dideoxy-1,4-   1,4-dideoxy-1,4-
                      (1,2-dideoxynojirimycin)   imino-D-arabinitol   imino-D-ribitol

Fig. 1. Chemical structures of components of the extractive from the leaves of *Morus alba*, 1-deoxynojirimycin and its derivatives

We have clarified that ELM competitively inhibits the activity of sucrase, maltase, and isomaltase using human and rat intestinal homogenates, and significantly suppresses the increment in blood glucose levels, when ELM is administered with sucrose to rats (Oku et al, 2006). In addition, we found that confections with ELM effectively suppress the post-prandial blood levels of glucose and insulin in healthy humans (Nakamura M et al, 2009). We suppose that confections with ELM can contribute to the prevention and the quality-of-life for pre-diabetic and diabetic patients.

To prepare the ELM solution, the leaves are extracted with 50% ethanol, and ethanol is removed with a rotary evaporator. ELM used in this study is kindly provided by Toyotama Healthy Food Co., Ltd. (Tokyo, Japan). The original extract solution contains 0.24% DNJ. A small amount of several types of DNJ derivative is measured using liquid chromatography-mass spectrometry (LC-MS). It has been clarified that this extraction is not associated with toxicity or hematologic, blood biochemical, or pathologic abnormalities in rats (Miyazawa et al, 2003).

3.2 Extractive from *Salacia chinensis* (ES)

The stems of *Salacia* species plants are pulverized and extracted with methanol for 3 h at 80°C. After filtration, the extract is evaporated to obtain a powder. The powder of the methanol extract is dissolved and purified using Sephadex LH-20 column chromatography. ES used in this study is kindly provided by Kobayashi Pharmaceutical Co., Ltd. (Osaka, Japan). Two compounds isolated from *Salacia* extracts, salacinol and kotalanol, strongly inhibit sucrase. Their structures are quite unique, bearing thiosugar sulfonium sulfate inner salt comprising a 1-deoxy-4-thio-D-arabinofranosyl cation and 1-deoxyaldosyl-3-sulfate anion (Fig. 2) (Shimoda et al, 1998; Yosikawa et al, 2001). It has been clarified that this extraction is not associated with toxicity or with blood biochemical or pathologic abnormalities in rats and other animals.

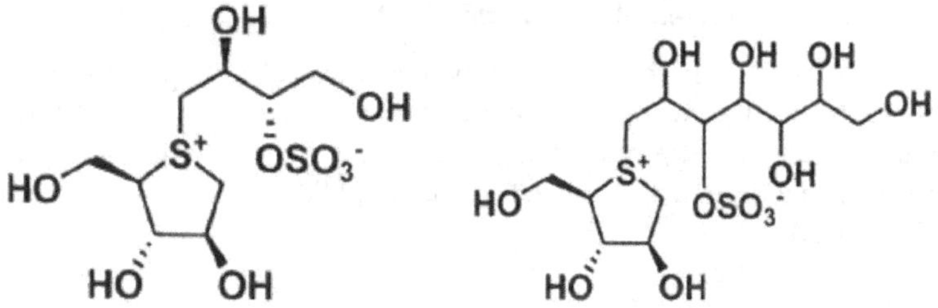

Salacinol   Kotalanol

Fig. 2. Chemical structure of components of the extractive from *Salacia chinencis* (ES)

3.3 Partially decomposed alginate by *Vibrio alginolyticus* SUN53 (Alg53)

Alginate, which is a copolymer of α-L-guluronate and β-D-mannuronate, is a gelling polysaccharide found in great abundance as part of the cell wall and intracellular material in brown seaweeds (Fig. 3) (Wong et al, 2000). We demonstrated that partially decomposed alginate by *Vibrio alginolyticus* SUN53 (Alg53) had a competitive inhibitory effect for sucrase of the vesicles of the intestinal brush border membrane of rats. The procedure for the preparation of Alg53 has been described (Nakamura S et al, 2008).

Alginate (0.5%) (mean M.W., 55,000) partially hydrolyzed by HCl is incubated with *Vibrio alginolyticus* SUN53 (10^6 CFU/mL) in culture medium (pH 7.0) containing 0.025% yeast extract, 0.05% peptone, 1% NaCl and 0.01% $FePO_4$ for 5 days at 25°C. After incubation, the supernatant is treated with 3 times-volume (75%) of ethanol to obtain low-M.W. hydrolyzed alginate. It is dried by freezing after ethanol is evaporated with a rotary evaporator. The

Inhibitory Effects of the Phytochemicals Partially Hydrolyzed Alginate, Leaf Extracts of Morus alba and Salacia
Extracts on Dental Caries

29

mean M.W. of partially decomposed alginate is approximately 1,000 by column chromatography using a Sephadex G-15 column. Tseng et al reported that alginate lyase isolated from *Vibrio alginolyticus* (ATCC17749) has specificity for polymannuronic blocks, and Haug et al reported that depolymerizing alginate by lyase yields a product containing deoxyuronic acid (Tseng et al, 1992; Haug et al, 1967). Therefore, it is considered that Alg53 also comprises penta- or hexa-mannuronic acid with deoxymannuronic acid as the non-reducing terminal moiety. The conversion ratio of Alg53 by *Vibrio alginolyticus* SUN53 is very low, so we could not obtain a sufficient amount of Alg53 for *in vivo* experiments using animals. We have to develop a culture condition in which Alg53 is produced effectively.

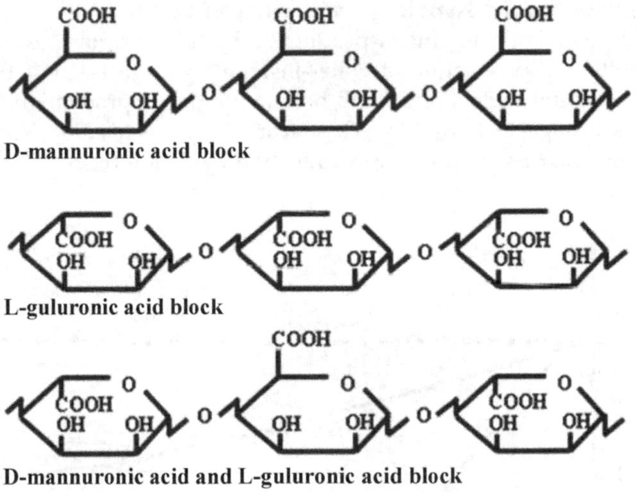

Fig. 3. Chemical structure of components of alginate

4. *In vitro* evaluation of the anticariogenic effects of phytochemicals

In this section, we introduce the anticariogenic effects evaluated using the three *in vitro* methods described above. The phytochemicals used in our experiments were Alg53, ELM, ES, and oolong as the positive control.

4.1 Effects of Alg53 on acid production by *S. sobrinus* 6715

The production of organic acids by *S. sobrinus* 6715 is illustrated in Fig. 4. The positive control maintained the initial pH. The results indicated that Alg53 disturbed the conversion of the substrate to organic acids. In contrast, the absence of Alg53 resulted in an immediate decline in pH after addition of the substrate, with the pH finally reaching 4.1. The addition of Alg53 suppressed pH decline and maintained a pH of 5.0. This suppressive effect for the production of organic acids was dependent upon the concentrations of Alg53 in the reaction mixture (Fig. 5). The inhibitory effect on pH decline was also investigated using ELM, ES and oolong, but these phytochemicals did not inhibit the pH reduction by *S. sobrinus* 6715.

4.2 Effects of ELM, ES, Alg53 and oolong on glucan production by GTase from *S. sobrinus* 6715 and *S. mutans* MT8148

Oolong has been used as a functional food to prevent dental caries. Oolong was therefore used to compare the inhibitory effects of other phytochemicals on glucan production by GTase. The inhibitory effect of phytochemicals on water-insoluble glucan synthesis by GTase from *S.sobrinus* 6715 is illustrated in Fig. 6A. The original ELM solution reduced the production of water-insoluble glucan to 66% of that of the control (ELM-free). ES also significantly reduced the synthesis of water-insoluble glucan. The inhibitory effect of ES was remarkable compared with that of ELM. The inhibitory effect of oolong on the production of water-insoluble glucan by GTase was stronger than that of ELM and of a similar level to that of ES. Fig. 6B shows water-insoluble glucan synthesis by GTase from *S. mutans* MT8148. ELM significantly inhibited the glucan production by GTase from *S. mutans* MT8148, and the ratio of inhibition of production of water-insoluble glucan was 64% that of the control (ELM-free). The inhibitory effect of ES and oolong on glucan production by GTase from *S. sobrinus* 6715 was stronger than that by GTase from *S. mutans* MT8148. The inhibitory effect of ELM was of a similar level on glucan production by GTase from *S. sobrinus* 6715 and *S. mutans* MT8148.

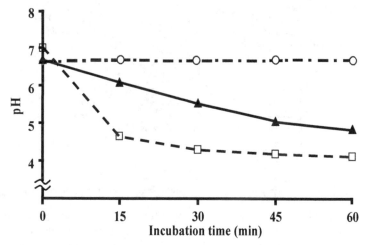

Open circle, positive control (no production of acid); open square, negative control (no inhibition); closed triangle, with Alg53
In the positive control (no production of acid), Stephan's buffer (pH 7.0) was added instead of glucose. In the negative control (no inhibition), distilled water was added instead of Alg53. Data are mean values of duplicate assays (Hashiguchi-Ishiguro et al, 2009).

Fig. 4. Time-course of pH decrease with acid production by *S. sobrinus* 6715 from glucose with and without partially decomposed alginate by *V. alginolyticus* SUN53

The inhibitory effect of Alg53 on water-insoluble and water-soluble glucan synthesis by GTase from *S.sobrinus* 6715 is illustrated in Fig. 7. The original Alg53 solution and a ten-fold dilution of Alg53 solution reduced the production of water-insoluble glucan to 21% and 23%, respectively. However, Alg53 barely affected the production of water-soluble glucan by GTase. These results demonstrated that Alg53 clearly inhibits the synthesis of water-insoluble (but not water-soluble) glucan by GTase from *S. sobrinus* 6715. Water-insoluble glucan is closely associated with the formation of biofilms on teeth surface. In addition, Alg53 has inhibitory effects on acid production and synthesis of glucan by mutans streptococci. That is, Alg53 has two types of anticariogenic effects. Accordingly, Alg53 may demonstrate considerable anticariogenic effects.

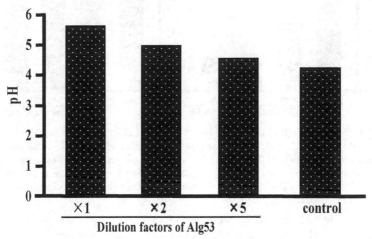

pH was measured after incubation for 1 h.
Control: water was added instead of Alg53
(Hashiguchi-Ishiguro et al, 2009)

Fig. 5. Inhibitory effect by different concentrations of partially decomposed alginate by *V. alginolyticus* SUN53 on acid production from glucose by *S. sobrinus* 6715

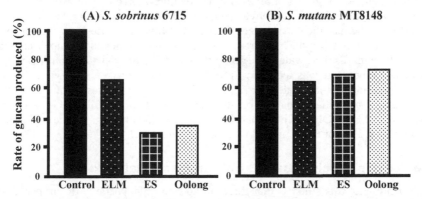

ELM, extractive from the leaves of *Morus alba*; ES, extractive from *Salacia chinensis*
Reaction mixture [GTase, 0.2 mL; sucrose solution, 0.31 mL (includes ^{14}C-sucrose, 20 μCi); test substance, 0.1 mL] incubated at 20° for 24 h at 37°C. The final concentration of sucrose in the reaction mixture was 1%. Glucan was expressed as the relative amount (%) of glucan produced as compared with the amount produced with the negative control (distilled water) (Hashiguchi et al, 2011).

Fig. 6. Inhibitory effects of the extractive from the leaves of *Morus alba*, *Salacia chinensis* and oolong on insoluble glucan produced by GTase

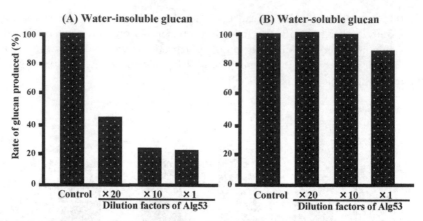

Reaction mixture [3% sucrose (final concentration, 1%) in 0.1 M phosphate buffer (pH 6.8), 1 mL; GTase from *S. sobrinus*, 0.3 mL; 0.1 M phosphate buffer (pH 6.8), 1.4 mL; Alg53, 0.3 mL] incubated at 20° for 24 h at 37°C. Glucan was expressed as the relative amount (%) of glucan produced as compared with the amount produced in the absence of Alg53. The amount of total carbohydrate was measured at 490 nm by the phenol-sulfuric acid method. Dates are expressed as mean values of duplicate assays (Hashiguchi-Ishiguro et al, 2009).

Fig. 7. Inhibitory effect of partially decomposed alginate by *V. alginolyticus* SUN53 on water-insoluble and water-soluble glucan produced by GTase from *S. sobrinus*

4.3 Effects of ELM and ES on sucrose-dependent cell adhesion on smooth surfaces

The inhibitory effect of ELM on sucrose-dependent adherence of cells onto the surface of glass test tubes was examined using growing cells of *S. sobrinus* 6715. Fig. 8A shows that cells adhered to the surface of glass test tubes after incubation. The cells grew well and adhered to the glass surface of the control (no phytochemical), ELM, ES and oolong. However, cells and glucan did not adhere to the glass surface of blank test tubes (sucrose-free). Fig. 8B shows the conditions of test tubes in which the reaction mixture was removed by pipetting, and then washed gently with distilled water. As shown clearly in Fig. 8B, cell adhesion was very strong in control test tubes, but was feeble in ELM, ES and oolong tubes; cells were removed by washing. The results demonstrate that ELM and ES inhibit the adhesion of cells to the glass surface. Adhered cells that remained on the surface of glass test tubes after washing were suspended with 1 N NaOH and absorbance measured at 550 nm (Fig. 9). The cell number was 60% for ELM and 21% for ES compared with that of the control.

5. Potential of phytochemicals as anticariogenic materials

The main finding of this study is that three phytochemicals, partially decomposed alginate by SUN53 (Alg53), the extractive from the leaves of *Morus alba* (ELM) and the extractive from *Salacia chinencis* (ES), have inhibitory effects on glucan synthesis by GTase. It may become a key point that certain phytochemicals have inhibitory effects on α-glucosidase when we screen natural materials which inhibit Gtase activity. However, the degree of inhibitory effect is not always similar for sucrase and GTase. The inhibitory effect of ELM and ES on sucrase was very strong. The inhibitory constant (Ki) of ELM and ES for sucrase was 2.1×10^{-4} mM and 6.7×10^{-4} mM, respectively (Oku et al, 2006).

Inhibitory Effects of the Phytochemicals Partially Hydrolyzed Alginate, Leaf Extracts of Morus alba and Salacia
Extracts on Dental Caries

33

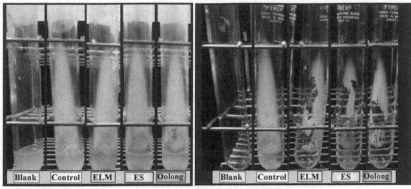

A: Right after incubation   **B: After washing**

ELM, extractive from the leaves of *Morus alba*; ES, extractive from *Salacia chinensis*
Reaction mixture [cell solution, 0.5 mL; 2% sucrose (final concentration, 1%) in BHI, 0.8 mL; test
substance 0.3 mL] incubated at 20° for 24 h at 37°C. In the blank, distilled water was added instead of
sucrose. In the negative control, distilled water was added instead of test substance (Hashiguchi et al,
2011).

Fig. 8. Adhesion of *S. sobrinus* 6715 and glucan on smooth surfaces of glass after incubation
with sucrose

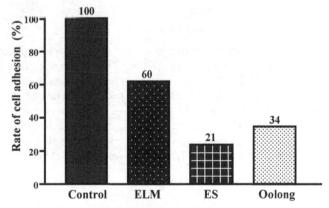

Fig. 9. Inhibitory effects of the extractive from the leaves of *Morus alba* and *Salacia chinensis*
on the adhesion of *S. sobrinus* 6715 and glucan (Hashiguchi et al, 2011)

In addition, Alg53 suppressed pH decline by the production of organic acids from glucose,
whereas ELM and ES could not suppress pH decline as well as oolong. For the prevention of
dental caries, Alg53 may be useful as a functional food that has two types of inhibitory
effects on the synthesis of glucan by GTase and acid production. Alternative sweeteners for
sucrose, such as sugar alcohols and oligosaccharides, are not used as substrates for acid
production by mutans streptococci, so pH decline does not occur. However, alternative
sweeteners cannot inhibit the production of organic acids from sugars. Therefore, we
recommend that ELM and ES are used in a combination of sugar alcohols or
oligosaccharides to prevent dental caries.

6. Future prospects of functional foods for the prevention of dental caries

In Japan, various types of functional foods have been developed and widely consumed for health promortion. Some of them have been advanced for prevention of dental caries. GTase inhibitors and sugar substitutes that are not the direct cause of dental caries are actively developed and utilized as preventive foods for dental caries. Recently, functional materials which enhance the defence system of host on dental caries are further added to those foods. For example, there are functional materials that promote re-mineralization of tooth and stimulate saliva excretion to block oral pH decline. The probiotics which improves oral bacterial flora may also be expected to be one of these functions. If functional materials that have different types of preventive effect for dental caries are combined in a functional food, the potential of functional foods may expand the food market for health promotion.

It is important that intraoral pH does not decline for prevention of dental caries among children, aduts and elderlies. So, sweeten confections between meals must have a resistance for utilization by mutans streptococci. However, dental caries cannot be completely prevented by the utilization of functional foods, although the risk of dental caries is decreased. Therefore, the combination of teeth brushing after meal and functional foods is very important for prevention of dental caries among all people. Furthermore, consumers need to pay attention, when they utilize some functional foods containing nondigestible oligosaccharide which improves the intestinal microbiota, because it produces acids to decrease oral pH.

7. Conclusion

We found that three phytochemicals that had inhibitory effects upon α-glucosidase also had inhibitory effects on glucan synthesis by GTase. This time we introduced partially decomposed alginate by SUN53, the extractive from the leaves of *Morus alba* and the extractive from *Salacia chinensis*. And Alg53 suppressed pH decline by the production of organic acids from glucose. Therefore, these phytochemicals are expected to be used as multiple functional food materials that can prevent the development of dental caries. Furthermore, these results may suggest that we propose the screening steps, another phytochemicals that have anticariogenic effects but haven't clarified yet.

8. References

Ariyo, B., Tamerler, C., Bucke, C. & Keshavarz, T. (1998). Enhanced penicillin production by oligosaccharides from batch cultures of penicillium chrysogenum in stirred-tank reactors. *FEMS Microbiology Letters*, Vol. 166, No. 1, (September, 1998), pp. 165-170, ISSN 0378-1097

Asano, N., Tomiola, E., Kizu, H. & Matsui, K. (1994). Sugars with nitrogen in the ring isolated from the leaves of *Morus bombycis*. *Carbohydrate Research*, Vol. 253, (February,1994), pp. 235-245, ISSN 0008-6215

Asano, N., Oseki, K., Tomioka, E., Kizu, H. & Matui, K. (1994). *N*-containing sugar from *Morus alba* and their glycosidase inhibitory activeties. *Carbohydrate Research*, Vol. 259, No. 2, (June, 1994), pp. 243-255, ISSN 0008-6215

Inhibitory Effects of the Phytochemicals Partially Hydrolyzed Alginate, Leaf Extracts of Morus alba and Salacia
Extracts on Dental Caries

35

Asano, N., Yamashita, T., Yasuda, T., Ikeda, K., Kizu, H., Kameda, Y., Kato, A., Nashu, RJ.,
Lee, HS. & Ryu, KS. (2001). Polyhydoxylated alkaloids isolated from mulberry trees
(*Morus ulba L.*) and silkworms (*Bombyc mori L.*). *Journal of Agriculture and Food
Chemical*, Vol. 49, No. 9, (September, 2001), pp. 4208-4213, ISSN 0021-8561

Baba, T., Ogawa, T., Okahashi, N., Yakushiji, T., Koga, T., Morimoto, M. & Hamada, S.
(1986). Purification and characterization of the extracellular D-glucosyltransferase
from serotype c *Streptococcus mutans*. *Carbohydrate Research*, Vol. 158, No. 1,
(December, 1986), pp. 147-155, ISSN 0008-6215

Beppu, H., Shikano, M., Fujita, K., Itani, Y., Hamayasu, K., Kishino, E., Ito, T., Ozaki, S.,
Shimpo, K., Sonoda, S. & Higashiguchi, T. (2006). Effects of single and 3-month
repeated ingestions of a Kothalahim granule preparation containing Kothala
himubutu extract on the glucose metabolism of humans. *Nippon Shokuhin Shinsozai
Kenkyuukaishi*, Vol. 8, No. 2, (2006), pp. 105-117, ISSN 1344-8935

Ci, SX., Huynh, TH., Louie, LW., Yong, A., Beals, BJ., Ron, N., Tsang, WG., Soon-Shiang, P.
& Desai, NP. (1999). Molecular mass distribution of sodium alginate by high-
performance size-exclusion chromatography. *Journal of Chromatography A*, Vol. 864,
No. 2, (December, 1999), pp. 199-210, ISSN 0021-9673

Draget, KI., Stokke, BT., Yuguchi, Y., Urakawa, H. & Kajiwara, K. (2003). Small-angle x-ray
scattering and rheological characterization of alginate gels. 3. Alginic acid gels.
Biomacromolecules, Vol. 4, No.6, (November-December,2003), pp. 1661-1668. ISSN
1525-7797

Drent, ML., Tollefsen, AT., van, Heusden, FH., Hoenderdos, EB., Jonker, JJ. & van, der,

Veen, EA. (2002). Dose-dependent efficacy of miglitol, an α-glucosidase inhibitor, in type 2
diabetic patients on diet alone: results of a 24-weeks double-blind placebo-
controlled study. *Diabetes, Nutrition & Metabolism*, Vol. 15, No. 3, (June, 2002), pp.
152-159, ISSN 0394-3402

Dubois, M., Gilles, K., Hamilton, JK., Rebers, PA. & Smith, F. (1956). Colorimetric method
for determination of sugars and related substances. *Analytical Chemistry*, Vol. 28,
No. 3 (March, 1956), pp. 350-356, ISSN 0003-2700

Flammang, AM., Erexson, GL., Mirwald, JM. & Henwood, SM. (2007). Toxicological and
cytogenetic assessment of a *Salacia oblonga* extract in a rat subchronic study. *Food
and Chemical Toxicology*, Vol. 45, No. 10, (October, 2007), pp. 1954-1962, ISSN 0278-
6915

Frostell, G. (1970). A method for evaluation of acid potentialities of food. *Acta Odontologica
Scandinavica*, Vol. 28, No. 5, (November, 1970), pp. 599-608, ISSN 0001-6357

Furiga, A., Lonvaud-Funel, A., Dorignac, G. & Badet, C. (2008). *In vitro* anti-bacterial and
anti-adherence effects of natural polyphenolic compounds on oral bacteria. *Journal
of Applied Microbioligy*, Vol. 105, No. 5, (November, 2008), pp. 1470-1476, ISSN 1364-
5072

Furuta, T., Koga, T., Nisizawa, T., Okahashi, N. & Hamada, S. (1985). Purification and
characterization of glucosyltransferases from *Streptococcus mutans* 6715. *Journal of
General Microbiology*, Vol. 131, No. 2, (February, 1985), pp. 285-293, ISSN 0022-1287

Gustafsson, BE., Quensel, CE., Lanke, LS., Lundquist, C., Grahnen, H., Bonow, BE. & Krasse,
B. (1954). The Vipeholm dental caries study. The effect of different levels of

carbohydrate intake on caries activity in 436 individuals observed for five years. *Acta Odontologica Scandinavica*, Vo. 11, No. 3-4, (September, 1954), pp. 232-264, ISSN 0001-6357

Hamada, S. & Torii, M. (1978). Effects of sucrose in culture media in location of *Streptococcus mutans* and cell adherence to glass surface. *Infection and Immunity*, Vol. 20, No. 3, (June, 1978), pp. 592-599, ISSN 0019-9567

Hamada, S., Horikoshi, T., Minami, T., Okahashi, N. & Koga, T. (1989). Purification and characterization of cell-associated glucosyltransferase synthesizing water-insoluble glucan from serotype c *Streptococcus mutans*. *Journal of General Microbiology*, Vol. 135, No. 2, (February, 1989), pp. 335-344, ISSN 0022-1287

Hashiguchi-Ishiguro, M., Nakamura, S. & Oku, T. (2009). Inhibitory effects of partially decomposed alginate on production of glucan and organic acid by *Streptococcus sobrinus* 6715. *Journal of Clinical Biochemistry and Nutrition*, Vol. 44, No. 3, (May, 2009), pp. 275-279, ISSN 0912-0009

Hashiguchi, M., Nakamura, S. & Oku, T. (2011). Inhibitory effects of extractive from leaves of *Morus alba* and *Salacia chinensis* on production of insoluble glucan from ^{14}C-sucrose and cell adhesion by Mutans streptococci. *Journal of Japanese Associaction for Dietary Fiber Research*, Vol. 15, No. 1, (July, 2011), pp. 13-19, ISSN 2186-4136 (in Japanese)

Haug, A., Larsen, B. & Smidsrod, O. (1967). Studies on the sequence of uronic acid residues in alginic acids. *Acta Chemica Scandinavica*, Vol. 21, No. 3, (1967), pp. 691-704, ISSN 0001-5393

Hayachibara, MF., Koo, H., Rosalen, PL., Duarte, S., Franco, EM., Bowen, WH, Ikegaki, M. & Cury, JA. (2005). In vitro and in vivo effects of isolated fractions of Brazilian propolis on caries development. *Journal of Ethnopharmacology*, Vol. 101, No. 1-3, (October, 2005), pp. 110-115, ISSN 0378-8741

Hinoide, M., Imai S. & Nisizawa, T. (1984). New artificial mouth for evaluation of plaque accumulation, pH changes underneath the plaque, and enamel demineralization. *Japanese Journal of Oral Biology*, Vol. 26, No. 1, (March, 1984), pp. 288-291, ISSN 0385-0137

Ito, K., Nakamura, Y., Tokunaga, T., Iijima, D. & Fukushima, K. (2003). Anti-cariogenic properties of a water-soluble extract from cacao. *Bioscience, Biotechnology, and Biochemistry*, Vol. 67, No. 12, (December, 2003), pp. 2567-2573, ISSN 0916-8451

Johnson, FA., Craig, DQ. & Mercer, AD. (1997). Characterization of the block structure and molecular weight of sodium alginates. *Journal of Pharmacy and Pharmacology*, Vol. 49, No. 7, (July, 1997), pp. 639-643, ISSN 0022-3573

Kawada, A., Hiura, N., Shiraiwa, M., Tajima, S., Hiruma, M., Hara, K., Ishibashi, A. & Takahara, H. (1997). Stimulation of human keratinocyte growth by alginate oligosaccharides, a possible co-factor for epidermal growth factor in cell culture. *FEBS Lettes*, Vol. 408, No. 1, (May, 1997), pp. 43-46, ISSN 0014-5793

Kawanabe, J., Hirasawa, M., Takeuchi, T., Oda, T. & Ikeda, T. (1992). Noncariogenicity of erythritol as a substrate. *Caries Research*, Vol. 26, No. 5, (November, 2009), pp. 358-362, ISSN 1421-976X

Inhibitory Effects of the Phytochemicals Partially Hydrolyzed Alginate, Leaf Extracts of Morus alba and Salacia
Extracts on Dental Caries

37

Keyes, PH. (1958) Dental caries in the molar teeth of rats. I. Distribution of lesions induced by high-carbohydrate low-fat diets. *Journal of Dental Research*, Vol. 37, No. 6, (November-December, 1958), pp. 1077-1087, ISSN 1544-0591

Keyes, PH. & Jordan, HV. (1964). Periodontal lesions in the Syrian hamsters. III. Findings related to an infections and transmissible component. *Archives of Oral Biology*, Vol. 9, (July-August, 1964), pp. 377-400, ISSN 0003-9969

Kimura, T., Nakagawa, K., Kubota, H., Kojima, Y., Yamagishi, K., Oita, S., Oikawa, S. & Miyazawa, T. (2007). Food-grade mulberry powder enriched with 1-deoxynojirimycin suppresses the elevation of postprandial blood glucose in humans. *Journal of Agriculture and Food Chemical*, Vol. 55, No. 14, (July, 2007), pp. 5869-5874, ISSN 0021-8561

Kojima, Y., Kimura, T., Nakagawa, K., Asai, A., Hasumi, K., Oikawa, S & Miyazawa T. (2010). Effects of mulberry leaf extract rich in 1-deoxynojirimycin on blood lipid profiles in humans. *Journal of Clinical Biochemistry and Nutrition*, Vol. 47, No. 2, (September, 2010), pp. 155-161, ISSN 0912-0009

Koo, H., Rosalen, PL., Cury, JA., Park, YK. & Bowen, WH. (2002). Effects of compounds found in propolis on *Streptococcus mutans* growth and glucosyltransferase activity. *Antimicrobial Agents and Chemotherapy*, Vol. 46, No. 5, (May, 2002), pp. 1302-1309, ISSN 1098-6596

Koo, H., Duarte, S., Murata, RM., Scott-Anne, K., Gregoire, S., Watson, GE., Singh, AP., & Vorsa, N. (2010) Influence of cranberry proanthocyanidins on formation of biofilms by *Streptococcus mutans* on saliva-coated apatitic surface and on dental caries development in vivo. *Caries Research*, Vol. 44, No. 2 , (March, 2010), pp. 116-126, ISSN 1421-976X

Leitão, DP., Filho, AA., Polizello, AC., Bastos, JK., Spadaro, AC. (2004). Comparative evaluation of in-vitro effects of Brazilian green propolis and *Baccharisdracunculifolia* extracts on cariogenic factors of *Streptococcus mutans*. *Biological & Pharmaceutical Bulletin*, Vol. 27, No. 11, (November, 2004), pp. 1834-1839, ISSN1347-5215

Li, Y., Huang, TH. & Yamahara, J. (2008). *Salacia* root, a unique Ayurvedic medicine, meets multiole targets in diabetes and obesity. *Life Sciences*, Vol. 82, No. 21-22, (May, 2008), pp. 1045-1049, ISSN 0024-3205

Lingström, P., van, Ruyven, FO., van, Houte, J. & Kent, R. (2000). The pH of dental plaque in its relation to early enamel caries and dental plaque flora in humans. *Journal of Dental Researc*, Vol. 79, No. 2, (February, 2000), pp. 770-777, ISSN 1544-0591

Makinen, KK., Bennett, CA., Hujoel, PP., Isokangas, PJ., Isotupa, KP., Pape, HR, Jr. & Makinen, PL. (1995). Xylitol chewing gums and caries rates: a 40-month cohort study. *Journal of Dental Research*, Vol. 74, No. 12, (December, 1995), pp. 1904-1913, ISSN 0022-0345

Miyazawa, M., Miyahara, T., Sato, S. & Sakai, A. (2003). Ninety-day dietary toxicity study of mulberry leaf extract in rats. *Journal of the Food Hygienic Society of Japan*, Vol. 44, No. 4, (August, 2003), pp. 191-197, ISSN 0015-6426 (in Japanese)

Nakahara, K., Kawabata, S., Ono, H., Ogura, K., Tanaka, T., Ooshima, T. & Hamada, S. (1993). Inhibitory effect of oolong tea polyphenols on glucosyltransferases of mutans streptococci. *Applied and Environmental Microbiology*, Vol. 59, No. 4, (April, 1993), pp. 968-973, ISSN 0099-2240

Nakamura, M., Nakamura, S. & Oku, T. (2009). Suppressive response of confections containing the extractive from leaves of *Morus alba* on postprandial blood glucose and insulin in healthy human subjects. *Nutrition & Metabolism* (Lond), Vol. 6, No. 29,(open access), (July, 2009), ISSN 743-7075

Nakamura, S., Aki, M., Hashiguchi-Ishiguro, M., Ueda, S. & Oku, T. (2008). Inhibitory effect of depolymerized sodium alginate by *Vibrio alginolyticus* SUN53 on intestinal brush border membrane disaccharidase in rat. *Japanese Association for Dietary Fiber Research*, Vol. 12, No. 1, (June, 2008), pp. 9-15, ISSN 1349-5437 (in Japanese)

Natsume, M., Kamo, Y., Hirayama, M. & Adachi, T. (1994). Isolation and characterization of alginate-derived oligosaccharides with root growth-promoting activities. *Carbohydrate Research*, Vol. 258, (May, 1994), pp. 187-197, ISSN 0008-6215

Newbrun, E., Hoover, CI. & Gwen, JW. (1983). Inhibition by acarbose, nojirimycin and 1-deoxynojirimycin of glucosyltransferase produced by oral Streptococci. *Archives of Oral Biology*, Vol. 28, No. 6, (June, 1983), pp. 531-536, ISSN 0003-9969

Oku, T., Nakamura, S. & Okazaki, M. (1997). Suppressive effects of alginic acids lowered molecule for the elevation of blood glucose and the insulin secretion in human subjects. *Journal of Japanese Associaction for Dietary Fiber Research*, Vo. 1, No. 1, (July, 1997), pp. 13-18, ISSN 2186-4136 (in Japanese)

Oku, T., Nakamura, S. & Okazaki, M. (1998). Effects of partially hydrolyzed sodium alginic acid on defecation and fecal conditions. *Eiyogakuzashi*, Vol. 56, No. 2, (February, 2010), pp. 31-41, ISSN 1883-7921 (in Japanese)

Oku, T. (2005). Digestion, fermentation, absorption and metabolism of non-digestible and/or non-absorbable saccharides and their maximum permissive dosage to produce transitory diarrhea. *Journal of Japan Society of Nutrition and Food Science*, Vol. 58, No. 6, (December, 2005), pp. 337-342, ISSN 0287-3516 (in Japanese)

Oku, T., Yamada, M., Nakamura, M., Sadamori, N. & Nakamura, S. (2006), Inhibitory effects of extractives from leaves of *Morus alba* on human and rat small intestinal disaccharidase activity. *British Journal of Nutrition*, Vol. 95, No. 5, (May, 2006), pp. 933-938, ISSN 0007-1145

Ooshima, T., Sobue, S., Hamada, S. & Katani, S. (1981), Susceptibility of rats, hamsters, and mice to carious infection by *Streptococcus mutans* serotype c and d organisms. *Journal of Dental Research*, Vol. 60, No. 4, (April, 1981), pp. 855-859, ISSN 1544-0591

Ooshima, T., Izumitani, A., Minami, T., Yoshida, T., Sobue, S., Fujiwara, T. & Hamada, S. (1992). Noncariogenicity of maltitol in specific pathogen-free rats infected with mutans streptococci. *Caries Research*, Vol. 26, No. 1, (November, 2009), pp. 33-37, ISSN 1421-976X

Ooshima, T., Minami, T., Aono, W., Izumitani, A., Sobue, S., Fujiwara, T., Kawabata, S. &Hamada, S. (1993). Oolong tea polyphenols inhibit experimental dental caries in SPF rats infected with Mutans streptococci. *Caries Research*, Vol. 27, No. 2, (November, 2009), pp. 124-129, ISSN 1421-976X

Pigman, W., Elliot Jr, HC. & Laffre, R. (1952). An artificial mouth for caries research. *Journal of Dental Research*, Vol. 31, No. 5, (October, 1952), pp. 627-633, ISSN 1544-0591

Inhibitory Effects of the Phytochemicals Partially Hydrolyzed Alginate, Leaf Extracts of Morus alba and Salacia
Extracts on Dental Caries

39

Raimbaud, E., Buleon, A. & Perez, S. (1992). Molecular modeling of acarviosine, the pseudo-disaccharide moiety of acarbose, and other inhibitors of α-amylases. *Carbohydrate Research*, Vol. 227, (April, 1992), pp. 351-363, ISSN 0008-6215

Shimoda, H., Kawamori, S. & Kawahara, Y. (1998). Effects of an aqueous extract of *Salacia reticulate*, a useful plant on Sri Lanka, on postprandial hyperglycemia in rats and humans. *Journal of Japan Society of Nutrition and Food Science*, Vol. 51, No. 5, (October, 1998), pp. 279-287, ISSN 0287-3516 (in Japanese)

Sreebny, LM. (1982). Sugar availability, sugar consumption and dental caries. *Community Dentistry and Oral Epidemiology*, Vol. 10, No. 1, (February, 1982), pp. 1-7 ISSN1600-0528

Stephan, RM. (1940). Changes in hydrogen ion concentration on tooth surfaces and in carious lesions. *Journal of American Dental Association*, Vol. 27, (1940), pp. 718-723, ISSN 0002-8177

Tseng, C-H., Yamaguchi, K., Nishimura, M. & Kitamikado, M. (1992). Alginate lyase from *Vibrio alginolyticus* ATCC 17749. *Nippon Suisan Gakkaishi*, Vol. 58, No. 11, (November, 1992), pp. 2063-2067, ISSN 0021-5392

Tsunehiro, J., Matsukubo, T., Shiota, M. & Takaesu, Y. (1997). Effects of a hydrogenated isomaltooligosaccharide mixture on glucan synthesis and on caries development in rats. *Bioscience, Biotechnology, and Biochemistry*, Vol. 61, No. 12, (December, 1997), pp. 2015-2018, ISSN 0916-8451

Yagi, M., Kouno, T., Aoyagi, Y. & Murai, H. (1976). The structure of moranoline, a piperidine alkaloid from *Morus species*. *Nippon Nogeikagaku Kaishi*, Vol. 50, No. 11, (1976), pp. 571-572, ISSN 0002-1369

Yanagida, A., Kanda, T., Tanabe, M., Matsudaira, F. & Oliveira, CJG. (2000). Inhibitory effects of apple polyphenols and related compounds on cariogenic factors of mutans streptococci. *Journal of Agricultural and Food chemistry*, Vol. 48, No. 11, (November, 2000), pp. 5666-5671, ISSN 0021-8561

Yasuda, K., Shimowada, K., Uno, M., Odaka, H., Adachi, T. & Shihara, N. (2003). Long-term therapeutic effects of voglibose, a potent intestinal α-glucosidase inhibitor, in spontaneous diabetic GK rats. *Diabetes research and clinical practice*, Vol. 59, No. 2, (February, 2003), pp. 113-122, ISSN 0168-8227

Yoshikawa, M., Nishida, N., Shimoda, H., Takada, Y., Kawahara, Y. & Matsuda, H. (2001). Polyphenol constituents from Salacia species: quantitative analysis of Mangiferin with α-glucosidase and aldose reductase inhibitory activities. *Journal of the Pharmaceutical Society of Japan*, Vol. 121, No. 5, (May, 2001), pp. 371-378, ISSN 1347-5231 (in Japanese)

Van, Loveren, C. (2004). Sugar alcohols: what is the evidence for caries-preventive and caries-therapeutic effects? *Caries Research*, Vol. 38, No. 3, (May, 2004), pp. 286-293, ISSN 0008-6568

Venkitaraman, AR., Vacca-Smith, AM., Kopec, LK. & Bowen, WH. (1995). Characterization of glucosyltransferaseB, GtfC, and GtfD in solution and on the surface of hydroxyapatite. *Journal of Dental Research*, Vol. 74, No. 10, (October, 1995), pp. 1695-1701, ISSN 0022-0345

Wong, TY., Preston, LA. & Schiller, NL. (2000). Alginate lyase: Review of major sources and enzyme characteristics, structure-function analysis, biological roles, and applications. *Annual Review of Microbiology*, Vol. 54, (October, 2000), pp. 289-340, ISSN 0066-4227

Effect of 1000 or More ppm Relative to 440 to 550 ppm Fluoride Toothpaste – A Systematic Review

Alexandra Saldarriaga Cadavid[1],
Rubén Darío Manrique Hernández[2] and Clara María Arango Lince[3]
[1]Faculty of Odontology, Pediatric Dentistry and Epidemilogy, Research Department,
[2]Department of Epidemiology,
[3]Faculty of Odontology, Pediatric Dentistry Department,
CES University, Medellín
Colombia

1. Introduction

During the last three decades a significant worldwide reduction – of dental caries has been observed. Experts agree that fluoride in its multiple presentations has played an important role, together with changes in oral hygiene habits among different populations. Fluoride toothpastes has gained interest as a relevant strategy in prevention because of its important role in dental caries reduction, that can reach up to 40% (7,8,14). However, at the same time, they have contributed to an increase in the prevalence of dental fluorosis in children. There is concern about dental fluorosis related to the chronic intake of excessive quantities of fluoride in children under 6 years of age. Some authors have reported that the early use of fluoridated toothpastes in young children is a very important risk factor (13,17,22,33,34). Beside fluoride concentration, the duration and age of exposure are important factors in fluorosis prevalence (2).

In order to reduce the risk of dental fluorosis, the use of toothpaste with 440 to 550 ppm F in children less than six years old has been recommended (5). The efficacy of these toothpastes in reducing dental caries is still unknown and controversialy among the scientific community (1,3). In Colombia, the fluoride concentration of toothpastes for preschool children below the age of 6 years was limited several years ago to 500 ppm in order to control dental fluorosis.

According to the Oral Health National Study (NSOH III)(13), the prevalence of dental fluorosis in Colombian children between 6 and 7 years old is 25.7%. The highest prevalence of moderate and severe dental fluorosis was found in Bogotá with 4.5% of the children being affected. Another study carried out in 2002 in four Colombian cities, to evaluate fluoride intake in 2 to 4 year olds from meals, beverages and toothpastes reported that in all cities except one, the total fluoride intake was above optimal limits (0.07 mgF/Kg of body weight) and even some were above the risk limit (0.1 mgF/Kg of body weight). From the three studied sources, the lowest fluoride intake was from beverages at 4.3%, followed by meals at 26%. The highest fluoride intake came from toothpastes which comprised 69% of the total ingested fluoride (15).

The use of 500 ppm fluoride pastes raised the question of how effective this toothpaste is compared with the 1000 or more ppm F toothpastes, in the prevention of dental caries.

Therefore, the aim of this study was to carry out a quantitative systematic review assessing the efficacy of toothpastes with low fluoride concentrations between 440 and 550 ppm in the reduction of dental caries in children under 14 years old compared to toothpastes that contain 1000 or more ppm F.

2. Methods

Search strategy: A literature search on Medline MeSH, Cochrane Library, Ovid, Sciencedirect and Embase databases between January 1970 to November 2003 was conducted, with the key words dental caries, toothpaste, fluoride, caries prevention or control, dentifrices, caries control, cariostatic agents, dental caries susceptibility.

The inclusion criteria were randomized controlled clinical trials, quasi-experimental and cohort studies in all languages, where all participants were less than fourteen years old and the main variable evaluated was dental caries reduction using the DMF or dmf index, comparing fluoride toothpaste concentrations between 440-550 ppm and toothpaste with 1000 ppm or more regardless of the initial dental caries level, treatment and nationality (see Table 1).

Author Year	Systemic Fluoride	Type	Participants	Intervention*
Reed 1973(27)	Non fluoridated comunity	RCT double blind	1525 children between 5 and 14 years	500 ppm 1000 ppm
Winter 1989(37)	Low (0.08 to 0.5 ppm) fluoridated community	RCT double blind	2177 children between 2 and 5 years	1055 ppm 550 ppm
Davies 2002(10)	Non fluoridated community	RCT blind	5028 children between 1 and 6 years	440 ppm 1450 ppm
Biesbrock 2003(6)	Non fluoridated community	RCT double blind	657 children between 9 and 12 years	500 ppm 1450 ppm

Only groups related with the meta-analysis objectives were included.

Table 1. Description of studies

Missing or unreported data were directly requested to the authors by e-mail. In the Reed (27) trial, the standard deviation was not reported, standard error was used to recalculate it assuming equal variances following the mean difference formula by Student's t-test.

Winter et al. (37) did not report the standard error or standard deviation; although one of the authors was contacted, the information could not be compiled. This standard deviation was calculated using the standard error which was obtained from confidence interval reported.

Ammari et al. (1) did not include both the Winter et al. (37) and Reed(27) trials. They argued high drop out percentages (29% and 28% respectively) and lack of explanation for these drop-outs. However, they included a drop-out percentage in their sample size estimation.

For the characteristic description of the studies found initially, the reviewers used an information extraction format, based on the format developed by Sally Hollis y Tina Leonard, Piel Cochrane Group(18).

The Chalmers criteria were used to evaluate the quality of these studies accepting those that had a score of 70% from 100 possible points (24).

The methodological procedure used to evaluate the studies consisted of an individual review by each examiner to verify the quality criteria of each study that complied with the inclusion criteria and graded them in a scorecard design for each of the different content indicators of the instrument. Afterwards, the research group evaluated as a team and assigned individual points to each study, trying to reach a consensus around those in which noticeable differences existed (assigned extreme values). A design format was used to total the final scores of each study. Studies that scored at least 70% were included in the final meta analysis. One trial could not be included in the meta-analysis (see Table2).

Study	Reason for exclusion
Holt, 1994(19)	Although groups to compare acomplished inclusion criteria, this study used the sample and data of a previous study (Winter, 1989). It was considered a secondary analysis of the mentioned study

Table 2. Excluded studies

This study was free of any conflict of interest, given that no company or pharmaceutical laboratory sponsored its execution, and its final result was not related to any commercial brand that distributes toothpastes in Colombia.

According to the Antioquia Health Secretary's resolution 008430 of 1993, this project was considered a "non risk investigation". It includes literature review techniques and no intervention or intended biological, physiological, psychological or social variable modifications were done on individuals.

3. Data analysis

In addition to the complete reading of each of the included articles and its quality evaluation, the following procedures were followed:

Mantel-Haenzel test of homogeneity was used to evaluate the null hypothesis that the included studies were homogeneous. Statistical calculations were carried out following the Mantel-Haenzel Q heterogeneity statistical formula. This test was compared with Chi square distribution with n-1 degrees of freedom and a confidence level of 95%, where n was the number of studies included in the meta analysis, which in this case was n=4. If under these circumstances the calculated Q_{MH} value was above the tabulated value of X^2, the homogeneity hypothesis was not rejected and no heterogeneity between the included studies was considered.

The estimated effect was measured in terms of average dental caries in each of the studied groups according to the dmf and DMF index. The final analysis evaluated the mean difference between the groups by applying the DerSimonian-Laird method for random effects.

A metaview graphics illustrated the estimated values of the individual studies and the combined estimated effect.

Once the first meta-analytic approach was completed after combining the results from the independent studies, a sensibility analysis was done to establish the solidity of the combined estimated effect after one or more studies with extreme high or low values were withdrawn from the meta analysis.

4. Results

The data presented in the dental literature to answer the question of the efficacy of toothpastes with fluoride concentrations between 440 and 550 ppm in dental caries prevention in children are very limited. Four randomized controlled clinical trial were selected from five references yielded by electronic and hand searches. The studies included in the meta-analysis are listed in chronological order in Table 1. The included trials comprised a total of 5657 participants under similar conditions regarding variables, such as no systemic fluoridation and positive participation in oral health programs. Baseline caries levels were reported in all studies. Winter et al.(37) did not report specific baseline caries data. they explained that they decided to conduct the trial on 2-year-old children based on the expectation that most would be caries free given that according to epidemiological evidence very few children aged 2 years or less have caries which would be limited to the main lesions affecting the upper incisors. Of the 2177 children examined only 32 (1.5 per cent) had caries of this type with a difference of only 2 children between the groups. As a further analysis on the validity of the approach, they repeated the analysis of data related to dental caries, omitting the 32 children, with no effect on the outcome.

5. Meta-analysis

The results of different estimations of the combined effect following the meta-analytic procedures with heterogeneous criteria, using the Dersimonian-Laird random effect model are shown in the metaview (7,8,14,17).

All procedures done to estimate the summary measure of effect, both as standardized mean difference and odds ratio, suggest that 440 to 550 ppm F toothpastes are not as effective in preventing dental caries in the primary and permanent dentition as pastes with 1000 ppm F or more.

Although the differences are statistically significant, the confidence intervals of all summary measures of effect are close to zero, both as standardized mean difference and odds ratio with the same results for the primary and permanent dentition.

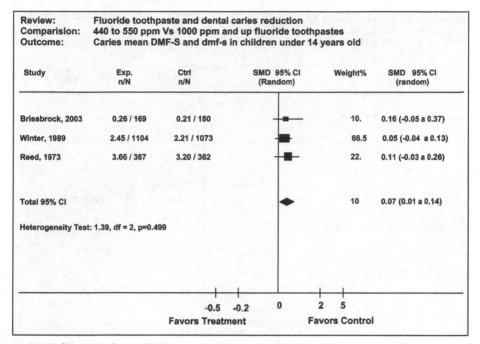

Review: Fluoride toothpaste and dental caries reduction
Comparision: 440 to 550 ppm Vs 1000 ppm and up fluoride toothpastes
Outcome: Caries mean DMF-S and dmf-s in children under 14 years old

Study	Exp. n/N	Ctrl n/N	SMD 95% CI (Random)	Weight%	SMD 95% CI (random)
Briesbrock, 2003	0.26 / 169	0.21 / 180		10.	0.16 (-0.05 a 0.37)
Winter, 1989	2.45 / 1104	2.21 / 1073		66.5	0.05 (-0.04 a 0.13)
Reed, 1973	3.66 / 387	3.20 / 362		22.	0.11 (-0.03 a 0.26)
Total 95% CI				10	0.07 (0.01 a 0.14)

Heterogeneity Test: 1.39, df = 2, p=0.499

-0.5 -0.2 0 2 5
Favors Treatment   Favors Control

Fig. 1. DMF-S and dmf-s in children under 14 years old: Metaview

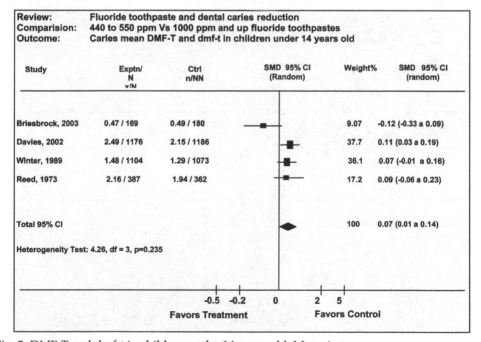

Review: Fluoride toothpaste and dental caries reduction
Comparision: 440 to 550 ppm Vs 1000 ppm and up fluoride toothpastes
Outcome: Caries mean DMF-T and dmf-t in children under 14 years old

Study	Exptn/N v/N	Ctrl n/NN	SMD 95% CI (Random)	Weight%	SMD 95% CI (random)
Briesbrock, 2003	0.47 / 169	0.49 / 180		9.07	-0.12 (-0.33 a 0.09)
Davies, 2002	2.49 / 1176	2.15 / 1186		37.7	0.11 (0.03 a 0.19)
Winter, 1989	1.48 / 1104	1.29 / 1073		36.1	0.07 (-0.01 a 0.16)
Reed, 1973	2.16 / 387	1.94 / 362		17.2	0.09 (-0.06 a 0.23)
Total 95% CI				100	0.07 (0.01 a 0.14)

Heterogeneity Test: 4.26, df = 3, p=0.235

-0.5 -0.2 0 2 5
Favors Treatment   Favors Control

Fig. 2. DMF-T and dmf-t in children under 14 years old: Metaview

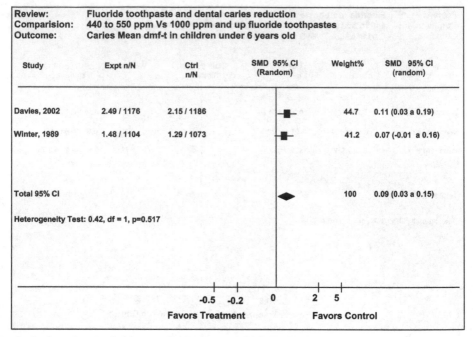

Fig. 3. dmf-t index in children under 6 years old: Metaview.

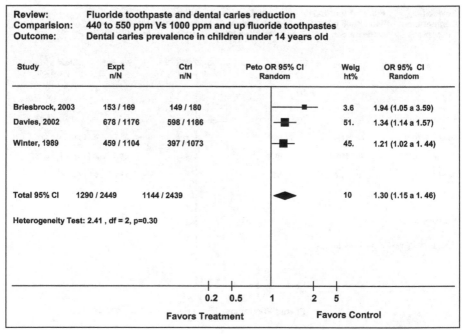

Fig. 4. Odds ratios to dental caries prevalence in children under 14 years old: Metaview.

Sensitivity Analysis: The study by Biesbrock et al.(6) was different in participation number with less weight than the other studies. Considering that this could influence the results, a sensitivity analysis was carried out by repeating the meta-analysis excluding this study. The odds ratio was not affected and the difference between the two groups was still significant (OR: 1.28 - $CI_{95\%}$: 1.13 to 1.44) in favor of toothpastes with 1000 ppm F or more.

Given that the results are in favor of toothpastes with 1000 ppm F or more, in dental caries prevalence reduction in children under 14 years old, the combined odds ratio was estimated again in order to determine the absolute risk reduction, assuming that these are more effective than those with 440 and 550 ppm F in dental caries prevention (see Table 3).

Groups	Dental caries		Total	OR - 95% CI
	Yes	No		
Fluoride > 1000 ppm	1144	1305	2449	0.76 (0.66 – 0.88)
Fluoride 440 to 550 ppm	1290	1159	2449	p value:
Total	2434	2464	4898	0.0002

Table 3. Summary estimate of odds ratio. random-effects model.

According to these results there is a lower proportion of caries in children treated with dental toothpastes with 1000 ppm F or more, with an attributable risk factor of 0.0596 (6%) (p<0.00001). This demostrates how children under 14 years old using toothpastes with 1000 ppm F or more have approximately 6 percent more protection against caries than when they use toothpastes between 440 and 550 ppm F. To learn more about the impact and efficacy of this therapy the number needed to be treated to prevent one event was calculated (NNT= 14.6 $IC_{95\%}$ 11 a 32).

6. Discussion

Fluoride concentrations used in toothpastes are an important factor concerning toothpaste efficacy in reducing dental caries. Literature reviews such as the one done by Richards et al.(28) conclude that the optimal fluoride concentration in toothpaste is 1000 ppm F. This concentration has shown to provide best benefits in reducing dental caries and fluorosis. Meanwhile with fluoride concentrations less than 1000 ppm the efficacy in the reduction of dental caries is diminished (29).

Recently, some meta-analysis has been published to describe the efficacy of different fluoride concentrations used in toothpastes to prevent dental caries in children and teenagers (1,20,21,33). However, none of them obtained conclusions regarding toothpastes with 440 and 550 ppm F.

There were a limited number of studies comparing low F (440 to 550 ppm) to high F (1000 or more ppm) toothpastes. For this meta-analysis only five studies were found, out of which four were selected.

The total sample size of children under 14 years old included in the 4 selected studies was 5657, the fluoride compounds in the toothpastes used were sodium fluoride in 440, 500, 550 and 1450 ppm; and sodium monofluorophosphate in 1000, 1055 and 1450 ppm, as they are the most used in general population.

Winter et al. (37) reported the first clinical controlled trial in children under 2 years old followed during three years. All included trials in comparison experienced relative high percentage of subjects at baseline who dropped out during the course of studies. However in all of these studies they considered this at the moment of the sample size estimation. Davies et al (10) were the only ones to report the reason for these drop outs.

In some cases it was necessary to contact the author to obtain additional data (DMF-T) such as the Biesbrock et al.(6) study in order to compare it with the other three studies.

The diagnostic system used in all the studies was the DMF and dmf indices at the level of cavity (D3) (16,25); The Biesbrock study was the only one that included opacity lesion with microcavity data in their analysis (D2) (16,25). Regardless of some authors considering that there may be some differences between primary and permanent enamel in reactivity to caries challenges (1,32), this is not clear. Thus we combined primary and permanent dentition.

Some clinical studies have shown that with 1000 to 2500 ppm F toothpaste an increase of 6% is obtained in dental caries protection for each 500 ppm (23,35).

Combined evidence from the included assay suggest that toothpastes with concentrations of 1000 ppm and more are more effective in caries reduction, showing a higher prevalence of dental caries in children under 6 years who used lower fluoride concentrations (440 to 550 ppm) toothpastes. It is important to note that precisely the group of children younger than 6 years is the main consumer of this toothpaste because this is the group in which traditional 1000 ppm F toothpaste is being replaced.

The results of this meta-analysis show that 440 to 550 ppm F toothpaste is less effective in preventing dental caries than 1000 ppm F toothpaste, and it is interesting to note that it is necessary to double the fluoride concentration to have a risk difference of only 6%. Similar results were reported by Amari et al.(1), as they found a caries Indexes Weighted Mean Difference of 0.6 between dental toothpastes with 250 ppm F and 1000 ppm F, and they emphasized that a fourfold increase in F concentration is necessary to obtain such a difference.

Twetman et al.(30) reported for daily use of fluoride toothpaste compared to placebo in the young permanent dentition (Prevented Fraction: 24.9%) and for toothpastes with 1500ppm F compared with standard toothpaste with 1000 ppm F in young permanent dentition(PF 9,7%), These were greater than the results of this meta-analysis where PF, expressed as percentage, was 6% in favor of 1000 ppm F as was expected.

Despite the fact that there were few studies included, it is important to note the homogeneity found between them as well as the quality even considering studies like Winter et al.(37) and Reed(27) which date back to 13 and 30 years respectively.

Similar conditions of the included studies related to variables as the non-public water or salt fluoridation and their participation in health supervised programs are in favor of the obtained results.

As there were a limited numbers of studies, asymmetry was difficult to asses, by funnel plot. However, comparing their sample size, the Biesbrock et al. (6) study, which had lowest sample size (n=349) did not alter the combined estimation of the effect when it was withdrawn from the sensibility analysis.

These results are an approach to answer the question of the efficacy of low fluoride toothpastes (considered for reducing fluorosis risk in children) in reducing dental caries incidence in a population in which dental caries is still a public health problem.

The fact that low fluoride concentration toothpaste is currently being recommended for children younger than 6 years old without enough scientific evidence must concern the scientific community, as the impact is greater in the population which does not have knowledge of these circumstances.

This study did not attempt to report possible adverse effects of fluoride toothpaste like dental fluorosis. Although some authors state that concentrations of 440 a 550 ppm F reduce the risk of developing dental fluorosis (19), there is a lack of clinical assays and cohort studies to confirm said hypothesis, leading to a lack of major clinical evidence in relation to the efficacy of low fluoride toothpaste in reducing dental caries in children younger than 6 years old and its impact on this population. This systematic review, increases the available evidence in this topic.

Recommendations for specific fluoride doses in toothpastes requires combined studies about dental caries incidence and dental fluorosis.

In order to learn the epidemiological significance of the clinical difference between these fluoride concentrations, it would be beneficial to promote community studies with different systemic fluoridation levels and high caries risk groups that would allow for the evaluation of fluorosis risk and caries risk, in order to more firmly establish if the use of low fluoride toothpastes is justified, in high caries risk children.

The concentration of fluoride in toothpaste is a protective factor for dental caries but is clear that in children less than 5 years is a risk factor for dental fluorosis. Dental caries is the most common chronic disease of childhood and continues been a public health concern (4,11,12,26,31). For dental caries management and disease control in children under 5 years the emphasis must be focus in other than fluoride concentration, is important to propos combined preventive approaches providing early access to dental services, medical approaches, no operative intervention and specific educational and informational actions for mothers and the newborn.

Recent Meta-analysis and clinical trials confirm the great effect of high concentration fluoride dental toothpaste (36). Although 6% sounds little its effect must not be underestimated, mainly in this age group when the relation between dental toothpaste quantity and fluoride concentration combination could be important and pertinent.

7. References

[1] Ammari AB, Bloch-Zupan A, Ashley PF. Systematic review of studies comparing the anti-caries efficacy of children´s toothpaste containing 600 ppm of fluoride or less with high fluoride toothpastes of 1000 ppm or above. Caries Res 2003;37:85-92.
[2] Burt BA, Keels MA, Heller KE. The effects of a break in water fluoridation on the development of dental caries and fluorosis. J Dent Res 2000;79:761-769.

[3] Bloch Zupan A. Is the fluoride concentration limit of 1500 ppm in cosmetics (EU Guideline) Still up-to date? Caries Res 2001;35(suppl 1):22-25.

[4] Beltán-Aguilar ED, Barker LK, Canto MT,Dye BA, Gooch BF, Griffin SO, et al. Surveillance for dental caries, dental sealants, tooth retention, edentulism, and enamel fluorosis-United States, 1988-1994 and 1999-2002. MMWR Surveil Summ 2005;54:1-43.

[5] Bentley EM, Ellwood RP, Davies RM. Fluoride Ingestion from toothpaste by young children. Br Dent J 1999;183:460-462.

[6] Biesbrock AR, Bartizek RD, Gerlach RW, Jacobs SA, Archila l. Effect of three concentrations of sodium fluoride dentifrices on clinical caries. Am J Dent 2003;16: 99-104.

[7] Bratthall D, Hänsel-Petersson G, Sundberg H. Reasons for the caries decline: What do the experts believe? Eur J Sci 1996;104: 416-422.

[8] Clarkson JJ, McLoughlin J. Role of fluoride in oral health promotion. Int Dent J 2000; 50:119-28.

[9] Saldarriaga cadavid A, Arango lince CM, Cossio Jaramillo M. Dental caries in the primary dentition of a Colombian population according to the ICDAS criteria. Braz Oral Res. 2010 Apr-Jun;24(2):211-6.

[10] Davies GM, Worthington HV, Ellwood RP, Bentley EM, Blinkhorn AS, Taylor GO, et al. A Randomised controlled trial of the effectiveness of providing free fluoride toothpaste from the age of 12 months on reducing caries in 5-6 year old children. Community Dental Health 2002;19:131-136.

[11] Dye BA, Tan S, SmithV, Lewis BG, Barker LK, Thornton-EvansG, et al.Trends in oral health status: United States, 1988-1994 and 1999-2004. Vital Health Stat 2007;11:1-92.

[12] Escobar-paucar G, Ramirez-Puerta BS, Franco-Cortez AM, Tamayo-Posada AM, Castro-Aguirre JF. Experiencia de caries dental en niños de 1 a 5 años de bajos ingresos. Medellin .Colombia. Revista CES odontologia 2009;22(1):21-28.

[13] Ellwood RP, O'Mullane DM. Dental enamel opacities in the groups with varying levels of fluoride in their drinking water. Caries Res 1995;29:137-142.

[14] Feyerskov O, Baelum V. Changes in prevalence and incidence of the major oral diseases. In: Oral biology at the turn of the century: misconceptions, truths, challenges and prospects. Guggenheim B, and Shapiro S. Editors. Institute of Oral Microbiology and General Inmunology. University of Zurich. Zurich;1998.

[15] Franco A, Martignon S, Saldarriaga A, Gonzales MC, Arbelaez MI, Ocampo A, et al. Total fluoride intake in children aged 22-35 months in four Colombian cities. Community Dent Oral Epidemiol. 2005;33:1-8.

[16] Fyffe HE, Deery C, Nugent ZJ, Nuttall NM, Pitts NB. Effect of diagnostic threshold on the validity and reliability of epidemiological caries diagnosis using the Dundee Selectable Threshold Method for Method for caries diagnosis (DSTM). Community Dent Oral Epidemiol 2000;28:42-51.

[17] Horowitz HS. The need for toothpastes with lower than conventional Fluoride concentrations for preschool-aged children. J Public Health Dent 1992;52:216-221.

[18] Hollis S, Leonard T. Cochrane Skin Group. Data extraction form. [updated 2004 sept 16; cited 2004 Jul 12]. Available from:
http://www.cochrane.org/crgprocedures/files/chapter4/attach9.doc

[19] Holt RD, Morris CE, Winter GB, Downer MC. Enamel opacities and dental caries in children who used a low fluoride toothpaste between 2 and 5 years of age. Int Dent J 1994;44:331-341.

[20] Johnson MF. Comparative efficacy of NaF and SMFP dentifrices in caries prevention: a meta-analityc overview. Caries Res 1993;27:328-36.

[21] Marinho VCC, Higgins JPT, Sheiham A, Logan S. Fluoride toothpastes for preventing dental caries in children and adolescents (Cochrane Review). In: The Cochrane Library, Issue 1, 2003. Oxford: Update Software.

[22] Mascarenhas AK, Burt BA. Fluorosis risk from early exposure to fluoride toothpaste. Community Dent Oral Epidemiol 1999;26:241-48.

[23] O´Mullane DM, Kavanagh D, Ellwood RP, ChestersRK, Shafer F, Huntington E, et al. A three-year clinical trial of a combination of trimetaphosphate and sodium fluoride in silica toothpastes. J Dent Res 1997;76:1776-81.

[24] Petitti DB. Meta-Analysis, Decision Analysis and Cost-Effectiveness Analysis. Methods for Quantitative Synthesis in Medicine. New York: Oxford University Press; 1994. p. 86.

[25] Pitts NB. Diagnostic tools and measurements - Impact on appropiate care. Community Dent Oral Epidemiol 1997;25: 24-35.

[26] República de Colombia. Ministerio de Salud. III Estudio Nacional de Salud Bucal Serie Documentos Técnicos Tomo VII. Ministerio de Salud. Bogotá, 1999.

[27] Reed MW. Clinical evaluation of three concentrations of sodium fluoride in dentifrices. JADA 1973;87:1401-1403

[28] Richards A, Fejerskov O, Larsen MJ. Fluoride concentrations in dentifrices in relation to efficacy, side-effects, and salivary clearence. In: Embery G, and Rolla G. Clinical and biological aspects of dentifrices. United States: Oxford University press1992. p. 73-90.

[29] Results of the Workshop. J Public Health Dent 1989;49(Spec Issue): 331-337.

[30] Twetman S, Axelsson S, Dahlgren H, Holm AK, Kallestal C, Lagerlof F, et al. Caries-preventive effect of fluoride toothpaste: a systematic review. Acta Odontol Scand 2003;61:347-355.

[31] Saldarriaga A, Arango CM, Cossio M,Arenas A, Mejía C, Mejía E, Murillas L.Prevalencia de caries dental en preescolares con dentición deciduas area metropolitana del Valle de Aburra. Revista CES odontologia 2009;22(2-):35-40.

[32] Sonju CA, Ogaard B, Duscher H, Ruber , Arends J, Sonju T. Caries development in fluoridated and non-fluoridated deciduos and permanent enamel in situ examined by microradiography and confocal laser scanning microscopy. Adv Dent Res 1997;11:442-447.

[33] Steiner M, Helfenstein U, Menghini G. Effect of 1000 ppm relative to 250 ppm fluoride toothpaste. A meta-analysis. Am J Dent 2004;17:85-88.

[34] StooKey GK. Review of fluorosis risk of self-applied topical fluoride: dentifrices, mouthrinses and gels. Community Dent Oral Epidemiol 1994; 22:181-6.

[35] Stephen KW, Creanor SL, Russell JI, Burshell CK, Huntington E, Downie CFA. A 3-year oral health response study of sodium monofluoro-phosphate dentifrice with and without zinc citrate: anticaries results. Community Dent Oral Epidemiol 1988;16:321-5.

[36] WalshT, Worthington HV, Glenny AM, Appelbe P, Marinho VC, Shi X. Fluoride toothpaste of different concentrations for preventing dental caries in children and adolescents. Cochrane Database Syst Rev.2010 Jan 20(1):CD007868.

[37] Winter GB, Holt RD, Williams F. Clinical trial of a low –fluoride toothpaste for young children. Int Dent J 1989;39:227-235.

4

Sealing of Fissures on Masticatory Surfaces of Teeth as a Method for Caries Prophylaxis

Elżbieta Jodkowska
Medical University of Warsaw,
Poland

1. Introduction

Tooth caries, which is regarded as a social disease in many countries, affects 100% of population. For many years both high prevalence and increasing intensity of caries have inspired researchers to find effective methods of fighting the disease. The quest for caries prevention methods has led to more and more widespread sealing of fissures of lateral teeth (premolars and molars), where sealants - thanks to mechanical protection from influence of oral cavity environment, thanks to reduction of retention sites and of bacterial flora in fissures - have effectively limited the development of carious disease.

Currently known methods of caries prevention can be deemed effective to the degree justifying their widespread application. Despite this fact, dentists across the world devote most of their working time to elimination of caries's results.

In permanent dentition, tooth decay most frequently affects masticatory surfaces of molars and, as numerous studies report, very soon after their eruption 2/3 of cavities are observed just there. This is confirmed by epidemiological studies, which have been conducted in Poland since 1987 under WHO supervision (29). The studies reveal that at the end of 1970s, over 50% of permanent molars were affected by caries in children aged 6-7 years, whereas children aged 9 years had almost all first permanent molars with carious cavities or filled. In the age group 13-15 years, the percentage of teeth affected by caries reached 80%, though occlusal surfaces of teeth constitute only 12.5% of all surfaces of teeth in the oral cavity. The aforementioned epidemiological studies indicate the importance of activities towards caries prevention on masticatory surfaces.

2. Morphology and microflora of intercusp fissures in teeth

Fissures on masticatory surfaces of lateral teeth are created during development of cusps in odontogenesis, which begins in the first weeks of fetal life with formation of deciduous tooth buds, and terminates about the age of 12 years, or 15-18 years with wisdom teeth. If some disturbances occur in the process of odontogenesis, they cause anomalies within forming dentine or enamel. During early dentinogenesis, insufficient supply of whole protein, amino acids and vitamins or introduction of chemical compounds such as multi-function phosphonic acids, diuretics, cytostatics results in impairment of odontoblast function, thus inadequate base substance for developing collagen matrix is produced.

During later dentinogenesis and biosynthesis of collagen, the above mentioned factors can cause a decrease of hydrolyzing enzyme's activity, thus lowering the amount of hydroxyproline in procollagen, which in turn results in production of defective organic dentine matrix. The created dentine has reduced number of dentinal tubules, which are sinuous along their length. If the harmful factors are active during mineralization of collagen matrix, predentine is formed. Odontoblast cells produce centers of intermediate tissue between dentine and bone; so-called osteodentin is formed.

Experimental studies proved that dentine mineralization emits an inductive signal for creation of soft protein enamel matrix. If dentine mineralization is disturbed, formation of primary protein enamel matrix is delayed. Stimulation by ameloblasts results in genetically conditioned activity of odontoblasts. If ameloblasts do not develop normally, development of odontoblast cells is inhibited and their function is impaired. Due to odontoblasts' impairment, enamel is subjected to underdevelopment, such as: hypoplasias and hypomineralization. During transition from amorphous to crystal phase, inadequate supply of elements such as calcium, phosphorus, fluorine and other microelements, or introduction of substances regarded as cytotoxic, disturb enamel mineralization. Disturbance of enamel mineralization proved to be a very complex process.

In properly structured and mineralized enamel, geometrical shapes of fissures are significantly diversified. Sizes and geometrical shapes of fissures also vary considerably in each individual. Shallow and deep irregularly shaped fissures are observed, narrow at the entrance and spreading near the base. The depth of fissures varies from a few to between 10 and 20 micrometers, depending on tooth's anatomical group. It happens that the central fissure reaches enamel-dentine junction, and sometimes even ends in dentine. However its bottom is usually covered by a thin layer of enamel (27). A fissure in an erupted tooth is filled with dental plaque with microflora changing with age, and residual food particles.

Longitudinal stripping of molars allowed assessment of mean sizes of fissures in those teeth. It was observed that the central fissure in molars has an average depth of 1.1mm, and its width at fissure entrance ranges from 0.2 to 0.5mm, and the width at fissure base has a mean value of 0.1 mm. Premolars indicate a larger diversity. According to Taylor and Gwinett (81) most commonly they are funnel-shaped with a narrowing at the middle of fissure's depth; inferior premolars have more varied shapes than superior ones. Generally in inferior premolars predominant fissures are narrow at the entrance and expanding at 1/3 of length towards the base. This creates conducive conditions for development of bacterial plaque and deposition of food remains, which leads to beginning and development of carious lesions. It was also observed that enamel covering fissures, especially on first permanent molars, demonstrates a smaller fluorine content than enamel on smooth surfaces of those teeth (16,72).

A lot of interesting information has been collected on the structure and composition of dental plaque residing in hollows of masticatory surfaces of teeth. The information comes from experimental studies carried out on gnotobiotic animals and from studies on people with the use of fissure models made of Mylar foil, placed in large amalgam fillings on molars' masticatory surfaces with the use of dentures as carriers for fragments of natural teeth (third molars). Dental plaque accumulating on smooth surfaces is different from plaque deposits in fissures. Plaque in fissures on masticatory surfaces is made of Gram positive cocci bacteria, which constitute 77-89% of total bacterial flora, short rods, a small amount of filiform microorganisms and blastomyces that are an almost regular ingredient of most plaque in intercusp fissures. Cocci form microcolonies, and bacterial plaque's matrix varies depending on the amount of culturable bacterial flora, plaque's thickness and its position in the fissure. *Streptococcus mutans* does not play any important role in early bacterial colonization of intercusp fissures. In one-day-old plaque this species can hardly be found. With time the number of these bacteria increases, but they constitute less than 10% of total streptococcus flora. Cocci are first to settle in fissures. As plaque ages, their content decreases from 62% on the first day to 46% after three days and down to 28% after eight days. After initial homing in fissures, probability of further addition of new microorganisms seems low. The structure of bacterial plaque in fissures differs from that of plaque accumulating on smooth surfaces. At fissure entrance, cocci are positioned in palisade arrangement, perpendicular to fissure's bottom, and they occur together with fusobacteria, which are considerably less numerous than in plaque on smooth surfaces. During colonization of smooth surfaces, a selection of homing microorganisms takes place. Only those microorganisms can settle which are capable of producing polysaccharides of increased viscosity. In case of fissure plaque, practically any microorganism can become its part. During early stage, the development of plaque on smooth surfaces results from bacterial cell divisions and by addition of microorganisms from saliva. Streptococci constitute almost 90% of bacteria in early plaque.

With development of methods for intercusp fissure sealing, there has been an increased interest in microflora status in carious cavities covered with sealant (75). Because of anatomical characteristics of masticatory surfaces of teeth, sealing material is introduced on bacterial plaque accumulated on the fissure's bottom. Therefore it is critical to obtain information about sealant's impact on microflora in the fissure. The sealant's impact on microflora of fissures not affected by caries has been the subject of numerous studies. Those studies were performed on implanted fragments of masticatory surfaces of teeth. Data indicate that after sealing, microflora in carious lesions becomes suppressed. However, under the sealant a presence of microorganisms capable of growing was observed, which are believed to be etiologically connected with carious processes. It was also demonstrated that sealing materials do not constitute a fully tight barrier separating fissures from oral environment, which occurs very soon after treatment.

Microbiological studies conducted by Jodkowska (32) showed that sealing of intercusp fissures not affected by caries led to a considerable reduction in the number of bacteria. The impact of this treatment on intercusp microflora varied depending on time elapsed after sealing and on the type of applied sealant. In a short time, which means 30 minutes after sealing with Nuva-Seal material, no bacteria growth was observed in 89% of examined samples. In further observation periods, after application of this material, a slow decrease of percentage of aseptic samples was observed, which reached the value of 17% after 18 months. After sealing with Concise BWSS (Brand White Sealant System) a reverse tendency was observed. Nuva-Seal material was more effective in fissure sealing than Concise (BWSS) in a short period immediately after treatment. The efficacy of sealing with this material decreased with time. On the other hand Concise (BWSS), which initially inhibited bacteria growth to a lesser degree than Nuva-Seal, proved more effective in later period of observation. After 18 months the activity inhibiting bacteria growth of both evaluated materials was similar. The most frequently isolated bacterial stains were *Streptococcus mutans* (25%), however more rarely strains classified as *Staphylococcus aureus* were obtained

(3,4%). In 71% of cases growth of only one strain was obtained, whereas in remaining cases various bacterial strains were isolated. Mixed bacterial flora was observed more frequently in material coming from teeth sealed with Nuva-Seal than from teeth sealed with Concise (BWSS).

The author also conducted microbiological studies on 30 first and second permanent molars in children whose condition of hard tissues in initial examination (visual - mirror and probe) in 16 cases suggested a suspicion of an early stage of initial caries and in 14 cases evident initial caries was diagnosed. Samples of material collected for bacteriological examination were collected after 30 minutes, two weeks, and also after two, eight, twelve and eighteen months from sealing. Samples were collected from occlusal surfaces of carious teeth covered with light-cured Nuva-Seal material and with chemically-cured Concise (BWSS). The research demonstrated that the highest reduction of culturable microorganisms in samples collected from fissures sealed with Nuva-Seal occurred 30 minutes after treatment. Then the reduction increased within the period from 2 weeks to 8 months and reached the level which was 300-fold lower compared to samples collected from control teeth. After 12 months of observation 70-fold less bacteria were cultured from sealed teeth, and after 18 months only 6.5-fold less than in samples collected from control teeth. On the other hand Concise (BWSS) material which initially inhibited bacteria growth to a lesser degree than Nuva-Seal, within the period from 2 to 8 months, indicated a 500-fold reduction of microflora compared to samples collected from control teeth. After 12 months of observation the number of culturable bacteria indicated a 100-fold reduction, and after 18 months the activity inhibiting bacteria growth of both assessed sealing materials was similar.

An analysis of isolation of individual bacteria strains and the number of isolated microorganisms in various periods of observation after sealing with both assessed materials indicated that Concise (BWSS) material had a more favorable effect on microflora of carious lesions than Nuva-Seal material. After application of Concise (BWSS) a less frequent development of bacteria etiologically associated with caries, belonging to *Streptococcus mutans* (*S. mutans*) species was observed. Microorganisms belonging to this species occurred solely in material collected from fissures sealed only during certain periods of observation. Numbers of *S. mutans* in material collected after sealing with Concise (BWSS) material were - in various periods of observation - generally much lower than numbers observed after application of Nuva-Seal material. After use of Nuva-Seal material, a less frequent development of mixed bacterial flora was observed. Clinical observations of carious teeth sealed with both assessed materials, which were performed during 18-month period, indicated that only in three cases, where sealant was damaged, slightly deepened carious cavities were observed under sealant. Studies by other researchers confirm the results obtained by the author and conform with the above results, while deepening of carious cavities, if it occurs, seems small (39). This is due mainly to the presence of a mechanical barrier which blocks an inflow of new microorganisms and of substrate for bacterial transformations. Moreover, acid etching of sealed teeth and regenerative capability of dentine may to some degree inhibit further progression of existing carious lesions in fissures (1). Study by Heller *et al.*, who assessed occurrence of caries in previously healthy teeth and in teeth with initial caries, where fissures were sealed in some patients of each group, observed after five years that among previously healthy teeth caries developed in 13% of not sealed teeth, whereas in case of sealed teeth the percentage was smaller and equaled 8% (28). After five years, in the group with previously diagnosed caries the condition of 52% of not sealed teeth and of 11% of sealed teeth deteriorated. According to the authors, sealing of teeth previously affected by caries was fully justified because through application of sealants - instead of conventional preparation and filling of cavities - one of the prophylactic methods against development of carious centers can be applied. Further research may bring more data on this issue.

Healthy enamel, especially its surface layer, however well mineralized during tooth eruption, undergoes continual chemical and physical changes throughout organism's life. Those changes may be favorable, yielding better mineralized, more mature enamel, or they may be unfavorable, especially when enamel is covered by bacterial plaque. Fermentable carbohydrates diffuse into dental plaque where they are metabolized and transformed into organic acids with low pH (lactic, formic, pyruvic acids) and with high pH (butyric, propionic, acetic acids). These acids may be buffered by various systems or they can diffuse into dental plaque or into oral fluid. However, they can also penetrate through the plaque-enamel surface and partly demineralize crystals on and immediately under the surface of enamel. The external surface of enamel is in the state of dynamic balance between demineralization and remineralization, which periodically follow each other.

Fissures in lateral teeth are particularly predisposed for caries development. Most typically caries starts in enamel of fissures. We know that it develops due to disturbances between demineralization and remineralization phases of enamel covered with bacterial plaque. Organic acids produced by bacteria penetrate through the plaque-enamel contact surface in a dissociated or non-dissociated form and diffuse in the liquid phase among enamel crystals or inside crystals. Continual elution of calcium and phosphorus ions, decrease of pH value, ion concentration and other factors have impact on diffusion, on amount of acids penetrating into enamel and on loss of majority of minerals from hydroxyapatites. Progression of carious processes in enamel of fissures depends on consecutive attacks of acids and further destruction of enamel's crystal structure. Early carious lesions are characterized by varied advancement of demineralization in the surface layer and inside the tissue, where the highest loss of non-organic compounds and degradation of prismatic structure is observed in the so-called subsurface layer. With a growing loss of non-organic components of enamel, its porosity increases. Demineralization of enamel in fissures starts at fissure entrance. The main demineralization center spreads sideways from isthmus of fissure along central fissure. Outside layer of enamel with early carious lesions observed on microphotographs indicated a considerably higher degree of mineralization compared to underlying areas of enamel and dentine. Conducted research confirms that in the beginning stage of carious lesion's development the degree of demineralization of fissures' enamel depends on topography and depth of fissures. The deeper and more diversified in shape the fissure, the higher the observable degree of demineralization. The degree of demineralization decreases towards fissure base. In wide fissures the degree of demineralization was smaller. The period of the first three years after tooth eruption is regarded to be of the highest susceptibility for caries development on masticatory surfaces. In dentine, demineralization period depends on the depth and width of fissures. At the entrance of all fissures, both narrow and wide, demineralization area was the largest. At fissure base the area of dentine was preserved and did not indicate symptoms of demineralization, whereas in deep fissures demineralization at fissure base was less pronounced. Narrow fissures indicated a smaller loss of non-organic compounds. In the narrowest fissures demineralization was deepest but in majority of fissures it was limited to the upper part, not reaching the fissure base. The described associations between dentine fissure morphology and range of tissue demineralization in conditions of experimental exposure to caries-inducing factor continued for eight weeks. However, the loss of minerals and dentine tissues was higher on the seventh day of the experiment compared to the loss observed eight weeks after the experiment (45).

3. Development of sealing methods and applied materials

Available methods for caries prophylaxis by means of fluorine compounds, limited consumption of carbohydrates and systematic removal of dental plaque - which effectively inhibit caries on smooth surfaces of teeth (from 35% to over 90%) - do not significantly impact the occurrence of caries on masticatory surfaces of teeth. Since 1965 the search for effective methods of prophylaxis against caries on occlusal surfaces of teeth has been considering individual anatomical characteristics of this surface and has been leading towards isolating of fissures in premolars and molars from the impact of oral environment (quot. after 37). The method which evoked special interest among clinicians consists in fissure and pit sealing on masticatory surfaces, i.e. in mechanical isolation of clinically healthy tissues from oral environment.

Attempts to control caries of masticatory surfaces of lateral teeth have a history of over one hundred years. The oldest concept was a removal of not lesioned fissures during preparation of carious cavities on masticatory surfaces. It was a so-called prophylactic dilatation, invented by Webb and strongly propagated by Black (quot. after 72). Nevertheless, as early as 116 years ago it was observed that prophylactic activities at the time of occurrence of carious events are frequently belated or insufficient. In 1895 Wilson performed prophylactic procedure of filling fissures of permanent molars with cement. Thus he realized Hunter's idea from 1778, who observed that fissure blocking may inhibit development of caries. In 1917 Hove introduced silver impregnation applying ammonia solution of silver nitrate, and in 1950 Ast applied zinc chloride (quot. after 78). Removal of healthy enamel (odontotomy, eradication, prophylactic dilatation) was especially controversial because most applied methods yield unsatisfactory caries reduction and masticatory surfaces turned brown-black.

Willingness to use less invasive methods led to search for new materials. The development of organic chemistry, especially polymers, greatly contributed to progress in prophylaxis of occlusal surfaces of teeth. In the course of performed studies, several chemical compounds were singled out which proved useful for fissure sealing. Generally they belonged to four groups (cyanoacrylates, polyurethanes, epoxy resins and bis-GMA resins).

Cyanoacrylates, which were first adhesive materials used for this procedure, did not gain clinical approval, because they clung to tooth surfaces for a very short time and frequently caused dentine complications. Polyurethanes, which demonstrated poor adhesion to enamel, were applied in caries prophylaxis mainly thanks to content of fluorine compounds. However the two groups of chemical compounds did not act up to expectations.

Only the introduction of epoxy resins by Schröder in 1953 and later of bis-GMA resins by Bowen in 1963 raised new hopes for clinicians. The new materials allow fissure isolation without disturbing healthy enamel. Apart from many advantages, such as: mechanical endurance, chemical resistance, relatively good adhesion, low contractility during polymerization, had one major disadvantage - lack of solid bonding to tooth's hard tissue, resulting in short-term retention of material on sealed teeth.

Only Buonocore in 1965, followed by Gwinett, Sharp and Silverstone demonstrated that permanent bonding of materials with enamel can be obtained after its etching. When etched enamel became a permanent element of clinical procedures with adhesive materials, adhesion and stability of bonding of compound materials with hard tissues of teeth increased on the principle of micromechanical retention. Sealing based on application of bis-GMA resins was introduced less than 50 years ago. Due to matrix type, content of filler particles, presence (or absence) of fluorine ions and efficacy of prophylactic sealant, they were divided into four generations.

Studies on first-generation sealants (sealants polymerized with UV light, started in late 60s) demonstrated diversified prophylactic efficacy of lateral tooth sealing. Their effectiveness depended on the number and type of sealed teeth (first molars, second molars and premolars), applied methodology of procedure, methodology of assessment and the fact that procedures were generally performed by doctors. Representatives of this generation were: Nuva-Seal, Alpha-Seal, Espe 717, Saga-Sealant, Lee-System. After 10-year-long observation, retention of material was 68.0% - 180 sealed teeth in children aged 7-8 years (31). Other authors after five years of observation obtained retention from 19.3% to 63.0% (70,72) and corresponding caries reduction from 57.9% to 43.0% (64).

Second-generation sealants (chemically polymerized, late 60s and early 70s) indicated a higher prophylactic efficacy compared to first-generation sealants (22). Their better effectiveness was due to introduced modifications, which resulted in improved physical-chemical properties (added filler particles) and improved retention to hard tissues of teeth, for example: Concise BWSS from 3M Kerr (PFS) Delton, Concise EBS (Enamel Bond System). Light-cured sealants, which also belong to the second generation, demonstrated lower microleakage (19-20%) compared to chemically cured sealants (50-67%). After 10 years 50% total retention of second-generation sealants was obtained, also a higher percentage of partial retention and of caries reduction (from 40 to 63%) compared to first-generation sealants (70,72). They were represented by light-polymerized Concise (BWSS), Prismashield resins.

Studies on third-generation sealants (polymerized with visible light - the first half of the 80s) demonstrated efficacy which was comparable with second-generation sealants as far as material retention and caries reduction are concerned. After five year of observation it was about 77% (65,66,67). This generation is represented by Concise LVC, Helioseal.

The fourth generation includes sealants with fluorine (late 80s). They are based on bis-GMA resin, urethane dimethacrylate, aliphatic methacrylates. Fluorine is released from fluosilicate glass (Helioseal F) or added in the form of sodium fluoride (Fluoroshield, Fissurit F, Ultraseal XT). The presence of fluorine in sealing material decreases caries risk on sealed surface, even when microcracks occur on sealant's surface. Lasting low concentration of this element in the oral cavity is especially significant. Fluorine level in dental plaque is from 6 ppm to 300 ppm, whereas in saliva it is from 0.001 ppm to 9.4 ppm. Sealants with fluorine such as: Helioseal F and Ultraseal XT were characterized by low viscosity, which enabled easy penetration of material into deep, narrow fissures. Moreover, they do not feature phase separation (i.e. sedimentation of ingredients), which makes them different from other fluorine sealants. Another advantage of Helioseal F and Ultraseal XT sealants is lack of air bubbles in material, which constitutes a common problem with sealing materials. Laboratory tests demonstrated that sealants with fluorine release twice as much fluorine ions within nine days compared to the number of fluorine ions released from glass-ionomer cements (68). In own experimental studies, the number of fluoride anions released from five sealants was determined by direct potentiometry method with the use of fluoride ion selective electrode. In order to obtain constant pH of contact solution and standard solutions, TISAB buffer was used, which eliminated any influence of alien ions. The potentiometer showed the potential of a given solution, while the amount of fluorine was calculated on the basis of calibration curve obtained for standard solutions. The study demonstrated that the value of fluorine ion emission level varied depending on the type of sealing material, type of fluorine compound in sealant, time of testing (short-term from 0.5 to 7 days and longitudinal during 15 study periods from 7 to 371 days). During the whole study period, the highest level of released fluorine ions was observed in Ultraseal XT (22.83 mgF/mm^2 after 12 months and 28.10mgF/mm^2 after 13 months of observation), and a much lower level in Fissurit F (from 13.04mgF/mm^2 after 12 months of observation and 9.30 mgF/mm^2 after 13 months of observation). The lowest level of released fluorine ions was observed for the three remaining sealants: Pentraseal, Ionoseal, Helioseal (4.40, 3.90, 3.40mgF/mm^2 respectively) and after13 months of observation for Helioseal, Pentraseal i Ionoseal (5.8, 4.0, 3.5mgF/mm^2 respectively). It was also observed that release of fluoride ions from sealants containing various fluorine compounds is a long-term process, though amounts of released fluoride ions are small (33).

Clinical studies comparing retention of sealants with fluorine to retention of sealants without fluorine, after one-year observation indicated a higher retention of sealants with fluorine. After three years of observation retention of materials with fluorine was similar. The obtained effect of reduced caries by application of sealants with fluorine was 83.9%, whereas with sealants without fluorine the result was 70% (30). The net gain index (which indicates the actual number of teeth saved from caries thanks to sealing) for 100 teeth sealed by application of sealants with fluorine was 30 teeth saved from caries, while only 15 teeth were saved by application of sealants without fluorine.

Another group of sealants which became a permanent part of caries prophylaxis are glass-ionomer cements (GICs). Thanks to their hydrolytic properties they are capable of forming solid and long-lasting bonds with hard tissues of teeth, non-etched enamel and dentine, and are characterized by similar release of active fluoride ions to surrounding fissures. However, it should not be forgotten that glass-ionomer cements used for sealing of lateral teeth are susceptible to impact of big masticatory forces, thus their application should be limited because of their low resistance to wear. Clinical studies showed low retention index for GICs used as sealants in observation periods from six months to seven years (73). Although a high percentage of sealant loss was observed , it was not directly related to development of caries (25,57,74,76). Examples of such sealants were: ASPA, Fuji III, Ketac Cem, Ketac Bond, Chemfil Superior.

At the beginning of the 90s the quality of glass-ionomer cements was improved by addition of bis-GMA and HEMA (2-hydroxyethyl methacrylate) resins. HEMA monomer was combined with a copolymer based on chains of itaconic acid, having - through amide groups - metacrylan groups polymerizing when exposed to light, which led to development of resin-modified glass-ionomer cements (RMGICs) and polyacid-modified resins which were tested as sealants. In *in vitro* studies, resin-modified glass-ionomer cements demonstrated the same or better adhesive properties and release of fluorine ions. Moreover, the addition of resins made glass-ionomer cements stronger and less brittle. As far as protection against secondary caries is concerned, no significant differences were observed between materials. A low retention index was obtained for Ketac GIC and Vitremer RMGIC after five years (57). The total retention index was less than 2% (1.6%) for both materials. The authors explained low retention with long-term use and insufficient resistance to abrasion of both materials. In another research Forss and Halme noticed 10% total retention after seven-year-long observation of conventional glass-ionomer cement (26). There have been numerous published reports comparing the efficacy of GIC sealants with efficacy of materials based on bis-GMA resins. They covered observation periods from one month to four years. However, due to various research methods, diversification of age groups, anatomical characteristics of observed teeth and number of repeated sealant applications, the results can not be compared, therefore their value is limited. Nevertheless the studies demonstrated decidedly worse retention among glass-ionomer cements compared to retention of sealants based on bis-GMA resins (25,62). Low retention of GICs was due to the fact that before application of sealant, tooth enamel was not subjected to any preparatory procedures aimed at improving retention, but only - according to instruction - teeth were cleaned of dental plaque, rinsed and dried. Probably the main cause of GIC loss may be its inadequate adhesion to enamel. Such explanation seems to confirm results of *in vivo* and *in vitro* studies on the impact of various preparatory procedures on GIC's adhesion to tissues of teeth. They indicate that adhesion can be improved by proper conditioning of enamel before application of cement. 30-second etching with 50% citric acid before application of cement or 10-second etching with 10% polyacrylic acid resulted in 26% retention after two years and 10% after seven years. The reasons for such unsatisfactory results are poor adhesion of cement to enamel, lack of procedures improving adhesion and brittleness of GICs. An improvement of cement's physical properties suggested by the authors, e.g. liquidity of cement which was created as a result of perfecting Fuji III, was not confirmed in two- and four-year studies reporting 4% retention, whereas with application of a comparable sealant based on bis-GMA resins - Delton - the values obtained after two and four years were respectively 79% and 61%. The discussed issue is GIS's ability to release fluorine, which enables anticarietic activity on neighboring tissues and facilitates remineralization of existing early carious centers in enamel. Observation of carious process after six and twelve months of observation in several cases in both study groups prevents formulation of an opinion on anticarietic activity of glass-ionomer cements. Mejer and Mjör after six and twelve months of study observed considerable loss of cement on 66% of masticatory surfaces sealed with Fuji III, however they did not observe carious lesions, whereas in case of sealing with bis-GMA resins (Delton and Concise), whose total retention after five years was as high as 90%, caries was present on 5% of masticatory surfaces (48). This suggests that even a small amount of cement which remains in fissures is enough for long-lasting caries prevention. *In vitro* studies demonstrated that fissures sealed with GIC are more resistant to demineralization than unsealed fissures, even if presence of sealant is not confirmed clinically, authors associate the anticarietic effect it with possible residue of cement remains at the fissures' bottom and continual release of fluorine by glass-ionomer cements. Some attention should also be paid to antibacterial activity of glass-ionomer cements against *S. mutans* and *S. sorbinus*. Suppression of colony growth is related to the ability to release fluorine ions. Therefore the choice of GIC as fissure sealant must result from other reasons than good retention or cariostatic property. Certainly it can be an alternative e.g. in the absence of proper humidity control, with partial tooth eruption or with mentally or physically handicapped patients. Apart from that, glass-ionomer cements have another advantage of simple application technique. Increased efficacy of sealing can be obtained by reapplication of sealant during routine visits, however this will increase cost of treatment. That is why only certain clinical situations can constitute an indication for such treatment, for example difficult children or those with a high caries risk (23).

It was observed that resin-modified cements demonstrate much stronger bonding forces with dentine (almost threefold) compared to conventional glass-ionomer cements, but considerably weaker than sealants based on bis-GMA resins. Retention of glass-ionomer cements after 6 months equaled 93%, after 24 months from 82.5% to 86%, and after four-year observation only 35% (50,51,86). Baseggio et al. assessed the efficacy of Vitremer modified glass-ionomer cement compared to Fluoishield conventional sealant based on bis-GMA resins containing fluorine. During three-year studies on sealants in second molars in 320 patients aged 2-16 years, retention of sealant modified with glass-ionomer cement was 5.10%, whereas retention of sealant based on bis-GMA resin equaled 91.08%, and total loss of retention was observed in 6.37% and 7.65% of sealed teeth respectively. Caries on masticatory surfaces was observed in 20.06% of teeth sealed with materials modified with glass-ionomer cement and in 8.91% of teeth sealed with materials based on bis-GMA resin (7).

Compomers, also called composite materials modified with polyfunctional acids, contain bis-GMA monomers, deionized glass which constitutes mechanical filler with 42-67% of volume and particle size 0.7-5µm, and monomers containing COOH acidic functional groups. Thanks to glass content they are capable of releasing fluorine contained in glass, but in a much lesser quantity than GICs or resin-modified GICs (63). A two-year assessment of sealants based on bis-GMA resins (Fissurit F, Fissurit FX, compomer Dyract Seal and ormocer Admira Seal) demonstrated that retention of the compomer (Dyract Seal) was much lower compared to the other sealants. However, no significant differences were observed in marginal tightness of assessed sealants and in caries presence on surfaces of sealed teeth (88). In research comparing two materials - one compomer and one based on bis-GMA resin - special emphasis was placed on advantages of compomers, which are easy to use, chemically and physically durable, and they release fluorine. No difference was observed between applied sealant and its retention and between the degree of caries reduction and material retention (quot. after 24). In another study in which GIC-based material with zinc and fluorine was used (Jonosit Seal DMG), after six years of observation in 77.5% of cases retention on occlusal surfaces of teeth was confirmed. Presence of caries was closely related to retention of material. In case of total retention of sealant, caries reduction was 99.6%, whereas with total loss of material after five years caries reduction was 69% (34). Other authors, such as Aranda et al. and deLuca-Froga et al., who assessed activity and preventive performance of resin-modified glass-ionomer cements (RMGICs) and composite materials modified with polyfunctional acids, observed that retention index changed after one-year observation, rising from 20% to 95.9% (4,18). An important factor which must be considered in case of glass-ionomer cements used as sealants is the fact that even after clinical loss of material, a small amount of sealant remains at the fissure's bottom with fluorine still being released, thus protecting masticatory surface. Higher grow of caries was observed in the control group compared to the group with applied sealant. Anticarietic protective effect of glass-ionomer cements remained even after their loss. Masticatory surface was protected in the period most susceptible to caries, i.e. during the first year after tooth eruption (82). In this period there is no contact of opposing teeth and children have difficulties with appropriate hygienic procedures. According to Forss and Halme, after this period the risk of caries is lower and consequences of sealant loss would be less significant (26). Therefore it was assumed that children from the study group would have a higher caries development than children from the control group, because the latter were older. However the research yielded opposite results. It should be stressed that glass-ionomer cements are recommended for sealing erupting teeth due to difficulties with proper isolation of teeth during application, while glass-ionomer cements are less sensitive to humidity, and because these teeth are susceptible to caries (62).

In a research where retention and efficacy of fissure sealing with glass-ionomer cements was assessed after reapplication of material, caries reduction on masticatory surfaces three years after sealing was 66.5% compared to untreated control group (42). This suggests that lost material should be supplemented in order to ensure the best protection of occlusal surface. The obtained results were better compared to sealing without supplementation of lost material (82). Repetitive application requires time an results in higher cost of treatment. Therefore such prophylactic program may be directed rather at patients from high risk groups, though it may also be applied for the whole population (55). With tooth eruption, all permanent molars should be sealed, which will prevent caries development and consequently will lead to a decrease in the value of the DMF score. However, costs of promoting such a program will be higher, because surfaces which probably would never be carious, would also be sealed (41). In case of sealing only teeth with high caries risk, occurrence of caries would decrease, as well as cost of treatment, which constitutes an important factor in public health protection (9). Thus it is necessary to establish which teeth indicate a higher caries risk and to choose appropriate material.

4. Aim and requirements for sealing materials

The aim of sealant application is:

- mechanical closure of anatomical fissures, crevices and pits on masticatory surfaces of lateral teeth, upper distal-lingual fissures, buccal surfaces of inferior teeth and blind pits in incisors,
- sealing of intercusp fissures from penetration of oral fluids, microorganisms and their substrates which start carious process,
- obtaining mechanical microretention of sealing materials,
- obtaining clinical efficacy in caries reduction on occlusal surfaces.

Requirements for sealing materials:

- appropriate period of activity, fast and easy application,
- fast bonding of material,
- fast curing,
- proper viscosity of material allowing deeper penetration into narrow fissures,
- good and long-lasting adhesion to enamel walls,
- thermal and mechanical properties similar to characteristics of hard tissues of teeth,

- low sorption and solubility in oral environment,
- resistance to abrasion,
- good tolerance by patient (must not disturb occlusion),
- topical and general non-toxicity of material,
- flexible equivalence with tooth tissues
- long-term anticarietic activity.

Appropriate period of activity, fast and easy application of sealants, fast bonding and curing should be within time limits accepted by the patient. Long curing may cause anxiety in a child, leading to moisturizing of treatment area, to outflow of material beyond the sealed site and thus to disturbance of proper polymerization (10). It occurs especially with little children, where sealed teeth are not yet fully erupted and covered with a fold of mucous membrane. Therefore chemically cured resins, which are cured from 45 to 90 seconds after initial mixing of material until completion of curing are not recommended. Materials polymerized with halogen light should be used, as they have a more favorable, unlimited activity time and are characterized by fast curing up to 20-40 seconds, depending on intensity of lamp-emitted light.

Constitution of materials for sealing fissures is generally similar to constitution of composite materials used to fill cavities in hard tissues of teeth. The difference is that fissure sealants have more liquid consistence than fillers, which allows penetration into etched fissures. Sealants based on bis-GMA formula contain amine accelerators and an initiator - benzoyl peroxide. Light-cured sealing materials require a lamp emitting wavelengths of 340-400 nanometers to initiate polymerization. Contemporary sealants are made of one ingredient which does not need mixing. It consists of three parts of viscous bis-GMA monomer, which is diluted with one part of MMA monomer (methyl methacrylate) in order to obtain material of relatively low viscosity. The activator is 2% methylbenzyl ether, which in the presence of 1-2% benzoyl peroxide and light initiates polymerization. Research on appropriate selection of monomer and diluent is very important and provides information about obtained physical properties of sealants. Replacement of methacrylate monomer with other monomers leads to changes of viscosity, impacts extension or shortening of curing time, and alters its hydrophilic character. Efficacy of sealing depends on resin's ability to penetrate fissures before its curing, i.e. on the ability to create a mechanical barrier for carious process. In order to produce an adequately strong bonding and secure proper retention, sealant has to flow over the surface of etched enamel and penetrate microfissures on etched surface. However, it is believed that resin's penetrative ability depends on etching pattern and enamel's moisture, surface tension of material, its viscosity and penetration index. Modifications in application of various monomers resulted in change of cuing time.

Studies on sealants' tightness confirmed the occurrence of microleakages for all assessed sealing materials (e.g. Epoxylite 9075, Nuva Seal, ESPE 717, Concise Enamel Bond, Kerr Fissure, Sealant Delton). Microleakage was observed on the sealant-enamel interface, and in case of glass-ionomer cements, dye penetrated through the whole surface of material. Nuva-Seal seemed the most resistant to dye penetration, though after two weeks some number of cases where dye penetration on the sealant-enamel interface occurred could be observed. In most studied cases ESPE 717 and Epoxylite 9075 materials demonstrated microleakage on the sealant-enamel interface and through the material. The occurrence of microleakage was related to hydrophobic structure of materials and their porosity, which constitutes a better barrier for dye penetration. The barrier resulting from material's hydrophobic properties is not stable and with time it deteriorates, which results in microleakage.

ASPA and Poly F glass-ionomer cements contain polyacrylic matrix, which is hydrophilic thanks to carboxyl groups. These materials are permeable to water and dye solutions. 24 hours after their application it was observed that aqueous dye solutions penetrated through the sealant-enamel interface and through the material. Another study on Concise, Delton, Kerr, Nuva-Seal sealants with the use of aqueous dye solutions with Ca45 and S35 radioactive isotopes did not show dye penetration when enamel was etched and sealant permanently and tightly adhered to enamel. Also extension of enamel curing time up to 30 seconds resulted in 32% decrease of microleakage occurrence compared to teeth etched for a shorter time.

Studies determining microhardness of sealants demonstrated varied degree of this parameter from initial 7.51±0.62 for Concise EB and 4.78±0.52 for ASPA cement, up to values increasing in time after three months: 16.49±0.29 for Concise EB and 55.28±1.31 for ASPA cement. Compared to sealants based on bis-GMA formula, ASPA cements after three months demonstrated higher stability and a higher flexibility factor. With increased amount of sealant, rigidity of material also increases along with susceptibility to deformation, that is Young's modulus. The best materials are those with Young's modulus below 10 GPa.

Solubility and disintegration of bis-GMA type sealing materials in oral environment is low and has no clinical significance. Compared to bis-GMA resins, glass-ionomer cements undergo dissolution and disintegration to a much higher degree. Water absorption of sealing materials is low, which is beneficial as it contributes to closure of marginal fissure created by polymerization contraction.

Sealants' resistance to abrasion depends on type of material, content, size and arrangement of filler's particles, as well as on anatomical conditions of sealed teeth. It is assumed that abrasion of sealants based on bis-GMA formula occurs due to impairment of silane bonding agent. Abrasion is a two-phase process: the first phase is characterized by abrasion of polymer and exposure of filler particles, whereas in the second phase they are torn out of the material. Abrasion of sealant on masticatory surface begins on fissure periphery in sites with the thinnest layer of material. Defects on fissure periphery are retention sites, where dental plaque accumulates. The rate of material abrasion also depends on the method of bonding basic ingredients and on the way of material application. Air bubbles trapped in material are sites with decreased resistance to abrasion. The degree of abrasion also depends on activity of separate tooth groups during mastication and on anatomy of tooth and its position in the arch. Sealant abrasion is observed in distal part of superior molars' masticatory surface twice as frequently as in medial parts of those teeth. Moreover, it has been proved that the highest abrasion occurs soon after sealant placement and it decreases with time. The lowest sealant loss was observed in inferior first premolars compared to the other premolar teeth. After 30 months mean value of material volume loss for premolars was 0.43±0.24mm^2, whereas mean depth of material loss was 221.8±115.1μm. In *in vitro* studies, abrasion, penetration and deformation four most commonly used bis-GMA resins sealants was assessed. It was proved, that materials were abraded to a different degree. The observed level of material wear increased as follows: Delton-21.5; Kerr-22.3; Nuva Seal-23.9; Carbimet -3.,0 (*10^{-4} mm^2/mm). The assessed sealants differed considerably in degree of penetration and formability, where the lowest values were observed for Kerr, and the highest values were observed for Nuva Seal, which was conditioned by material composition. For example, Kerr had 40% of quartz filler particles by volume, which increased its resistance to abrasion and decreased the risk of damaging the surface layer of resin susceptible to abrasion. Due to the necessity of avoiding mastication impairment, sealing material should be present only in anatomical fissures and crevices. Therefore its excess should be removed from occlusal surface.

Every substance of foreign origin which is introduced into oral environment may have an adverse impact and induce certain biological or health effects. Almost all organic ingredients can be washed out from polymerized sealing material by organic solvents, e.g. methanol, ethanol or water. Released formaldehyde and metacrylic acid are particularly dangerous, the latter creating an inhibitory oxygen layer in the surface layer of sealant after polymerization and it can release into oral environment for a long time (up to 115 days after polymerization). Admittedly it does not cause toxic effect, but it may contribute to a local allergic reaction. During monomer particle disintegration, alcohol may be formed (e.g. from bis-GMA resin - bivalent alcohol). Further metabolism of alcohol occurs in digestive tract, leads to release of bisphenol A (BPA), which is a constituent of many compounds, such as bis-GMA, bis-EMA (bisphenol ethoxylate dimethacrylate), TEGDMA (triethylene glycol dimethacrylate), applied in sealing materials. Bisphenol A was detected in saliva of patients subjected to prophylactic fissure sealing. The substance belongs to the group of chemical compounds called xenoestrogens, which - joining with estrogen receptors - imitate the activity of natural hormones, thus they may impact human health. In a study by Olea et al. (56) on the presence of bisphenol A, it was detected at the level of 90-931μg/ml in saliva samples collected from patients one hour after sealing. The study also demonstrated that sealing material exposed to 100ºC temperature for 30 minutes in buffers with pH 1 and pH 13, released bisphenol A in concentrations causing increased proliferation of MCF-7 cells up to one hour after application, which indicates induction of para estrogenic activity. In other studies authors assessing seven different sealants in vitro did not confirm the presence of bisphenol A in any of the assessed materials. However, determinable amounts of TEGDMA were detected in all studied sealants. It can also be supposed that with proper proceeding, bisphenol A will not be released if substances reacting with each other have a sufficient degree of purity. Only in products containing bis-GMA, small amounts of bisphenol A are released, and it occurs only directly after material curing. In most studies bisphenol A was detected in saliva only directly after application of sealant, and this was the case especially with "older" generation of Delton sealant, which still contained bis-DMA (bisphenol A dimethacrylate) in concentrations not affecting the organism. Approximate calculations of bisphenol A released from sealants showed that its level is lower than 1.5%, and such concentrations are too small to cause carcinogenic effect. A study assessing the presence and concentration of BPA (bisphenol A) in blood serum and saliva in 30 individuals aged 18-40 years before sealing and one, three and twenty-four hours after sealing (Delton Pit&Fssure Sealant Dentsplay) indicated the presence of bisphenol A in all examined patients before sealing at the level from 0.07 to 6.00 ng/ml. The level of bisphenol A three hours after sealing had the highest value and after twenty-for hours it returned to the same value as before sealing. The highest recorded concentrations of bisphenol A after a single application and after four subsequent applications were 3.98mg/ml and 9.08mg/ml respectively. Bisphenol A was not observed in blood serum at any stage of the study (89). Exposures to BPA from other sources than resins contributed to a change of BPA level in saliva. What is more, the amount of sealant's dose used in the study did not impact BPA concentration in blood serum. Further research is necessary to establish the impact of BPA from sealants on estrogen balance.

Chemical compounds contained in sealing materials may have a destructive influence on genetic material in DNA and RNA; it was proved that as many as 14 components of composite materials indicate genotoxicity. On the other hand it was not demonstrated if materials based on bis-GMA and UDMA (urethane dimethacrylate) indicate mutagenicity. It is known that TEGDMA (triethylene glycol dimethacrylate) used as componomer in nontoxic concentrations has mutagenic properties, it impairs proper cell structure, e.g. through interactivity with cell membrane, and its functionality, e.g. decreasing cell's glutathione level, which is responsible for cell structure protection and detoxication. Apart from that it changes expression level of many genes which are important for proliferation processes, control of cell cycle and cell death as well as for DNA replication and repair.

Dentine bonding systems, used to increase adhesion of sealant to hard tissues of teeth, including glutaraldehyde, proved mutagenic and genotoxic in some *in vivo* studies (89).

Data from available studies indicate that concentrations necessary to evoke mutagenic reaction in *in vivo* conditions are much higher than those which evoke a reaction in a patient. Data on mutagenic impact of materials show that their components act mainly in *in vitro* conditions. Such situation occurs especially in case of dentine bonding systems and light-activated glass-ionomer cements. It was proved that resin-modified glass-ionomer cements (Vitrebond) evoked genotypic reactions. The cause was 2-phenylindole chloride which had cytotoxic effect on cell cultures.

Therefore all materials introduced into oral cavity in certain conditions may harmfully impact the organism through releasing specific doses of chemical compounds.

4.1 Technique of sealing procedure

4.1.1 Tooth selection

Sealing procedure should be performed not later than four months after eruption of first permanent molars, at the age of 5-6 years, but practically even after 10 years of age - premolars at the age of 8-12 years, especially if caries is observed in deciduous teeth and first permanent molars, second permanent molars at the age of 11-13 years, and the procedure can be performed up to the 15th year of age. In a population with a high caries risk, also deciduous molars and permanent premolars should be sealed.

Sealant should be applied in teeth with narrow and deep fissures and in teeth with developmental abnormalities on masticatory surfaces. Sealing depends mainly on meticulousness during clinical procedure, i.e. isolation of teeth from moist oral environment, thorough cleaning of occlusal surfaces, etching, rinsing, drying and application of sealant.

4.1.2 Isolation of teeth to be sealed

This is a very important stage of the procedure. Maintaining the area dry is critical for successful sealing procedure. Usage of dental dam, saliva ejector and alternatively lignin rolls is recommended.

Difficulties with proper procedure occur during sealing of molars in maxilla (neighboring parotid gland) and in fissures of freshly erupted molars in maxilla and mandible, when a fold of mucous membrane covers tooth crown which is not fully erupted.

4.1.3 Cleaning of masticatory surface

Masticatory surfaces should be carefully cleaned of bacterial plaque with the use of a hard rotating brush with paste containing a small amount of pumice but no fluorine compounds. Many published reports assess various of cleaning masticatory surfaces before procedure and techniques of applying sealant. One of suggestions is to use a brush dampened with hydrogen peroxide, without pumice. Research demonstrated that after cleaning with pumice, its particles are forced into fissures, which may impair resin's penetration into fissures. Botti et al. assessed cleaning of occlusal surfaces from dental plaque with the use of a synthetic fiber brush and PROPHYflex 3 device (11). The results suggest that the assessed device was the most effective in removing dental plaque compared to cleaning by synthetic fibers. Preparation of masticatory surface by air abrasion was conducted with Air Flow sandblaster at 4.5-7 bars of pressure and at 90° angle from a distance of 1 mm. The abrasive material is aluminum trioxide. The high value of kinetic energy of particles ejected as a stream enables effective preparation of hard tissues. It is recommended to use grains below 50 microns and to abrade intermittently (35,54). Sound systems are based on pneumatic scaler working within the range 6000-6500Hz, vibration amplitude 60-1000 microns. The correct pressure should not exceed 1.5N. Diamond drill bits with 25 and 40 micron coating.

Laser etching with Er Cr:YSGG, 2W and 40Hz laser (8) and erbium laser Er:YAG 7W, Er:YAG (5.5W) (49,70,71). Er:YAG laser demonstrates a 15-fold higher water absorption than CO_2 laser and 20,000-fold higher than Nd:YAG laser. Activity time is thousandths of a second with a minimal energy dose. The energetic level for enamel ablation is $3.3J/cm^3$ and for dentine ablation it is $2.8J/cm^3$. Carisolv system and sodium hypochlorite demonstrated not only effective cleaning of fissures but also antibacterial properties (49,87). Fissure surface preparation with compressed air was assessed by Kramer N *et al.* (43), whereas Mosemi *et al.* studied the impact of masticatory surface preparation with Er Cr YSGG laser and air abrasion, as well as with 37% phosphoric acid on bonding strength on the wall with INSTRON servohydraulic machine. Samples were divided into three groups. In group A, masticatory surface was etched with acid only, in group B air abrasion and acid were applied, and in group C initial etching with laser and phosphoric acid was performed (53). The results indicate that bond strength was highest in the group where air abrasion and acid etching were applied, compared to the group with acid only etching or initial preparation by means of a laser and phosphoric acid etching (43).

4.1.4 Etching

After protecting a site from access of saliva, after cleaning and drying, etching procedure can be started. In order to obtain enamel etch, acid solution has to be spread on intercusp fissure surface for 15 seconds. The recommended concentration of phosphoric acid is 37%. The introduction of gel etches allowed to limit the impact of acid used to prepare enamel surface before application of sealant and to decrease the risk of uncontrollable contact of etch with dentine. Gels are applied only once, whereas liquid solutions of acids require multiple application. Etches in the gel form penetrate fissure enamel to the same degree as liquid etches. Acid penetration is hampered by impurities left over after mechanical cleaning of fissures.

It is advisable to repetitively moisten enamel with acid solution during etching, in order to unblock dentine microtubules by removal of calcium salts precipitated during chemical reaction, which limit the effect of etching. After introduction of one-stage etching (of enamel and dentine), dentists have been using self-etching systems based on non-washable acid monomers (low-concentration acids, 10% phosphoric or maleinic acid, 2.5% nitric acid or their mixtures including extra ingredients such as metal ions, glycerin) (2), which eliminate the rinsing phase thus shortening application time and greatly limit the risk of infection of the operative site by saliva and the risk of a mistake during application, which makes the procedure insusceptible to operator's manual "skills".

A soft brush is recommended for etch application, whereas cotton wool balls are not advisable as they contain bubbles of trapped air hampering even spreading of etching solution. Acid solution leads to creation of microfissures in enamel, whose presence enables sealant's penetration deep into tissues. Microscopically, enamel surface becomes rough and appears matt, in electron microscope view - pits of various shapes are visible which were created by a loss of some enamel prisms. The pits are 50-52µm deep.

4.1.5 Rinsing

After etching, the etched surfaces of teeth are rinsed with high pressure water for 10-20 seconds in order to remove acid and residue after the chemical reaction of etching. If etching was performed with an acid in gel form, rinsing time should be doubled.

4.1.6 Drying of etched surface of teeth

After rinsing the tooth's surface should be dried with compressed air for about 15 seconds and isolated from saliva by dental dam which constitutes a simple and effective method of protecting operative field against infection by microorganisms from saliva. This is necessary because any water remaining after rinsing as well as organic impurities from saliva left on the etched surface, impair sealant's penetration into microfissures, thus decreasing the strength of bonding between sealant and enamel. In case of contact with saliva, etching should be repeated for 15 seconds with subsequent rinsing and drying of the tooth. It should be checked with special attention that the compressed air is not polluted by water or oil.

4.2 Application of sealant

Sealant is applied on tooth's surface with delicate brushes made of camelhair, by means of special applicators with a plastic ball or with a cannula resembling a syringe needle. The time required for sealant application and its quantity depend on material type. Chemically cured sealants have a limited curing time and have to be mixed and placed before hardening commences. Otherwise they become too dense and do not reach the required depth in microfissures created by etching. Light-cured sealants have unlimited bonding time, which allows placing of resin when its viscosity is lowest. Too little sealant may cause early material loss, because it cannot cover the whole etched surface, which results in low retention. Too much sealant may impair occlusion or cause unsatisfactory retention due to break-off or abrasion of material. If a loss or inaccuracy in covering of surface is observed, excess material should be removed with a coarse and fine coated diamond drill with subsequent polishing until smooth (58,60). Surveys among children and their parents on acceptance of colored sealants (red, pink, yellow, white, opalescent) indicated that a great majority of individuals prefer - for aesthetic reasons - white and opalescent sealants.

4.3 Factors impacting effective sealing

Efficacy of sealing procedure is determined by: retention of sealant and obtained caries reduction. Factors impacting retention of sealing materials are:

- condition of tooth surface before sealing,
- morphology of fissures,
- degree of tooth eruption (and probably the time of tooth exposure to oral environment before sealing),
- anatomical features characteristic for an anatomical group,
- individual susceptibility to caries,
- type of sealing material,
- precision of sealing procedure.

Varied morphology of fissures in lateral teeth makes diagnostics of caries in fissures by means of dental mirror and probe ineffective (about 25% probability of caries detection). Fissure penetration with a sharp dental probe causes iatrogenic damage of enamel surface, often affected by demineralization processes. As literature reports, a less invasive method is diagnosing with the use of (5,59) electrical conductivity measurement (ECM), quantitative light-induced fluorescence (QLF) (5) and DIAGNOdent (58,68) in order to assess sensitivity and specificity of caries detection on occlusal surfaces (5,59). ECM demonstrates high sensitivity of between 93% and 96%. However specificity of this method is relatively low - less than 80% (71-77%). Specificity at the average level of about 75% means that 25% of healthy tooth surfaces is recognized and diagnosed as diseased and qualified for treatment, including invasive therapy. The ECM method enables long-term observations of carious lesions.

The FOTI method (fiber-optic-transillumination) serves to diagnose carious lesions, primarily on masticatory surfaces. The sensitivity of the test does not exceed 57%. In laser diagnostics the phenomenon of QLF and DIAGNOdent device are used. The sensitivity of the laser method enables detection of tiniest fluorescence changes related to demineralization of hard tissues. Research indicates the advantage of laser measurement compared to bitewing radiogram in examining occlusal surface lesions. The probability of caries detection in fissures by means of electric conductivity measurement is 93%, whereas the accuracy of X-ray diagnostics (bitewing radiogram) is 75% (46). Sensitivity of microbiological tests (determination of *Streptococus mutans* count) is 67% (40,84). Comparison of clinical test results with radiological results indicated that during clinical study 15% of teeth did not demonstrate any carious centers in fissures which were detectable by means of radiological examination. During repeated clinical tests performed by the same team on individuals aged 14, 17 and 20 years, no carious centers were observed, whereas during radiological examinations carious centers in enamel and dentine were observed respectively in 26.0%, 37.5% and 50.0% of examined teeth. Application of the radioluminescence method showed carious centers in 32.4% of sealed teeth which during previous clinical tests were deemed healthy (85). In 58% of teeth caries was observed in fissures, which included enamel and dentine (19).

The impact of fissure morphology on sealant's retention is associated with conditions of mechanical retention of material. Sealant is retained better in deep fissures than in shallow ones, and also better in fissures with initial caries, where fissure surface is uneven, than in fissures free from caries.

The degree of tooth eruption and tissues' exposure time to oral environment under sealant have a significant impact on the prophylactic effect of sealing (6). Healthy enamel during tooth eruption is relatively well mineralized, however the process of forming the non-organic composition of the tissue is not yet finished and is subjected to constant physical and chemical changes. Physical changes are various types of abrasion, microcracks and fractures of enamel which occur when crystals of enamel surface layer become fully etched by acids from consumed food. Chemical changes include enamel maturing, which results from continuous dynamic exchange of ions between plaque and fluid in oral cavity on one hand and enamel surface on the other one. Study results indicate that anatomical group of teeth, their position in the dental arch (superior, inferior) may also impact prophylactic efficacy of tooth sealing. It has been proved that sealing of inferior teeth yields better results than sealing of superior ones. Higher efficacy of sealing of inferior teeth is caused by better access of the operator to masticatory surfaces being sealed, better penetration of viscous sealant into fissures due to pressure gradient. An analysis of available literature and own studies indicates that the lowest results are obtained in case of sealing superior second premolars. It is connected - among other things - with small occlusal surface, short fissures and proximity of the parotid gland. A comparison of sealant retention on premolars and molars shows that sealing materials demonstrate better retention on molars. Caries reduction in premolars is also lower compared to reduction on molars after sealing procedure. Lower caries reduction in premolars may be associated with later eruption of those teeth and their generally lower susceptibility to caries compared to molars (36).

Type of sealing material has been deemed a particularly important factor which may impact the effect of sealing procedure to a greater degree than other factors. In caries prophylaxis of lateral teeth various methods and materials are used, e.g. fluoride varnish, resins based on bis-GMA formula (reinforced or not by microfiller particles) enriched or not by fluoride ions (44) and conventional glass-ionomer cements (chemically cured) (77,38), reinforced by silver filings (cements) and HEMA resin-modified cements (7), resins modified with polyacid (7), semi-fluid materials (13,14), ormocers (12,15). Sealing materials are characterized by liquid consistence which allows their inflow into fissures, however it is believed that sealant bonds with etched enamel on cuspal slopes and not at fissure bases (3).

Results of studies on fluoride varnishes showed that despite their efficacy in suppression of caries on flat surfaces of teeth, they are less effective in suppression of caries on masticatory surfaces. This is due to the fact that compared to bis-GMA resins and glass-ionomer cements, fluoride varnishes are retained at the most for a few days only, therefore their prophylactic effect depends on the number of fluoride ions released while the varnish remains on the tooth. Fluoride varnishes reduce caries from 50 to 70% depending on frequency of application. In case of three applications during one year, caries reduction on masticatory surfaces is from 50 to 56%, whereas with three yearly applications during three years the value increases to 70% (61). It seems that the long-term prophylactic effect of sealing procedure depends not only on the above mentioned factors - with reference to sealed masticatory surface and whole dentition - but also other factors, such as: type of fluoride compounds and frequency of its application, level of oral infection in a given individual, number of microorganisms from *Streptococcus mutans* group in saliva and person's dietary and hygienic habits. All mentioned factors may also be subjected to change in a certain period of time as a result of carious process activity modifications in a given individual. Matalon *et al.* (47) assessed antibacterial properties of sealing materials which contained fluorine. Four sealants were used: Helioseal F, Ultraseal XT, Dyract Seal and GC Fuji Triage. Samples of materials were "aged" for 30 days and rinsed daily with 0.05% solution of NaF for 14 days. After the last rinsing, a culture of *Streptococcus mutans* was added (about 1×10^6), which was placed on the surface of each sample and cultured for one hour at 37°C. Results indicated that GC Fuji Triage and Dyract Seal had antibacterial properties for 24 hours after the last exposure to fluorine. GC Fuji Triage maintained strong bactericidal activity up to 48 hours after fluorine rinse. After 72 hours none of the materials demonstrated antibacterial properties. The 30-day aging process resulted in total elimination of their antibacterial properties, but two-week daily rinsing with 0.05% solution of NaF restored antibacterial capability for glass-ionomer cement and compomer (47).

Increased efficacy of sealing of masticatory surfaces can be obtained by improving sealant's retention, elimination of marginal leakage, which prevent caries development under sealant (14,15,33,52,83). Original laboratory research on improving efficacy of sealing by modification of etching time (23, 30, 60 seconds) and application of intermediate system of dentine bonding indicated, that bonding systems applied on enamel etched with acid fill spaces created by partly dissolved enamel and penetrate deeper. After polymerization a hybrid layer is created. Application of bonding systems (Concise LCWS and Helioseal) showed that depending on etching time and type of sealing material with or without bonding system (Schotbond MP i Dyract) it was observed that with extended etching time the bonding strength of Concise LCWS on enamel wall without bonding system decreased, whereas the bonding strength of Heliosal increased. After application of bonding systems appropriate for a given sealing material, with extended etching time, strength of bonding on enamel wall decreased for Concise LCWS sealant with Schotbond MP intermediate bonding system and increased for Helioseal with Syntac intermediate system. In case of etched dentine covered directly with sealant, bonding strength on enamel's wall was insignificantly different, whereas with the use of intermediate systems (appropriate for a given sealing material) an increased bonding strength on the wall was observed. In case of Concise LCWS with Schotbond MP - 2.7-fold, in case of Heliomolar with Syntac > threefold (33).

Studies on morphology of Concise LCWS and Helioseal jonts with hard tissues of teeth indicated occurrence of two types of joints: gapless (adhesion on all surface), and with microfissure between tooth tissues and sealing material. The width of microfissures varied depending on sealing material - in case of Helioseal, microfissures were 30-90μm wide with dominating width of 30μm, whereas in case of Concise LCWS from 10-50μm with dominating width of 25μm. Moreover, micropores with diameter of up to 8μm were observed in Helioseal material, whereas in Concise LCWS material - vertical and horizontal microcracks of sealant extending to dentine were observed. After application of intermediate bonding systems and sealants, gapless joints were observed, however few had microfissures, which were from 1-50μm wide.

o szerokości ~ 20 μm.

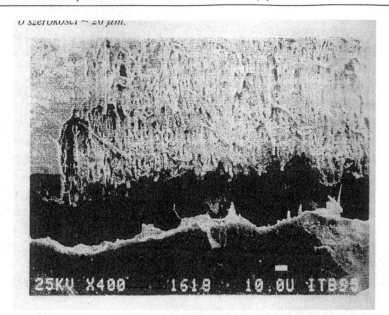

Fig. 1. The SEM microphotograph of the section of etched dentin coated directly with H sealer (horizontal level section). Visible (from the top) microstructure of the dentin and the fissure between the dentin and the sealer ~ 20 μm broad.

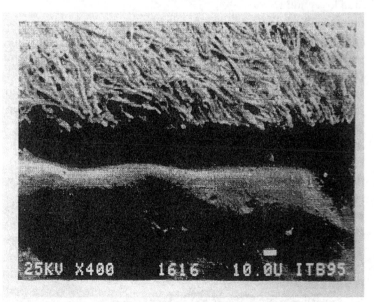

Fig. 2. The SEM microphotograph of the section of etched dentin coated directly with H sealer (horizontal level section). Visible (from the top) microstructure of the dentin and the fissure between the dentin and the sealer (30 - 90 μm broad). Clearly seen micro-pores in the sealer reaching the breadth of 8 μm.

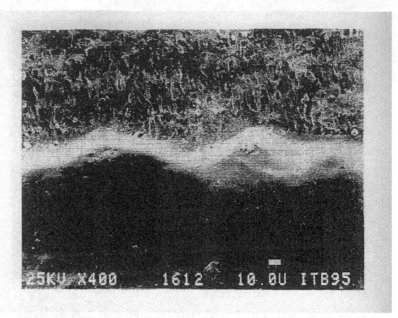

Fig. 3. The SEM microphotograph of the section of etched dentin coated directly with Sy and H sealer (horizontal level section). Visible (from the top) microstructure of the dentin and the fitting hybrid layer and sealer.

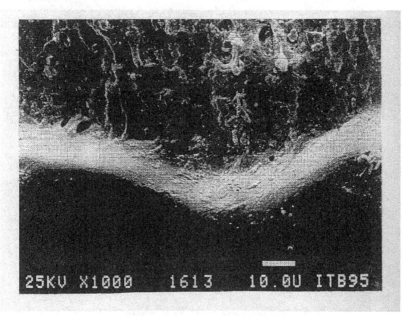

Fig. 4. The SEM microphotograph of the section of etched dentin coated by indirect bonding system Sy and H sealer. Visible magnified fragment of middle part of photography fig. 3.

In vitro and *in vivo* studies on application of X-ray microanalysis for assessment of penetration of selected elements included in sealing materials penetrating into dentine indicated that independent of type of conditions - *in vitro* or *in vivo* - an increased value of elements included in sealants and intermediate materials bonding to dentine was observed. Depth of penetration and concentration of elements in dentine depended on the method used for preparation of tissues. The highest concentration of elements on much wider and deeper surface was observed in *in vivo* samples, i.e. when tissue was etched, covered with intermediate material and then sealed, which shows that sealant infiltrated into sealed tissues, improving adhesion and tightness of the joint (33).

One of the most decisive directions of research is improvement of adhesion of sealing materials to tooth's hard surface, because in that way a microleakage of microorganisms or their substrates can be eliminated. The main disadvantage of contemporary adhesive materials is their limited stability *in vitro*. The most frequently quoted reason for clinical failure is loss of retention and marginal tightness, thus in order to extend clinical period of sealant use, one should focus on improvement of bonding stability of those biomaterials with tooth's tissues. The effectiveness of direct bonding of modern sealants is quite good, independent of their type, however during clinical trials bonding efficacy of some materials decreases dramatically, whereas others demonstrate higher stability (20). Results of clinical studies depend not only on patients and used materials but also on external factors, such as operator's skills, type of light source, isolation method, type of instruments used for finishing of sealing material. Factors connected with the patient, such as age, oral hygiene, have a higher impact than any properties of sealing material. Also occlusal tension, eccentric stress is one of the main reasons for sealant loss. Additionally, apart from occlusal load, temperature changes in oral cavity may have a negative impact on tooth/material interface, which is associated with repeated contractions/expansions of filling material resulting from higher expansion factors of thermal contraction than those for tooth's tissues.

Tooth/sealing material interface may also be destroyed by its exposure to water and human bacterial enzymes present in saliva. Penetration of water into hybrid layer and subsequent release of resin components leads to ineffective polymerization *in situ* and to their degradation. Hydrolysis of remaining hydroxyapatites and collagen fibers insufficiently covered with resin additionally impairs long-term efficacy of bonding. Interfacial junction sealing material/tooth is subjected to both chemical and mechanical degradation. Chemical degradation is hydrolysis and plasticization of resin components, also associated with water penetration. Hydrolysis may disrupt a conventional bond, join different units of collagen fibers as well as resin polymers. The process can be aided by bacterial enzymes and by dentine itself. Then in turn catabolites are released together with residual monomers which may weaken the bonding mechanics and promote more water penetration. Water may also decrease fiction forces between polymer chains, which is called resin plasticization. Repetitive mechanical loads can also damage bonding cohesion. During each mastication cycle, the interfacial junction is strained. At some sites, concentration of tension may exceed the bond's resistance to disruption, which results in formation of cracks that spread and lead to damage of material cohesion. A bond is more resistant to cracking in adhesive systems with microfiller particles compared to systems without microfiller particles (21,80).

All resin-based adhesive materials while shrinking induce tensions on interfacial junction, which may lead to crack formation and consequently to microleakage. It was proved that a microleakage may appear between the hybrid layer and dentine even when no crack is observed (2,79).

5. Summary

Taking into consideration a high prevalence and intensification of caries of lateral teeth in children, apart from other methods of caries prophylaxis, such as contact fluorization, which protects flat and contact surfaces of teeth - it is advisable to apply fissure sealants of lateral teeth, i.e. molars and premolars, starting with freshly erupted permanent first molars through subsequently erupting posterior teeth. In order to decrease caries prevalence in our population, it is necessary to conduct awareness-forming oral hygiene training, to create motivation for proper tooth brushing, to advise a diet aimed at reduction of carbohydrate consumption and elimination of additional meals.

Results of numerous laboratory tests indicated that extension of enamel etching time significantly increased the stability of bonds with sealing material. Application of intermediate adhesive systems on enamel increased the strength of enamel bonding with sealing materials only slightly, whereas their application on dentine significantly improved bonding stability (about threefold) compared to dentine coated with sealant alone. An assessment of morphology of dentine joints where dentine was coated with bonding agents and sealant demonstrated occurrence of gapless joints, whereas when sealant was applied directly on dentine, joints with microcracks were formed. Elements included in sealing materials and adhesive systems penetrate into dentine deep and wide, improving retention and tightness of bonding with hard tissues of teeth.

Sealants with fluorine release it into hard tissues of teeth. The level of emission depends on type of fluorine compound and its concentration in sealant. On the basis of literature analysis and own longitudinal clinical studies as well as laboratory tests I confirm the advisability of sealing procedure, expanding it not only on permanent first molars, but including also second molars and - in children requiring special care and having a high caries risk - premolars. Laboratory tests confirmed that that adhesion and tightness of joints between sealants and tooth's hard tissues can be increased, and microleakage can be minimized.

6. References

[1] Abuchaim C., Rotta M., Grande RH., Loquercio AD., Reis A.: Effectiveness of sealing active proximal caries lessions with an adhesive system:1-year clinical evaluation. Braz. Oral. Res. 2010, Jul-Sep;24(3):361-367.

[2] Al-Sarheed MA.: Evaluation of shear bond strength and SEM observation of all-in-one self-etching primer used for bonding of fissure sealants. J Contem Dent Prac 2006, 7, 2, 1-8.

[3] Andjelie P. i wsp.: Fissurenversiegoelungen als primare Verbungunosomassnahme: Eine vierjähringe Bewertungsstudie In Stara Pazova, Oralphropylaxe 1991, 13, 3-10.

[4] Aranda M., Garcia-Goday F.:Clinical evaluation of the retention and wear of a light-cured pit and fissure glass ionomer sealant. J.Clin Pediatr Dent.1995, 19, 273-277.

[5] Askaroglon E., Kavvadia K., Lagouvardos P., Papagiannoulis L.:Effect of sealants on laser fluorescence caries detection in primary teeth. Laser Med. Sci.2011 Jan;26(1) 29-34.

[6] Barja-Fidalgo F., Maroun S., de Oliveira BH.: Efecteviness of a glass ionomer cement used as a pit and fissures sealant in recently erupted permanent first molars. J Dent Child (Chic) 2009 Jan-Apr, 76 (1):34-40.

[7] Baseggio W., Naufel FS., Davidoff DC., Nahsan FP., Flury S, Rodriques JA.: Caries-preventive efficacy and retention of a resin-modified glass ionomer cement and a resin-based fissure sealant:a 3-years split-mouth randomized clinical trial. Oral Health Prev.Dent.2010, 8 (3):261-268.

[8] Baygin O., Korkmaz FM., Tüzuner T., Tanriver M.: The effect of different enamel surface treatments on the microleakage of fissure sealant. Laser Med Sci.2011, Apr.8, laser erbowy Er:Yag 7W, Er:YAG (5, 5W).

[9] Berger S., Goddon I., Chen CM., Senkel H., Hickel R., Stösser L., Heinrich-Wettzier R., Kühnisch J.: Are pit and fissure sealants needed in children with a higher caries risk? Clin Oral Investig.2010, 14(5) :613-620.

[10] Borges BC., Bezerra GV., Mesquita Ide A. , Pereira MR., Aguiar FM., Santos AJ, Pinheiro.: Effect of irradiation times on the polymerization depth of contemporary fissurce scalant with different opacities. Braz Oral Res.2011, Apr;25 (2):135-142.

[11] Botti RM., Bossu M., Zallocco N., Vestri A., Polimeni A.: Effectiveness of plaque indicators and air polishing for the sealing of pits and fissures. Eur J Paediatr.Dent.2010, 11(1):15-18.

[12] Cehreli SB., Arikan S., Gulsahi K., Arhun N., Arman A., Sargon M.: Effect of LED curing on marginal integrity of an ormocer-based sealant. J. Dent Child (Chic) 2009 Jan-Apr; 76(1):53-57.

[13] Chaitra TR., Subba Reddy VV., Devarasa GM., Ravishankar TL.: Flowable resin used as a sealant in molars using conventional, enameloplasty and fissurotomy techniques an in vitro study. J Indian Soc Pedod Prev Dent.2010, Jul-Sep:28(3):145-150.

[14] Chaitra TR., Subb RV., Devarasa GM., Ravishankar TL.: Microleakage and SEM analysis of flowable resin used as a sealant following three fissure preparation techniques –an in vitro study. J. Clin Pediatr Dent., 2011 Spring;35(3)277-282.

[15] Cohreli ZC., Gungor HC.: Quantitative microlakage evaluation of fissure sealants applied with or without a bonding agent; resultats after four-year water storage in vitro. J. Adhes Dent.2008 Oct;10 (5): 379-384.

[16] Condeli A, Scavizzi F, .Marci F.: The relationship between fluoride concentration and the caries frequency of different tooth surfaces in a hight fluoride area. Caries Res., 1970, 4, 1, 69-77.

[17] Cohreli SB., Arikan S., Gulsahi K., Arhun N., Arman A., Sargon M.: Effect of LED curing on marginal integrity of an ormocer-based sealant. J Dent.Child (Chic) 2009, Jan-Apr; 76 (1):53-57.

[18] de Luca-Fraga LR., Freire Pimenta LA. : Clinical evaluation of glass-ionomer /resin-based hybrid materials used as pit and fissures sealants. Quintessence Int.2001, 32, 463-468.

[19] Deery C i wsp.: Clinically undetected occlusal dentine Caries : a radiographic comparison. Caries Res., 1992, 26, 305-309.

[20] De Munck J., Van Landayt K., Peumans M., Poitevin A., Lambrechts P., Bream M., van Meerbreek B.: A critical review of the durability of adhesion to tooth tissue method and results. J Dent Res., 2005, 84 (2):118-132.

[21] Destoop V.: The cracking resistance and adhesion to dentine of dental restorative materials; a fracture mechanics, approach (Doctoral tesis) Leuven:Universite Catolique de Louvain, Belgium.

[22] Doyle WA., Brose JA.: A five-year study of the longevity of fissure sealants. J Dent Child 1978, 45:23-26.

[23] Duffin S.:Managing caries in the high-risk child. Compend Contin.Educ.Dent.2009, 30 (2) 106-108.

[24] .Fidecki M., Jodkowska E.:Evaluation of the effectiveness of fissure sealing as presented by Polish autors. Polish Dental Society 2008, 61, 11, 784-796.

[25] Forss H., Halme E.: Retention of a glass ionomer cement and a resin-based fissure sealant and effect on carious outcome after 7 years. Community Dent Oral Epidemiol.1998;26, 21-25.

[26] Forss H., Williams B., Winter GB.:Fissure sealants further results at 4 years. Br. Dent J 1981, 150:183-187.

[27] Gillianqs B., Buonocore M.: Thickness of enamel at the base of pits and fissures in human molars and biscuspids. J Dent Res., 1961, 40, 2:119-123.

[28] Heller KE., Reed SG., Bruner FW., Eklund AS., Burt BA.:Longitudinal evaluation of sealing molars with and without incipient dental caries in a public health program.J.Public Health Dent.1995, 55, 148-153.

[29] Jańczuk Z.: Results of national Polish epidiomedical examination of masticatory organ. Mag.Stomat., 1991, I, 1, 28-31.

[30] Jensen OE., Billings RJ., Featherstone DB.: Clinical evaluation of Fluoroshield pit and fissure sealant. Clin.Preven.Dent., 1990, 12, 4, 24-27.

[31] Jodkowska E.: Long time clinical observations on prophylactic efficacy of intertubular grooves sealing up. Magazyn Stomat., 1991, I, (5):9-11.

[32] Jodkowska E. :Mikrobiological aspects of sealing of intercuspidal grooves in the light of own investigations.Czas.Stomat.1986, XXXIX, 9, 577-582.

[33] Jodkowska E.: Efficacy of fissure sealing in the light of long-term clinical observations and clinical evaluation. Habilitation dissertation. Medical Academie Warsaw 1999.

[34] Jodkowska E., Raczyńska M.: Five-year clinical observations of the efficiency of Ionosit-Seal pit and fissure sealant in caries prevention in permanent molars and premolars. Stomat.Współczesna 2003, vol.10, 5:31-33.

[35] Jodkowska E., Raczyńska M., Sobczak M., Remiszewski A.:The evaluation of the air-abrasive method as treatment pit and fissure carious lesion In permanent teeth-preliminary report. Dent.Med.Probl.2003, 40, 2, 295-298.

[36] Jodkowska E.: Efficacy of pit and fissure sealing –long-term clinical observations. Quintessence Int.2008 July/August, 39(7):395-602.

[37] Judit S.: Fissure sealing. A review. Fogorv Sz.2008 Aug:101(4) 137-146.

[38] Kamala BK., Hegde AM.: Fuji III vs Fuji VII glass ionomer sealants a clinical study. J. Clin Pediatr Dent.2008 Fall;33 (1):29-33.

[39] Kantovitz KR., Pascon FM., Nobre-dos-Santos M, .Puppin-Rontani RM.: Reviev of the effects of infiltrants and sealers on non-cavitated enamel lesions. Oral Health Prev.Dent., 2010, 8, (3):295-305.

[40] Kay E., Nuttall N.: Relationship between dentistis treatment attributes and restorative decision. Made on the basic of simulated bitewing radiographs. Community Dent Oral Epidemiol., 1994, 22, 71-74.

[41] Kielbasa AM., Muller J., Gernhardt CR.: Closing the gap between oral higiene and minimalny invasive dentistry: a review on the resin infiltration technique of incipient (proxymal) enamel lesions. Quintessence Int.2009, 40 (8) 663-681.

[42] Komatsu H., Shimokobe H., Kawakami S., Yoshimura M.: Caries-preventive effect of glass-ionomer sealant reapplication. Study presents 3-year results.J. Am Dent Assoc., 1994;125:543-549.

[43] Kramer N., Garcia-Goday F., Lohbauer U., Schneider K., Assmann I., Frankenberger R.: Preparation for invasive pit and fissure sealing: air-abrasion or bur? Am J Dent.2008 Dec; 21(6):383-387.

[44] Kusgoz A., Tuzuner T., Ulker M., Kemer B., Saray O.: Conversion degree, microhardness, microleakage and fluoride release of different fissure sealats.J Mech Behav Biomed Mater 2010 Nov 3 (8) 594-599.

[45] Lagerweij MD., Damen JJM., ten Cate JM.: Demineralization of dentin grooves in vitro. Caries Res., 1996, 30, 231-236.

[46] Lussi F.: Validity of diagnostic and treatment decisions of fissure caries. Caries res., 1991, 25, 296-303.

[47] Matalon S., Peretz B., Sidon R., Weiss EL., Slutzky H.: Antibacterial properties of pit and fissure sealants combined with daily fluoride month rinse. Pediatr.Dent 2010;32 (1):9-13.

[48] Mejäre J., Mjör JA.: Glass-ionomer and resin-based fissure sealants: a clinical study. Scand.J Dent. Res 1990, 98:345-350.

[49] Markovic D., Petrovic B., Peric T., Miletic J., Andjelkovic S.: The impact of fissure depth and enamel conditioning protocols on glass-ionomer and resin-based fissure sealant penetration. J. Adhes Dent.2011, 13 (2):171-178.

[50] Mc Kenna EF., Grundy G.: Glass ionomer fissure sealants applied by operative dental auxiliaries.Retention rate after on year. Aust.Dent.J 1987, 32, 200-203.

[51] .Mc Lean JW., Wilson AD.: Fissure sealing and filling with an adhesive glass-ionomer cements. Br Dent J..1974, 136, 269-276.

[52] Michalaki MG., Oulis CJ., Lagouvardos P.: Microleakage of three different sealants on sound and questionable occlusal surface of permanent molars: an in vitro study. Eur Arch Paediatr Dent 2010 Feb; 11(1):26-31.

[53] Moslem M., Erfanparast L., Fekrazed R., Tadayon N., Dadjo H., Shadkar MM., Khalili Z.: The effect of Er, Cr:YAG laser and air abrasion on shear bond strenght a fissure sealant to enamel. J Am Dent Assoc.2010, 141 (2) 157-161.

[54] Moyaho-Bernal A., Vaillard-Jimenez E., Montiel-Jarquin AJ., Martinez-Fernandez RG.:A comparative study between two different technics for retention the pit and fissure sealant. Rev.Med Inst.Mex Sequro Sol.2011, January-February 49 (1) 13-16.

[55] Ouks CJ., Berdouses ED.:Fissure sealant retention and caries development, after resealing on first permanent molars of children with low moderate and high caries risk. Eur.Arch Paediatr Dent 2009, 10 (4):211-217.

[56] Olea N., Pulgar R., Olea-Serrano F., et all.: Estrogenicity of rersin-based composites and sealants used in dentistry. Env.Health Persp., 1996, 104:298-305.

[57] Pardi V., Pereira AC., Mialhe FL., Meneghin MC., Ambrosano GMB.: A 5-years evaluation of two glass-ionomer cements used as fissure sealants. Community Dent Oral Epidemiol., 2003, 31, 386-391.

[58] Pelka MA., Altmaier K., Petschelt A., Lahbauer U.:The effect of air-polishing abrasives on wear of direct restoration materials and sealants.J Am Dent Assoc.2010 Jan, 141(1):63-70.

[59] Perreira AC., Eggertsson M., Martinez-Mier EA., Mialhe FL., Eckert GJ., Zero DT.:Validity of caries dedection on occlusal surfaces and treatment decisions based on results from multiple caries-detection methods. Eur.J Oral Sci.2009, Feb;117(1):51-57.

[60] Perez C dos R, Hirata RJ., da Silva AH., Sampaio EM., de Miranda MS.: Effect of a glaze /composite sealant on the 3D surface roughness of esthetic restorative materials. Oper.Dent 2009, Nov-Dec., 34(6):674-680.

[61] Petersson LG.: Fluoride mouth rinses and fluoride varnishes. Caries Res., 1993, 27, suppl 1, 35-42.

[62] Poulsen S., Beiruti N., Sadat N.: A comparison sealing of retention and the effect on caries of fissure sealant with a glass ionomer and a resin-based sealant. Community Dent Oral Epidemiol.2001, 29:298-301.

[63] Preston AJ., Agalamanyi EA., Higham SM., Mair LH.: The recharge of esthetic dental restorative materials with fluoride in vitro –two years` results. Dent.Mat.2003, 19:32-37.

[64] Richardson BA., Smith DC., Hargreaves AJ.:A 5-year clinical evaluation of the effectiveness of a fissure sealant in mentally retarded Canadian children. Community Dent Oral Epidemiol.1981, 9, 4:170-174.

[65] Ripa LW.: Sealants revisited.An update of the effectiveness of pit and fissure sealants Caries, Res.1989, 27 (Suppl 1) 77-82.

[66] Ripa LW.: Retionale and review of clinical trials. Jnt Dent Assoc.1989, 2, 341-344.

[67] Ripa LW.: The current status of pit and fissure sealants. A review J Can Dent Assoc.1993, 5, 367-379.

[68] Rock WP.: A comparative study of fluoride-releasing composite resin and glass ionomer materials used as fissure sealants. J.Dent 1996, 24, 4, 275-280.

[69] Rodriques JA., Diniz MB., Hug J., Cordeiro RC., Lussi A.: Relationship between DIGNOdent values and sealants penetration depth on occlusal fissures. Clin.Oral Investig.2010 Dec;14 (6):707-711.

[70] Romcke RG.: Retention and maintenence of fissure sealants over 10 years. J.Can Dent.Assoc.1990, 56, 235-237.

[71] Sancakli HS., Erdemir W., Yildiz E.: Effects of Er:YAG laser and air abrasion on the mikroleakage of a resin-based fissure sealant material. Photomed Laser Surg.2011 Feb.9

[72] Simonsen RJ.: Retention and effectiveness of dental sealants after 15 years. J.Am.Dent.Assoc., 1991, 122, 34-42.

[73] Simonsen RJ.:Glass ionomer as fissure sealant a critical review. J.Public Health Dent.1996, 56 (3):146-149.

[74] Simonsen RJ.: A review of the clinical application and performance of pit and fissure sealant.Aust.Dent.J., 2011, Jun 56, suppl.1:45-58

[75] Simonsen RJ.: A review of the clinical application and performance of pit and fissure sealants. Aust.Dent J., 2011 Jan 56 Suppl 1:45-58.

[76] Skartveit I., Tveit AB., Tötdal B., Ovrebo RC., Raadal M.: In vivo fluoride uptake in enamel and dentin from fluoride containing materials. ASDC J Dent Child 1990, 57, 97-100.

[77] Sly EG., Kaplan AE., Missana L.:Clinical evaluation of glass ionomer for pit and fissure sealing of fully erupted molars. Acta Odontol Latinoam 2010, 23 (1):3-7;

[78] Stanley RT., Hagman FT., Itkoff DA., Pryor HG.:A clinical raport on preventive resin restorations. Ohio Dent.J., 1986, 60, 5, 10-18.

[79] Suppa P., Breschi L., Ruggeri A., Mazzotti G., Prati C., Chersoni S., et all.: Nanoleakage within the hybryd layer a correlative FEISEM, TEM investigation. J.Biomed Mater Res.B.: Appl Biomater 2005, 73:7-14.

[80] Tam LE., Khoshand S., Pillar RM. :Fracture resistance of dentin-composite interfaces using different adhesive resin layers. J.Dent 2001, 29:217-225.

[81] Taylor CL., Gwinett AJ.: A study of the penetration of sealants into pits and fissures. J. Am Dent Assoc., 1973, 87:1181-1188.

[82] Tianvivat S., Chonqurivatwong V., Sirisakulveroj B.: Loss of sealant retention and subsequent caries development. Community Dent Health 2008, 25 (4):216-220.

[83] Topaloglu AKA., Riza Alpoz A. :Effect of saliva contamination on microleakege of three different pit and fissure sealants. Eur J Paediatr.Dent 2010, Jun; 11 (2):93-96.

[84] Weerheijm KL. i wsp.: Sealing of occlusal hidden caries lesions; an alternative for curative treatment ? ASDC J Dent.Child., 1992, 59, 263-268.

[85] Weerheijm KL. i wsp.: Clinically undetected occlusal dentine caries: a radiographic comparison. Caries Res., 1992, 26, 305-309.

[86] Williams B.: Fissure sealants: a 4-year clinical trial comparing en experimental glass-polyalkenoate cement with a bis glycidyl methacrylate resin used as fissure sealants. Br Dent J.1996, 180, 104-108.

[87] Yamada Y., Hossain M., Kimura Y., Masuda Y., Jayawardena JA., Nasu Y.:Removal of organic debris from occlusal fissures:advantage of Carislov system over sodium hypochlorite.J.Clin Pediatr Dent.2010, Fall 35 (1):75-79.

[88] Yilmaz Y., Beldüz N., Eyüboglu O.:A two-year-evaluation of fluor different fissure sealants. Eur.Arch Paediatr Dent.2010, 11 (2) 88-92.

[89] Zimmerman-Downs JM., Shuman D., Stull SC., Ratzlaff RE.: Bisphenol A blood and saliva levels prior to and after dental sealant placement in adults. J Dent. Hyg.2010;84(3):145-150.

5

Probiotics and the Reduction of Dental Caries Risk

Arezoo Tahmourespour

Islamic Azad University, Khorasgan- Isfahan Branch,
Iran

1. Introduction

Dental caries and periodontal disease are major public health problems that bother all countries in the world. Dental carie is an infectious, communicable disease that acid-forming bacteria of dental plaque can destroy tooth structure in the presence of fermentable carbohydrates such as sucrose, fructose, and glucose. The mineral content of teeth is sensitive to increases in acidity from the production of lactic acid. So, the infection results in loss of tooth minerals from the outer surface of the tooth and can progress through the dentin to the pulp, finally compromising the tooth vitality. Industrialized nations have controlled the problem with fluoride enriched water and personal hygiene products since early in the 1960s, but cariogenicity remains a crisis that economically burdens the health care system. Dental disease remains a "silent epidemic" in the world that threatens children and adults. The oral streptococci especially mutans Streptococci are related with the development of caries in humans and animals (Caglar et al., 2001; Natcher, 2001; Kargul, 2003). For the past 150 years, the predominant mode of caries management has been the surgical approach, predating our current understanding and reliable with the original concept that dental caries was a gangrenous process resulting in extraction of carious teeth. Later, just the demineralized portions of the tooth were removed and replaced with an inert restorative material. This mechanical solution for a biological problem prevailed.

Today, dental practitioners still teach the removal of diseased tooth structure which suggests we should expect a "cure". The insight however, is that it has repeatedly been shown not to remove the causative infection. There is a paradigm shift in the management of dental caries. Research in cariology is sky-rocketing, bringing out hidden facts of this age-old disease, but education and clinical practice are adopting them at a snail's pace. In clinical practice dental caries is still being treated symptomatically, just like the common cold. Clinicians have adopted a comfort level from many years of practicing 'restorative' dentistry, but unlike the common cold that does not have a cure, dental caries has abundant options to be cured and eradicated (Anderson and Shi, 2006; Carounanidy, 2010).

Throughout the past few decades, changes have been observed not only in the incidence of dental caries, but also in the distribution and pattern of the disease in the population. These changes have main hints for diagnosis and management of early lesions, predicting caries risk, and conducting effective disease prevention and management programs for populations. In order to make continued progress in eliminating this, new strategies will be required (Natcher, 2001).The broad management of dental caries should involve the management of disease as well as the lesion. There is now an intense focus on preventive strategies. Essentially, all preventive treatment strategies either alter or modify the causative factors in dental caries etiology, such as diet, host, salivary, and microbial factors.

Numerous anti-plaque agents available in the market have been tested for their ability to interfere dental biofilm formation or metabolism. However, due to several undesirable side effects associated with these agents, going along with the increasing global problem with antimicrobial drug resistance, the search for alternate agents is necessary (Tahmourespour, 2011). Targeted agents are so expected to be highly specific, to pose an insignificant resistance development problem, and to have minimal effects on vital human cell functions. A suggested approach to overcome the limitations of the traditional disease management strategies is using inexpensive, effective, stable, novel and natural products as anti biofouling agent. Whole bacteria replacement therapy or using natural products of some bacteria such as the secondary metabolites of them for decreasing of oral cavity pathogens must be investigate.

2. Biofilm formation, a pioneer step of dental caries

Dental plaque has been discussed as a biofilm (figure 1). Donlan and Costerton (2002) presented the most relevant description of a biofilm.

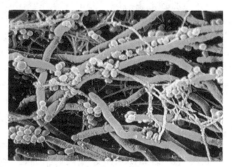

Fig. 1. Colored scanning electron micrograph of dental plaque (*Streptococcus mutans* bacteria are pink).

They declared that a biofilm is "a microbially derived sessile community characterized by cells that are attached to a substrate or to each other, are embedded in a matrix of extracellular polymeric substances that they have produced, and exhibit an altered phenotype with respect to growth rate and gene transcription."

A biofilm is structured to maximize energy. Degree of organization and multispecies organization characterize the four stages of biofilm growth (Figure 2). There are four stages in the lifecycle whether the organism is planktonic or as member of a biofilm. Stage I is the inactive or least metabolically active state. Transformation from Stage I to Stage II needs significant genetic up-regulation. Stage III involves maturity of the biomass, and total organism concentration can come near 10^{11} or 10^{12} colony-forming units per milliliter. At this phase, new antigens may be expressed, genetic exchange enhanced and membrane transport maximized. Stage IV (apoptosis or death) signals detachment or sloughing from the biofilm (Donlan & Costerton, 2002; Thomas et al., 2006).

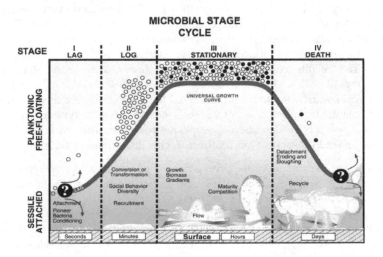

Fig. 2. Four stages of dental plaque biofilm growth: Stage I attachment (lag [not inert, but metabolically reduced]), Stage II growth (log [exponential growth]), Stage III maturity (stationary) and Stage IV dispersal (death) (Thomas et al 2006).

3. Dental plaque biofilm management

For therapeutic purposes, it is necessary to attack the formed biofilm. For prophylactic purposes, it seems reasonable to target processes involved in the actual biofilm formation of single- or mixed-bacterial communities that have the potential to cause or support disease, without disturbing the balance of the normal flora. It is known that the mature oral biofilm is the result of a well regulated series of processes, which begins by adhesion of planktonic cells to the surfaces and could represent potential targets for biofilm control.

The shift in the treatment paradigm incorporates the ecological plaque hypothesis, which states that prevention of disease should not only focus on the putative pathogens inhibition, but also on interference with environmental factors that drive selection and enrichment for these bacteria as reported by Marsh(2005). One of the key characteristics of biofilm that could be targets for dental plaque management includes its behavior as an adhesive mass.

The environmental key factors in concerned with biofilm formation are the fermentable dietary carbohydrates and Streptococci, as pioneer strains, depend on them as an energy source (Tahmourespour et al., 2010). The cariogenicity of sugar-containing foods can be modified by many factors including the amount and type of carbohydrates, protective components (proteins, fats, calcium, phosphate, fluoride) and physical and chemical properties (liquid vs. solid retentiveness, solubility, pH, buffering capacity). The fact that sugars are readily metabolized by oral bacteria, leading to the production of organic acids and extra cellular polysaccharides such as glucan and fructan was shown repeatedly in clinical studies (Zero, 2004; Touger et al., 2003). Numerous studies have established the role of sugars in caries etiology and the importance of sugars as the principal dietary substrate that drives the caries process (Caglar et al., 2005; Touger et al., 2003; Loo et al., 2003).

In a study, the ability of Mutans Streptococci to form biofilm measured in the presence of some sugars. The biofilm formation (percentage of strongely adherent strains in Fig. 3) in the presence of sucrose was higher than other carbohydrates significantly (p < 0.05). It is also revealed that the number of attached bacteria increased with the increase of sucrose concentration. The results corresponded to a non linear increase of attached bacteria (Tahmourespour et al., 2010). Therefore, among the various tested carbohydrates in this study and other different researches, sucrose is considered the most cariogenic dietary carbohydrate, because it is fermentable, and also serves as a best substrate for the synthesis of extracellular and intracellular polysaccharides and dental plaque formation (Brown et al., 2005; Bowen, 2002; Cury et al., 2000; Pecharki et al., 2005; Ribeiro et al., 2005; Leme et al., 2006).

Evidences show that expression of required genes for glucan and fructan synthesis, such as gtfB, gtfC and ftf, is well-regulated after initial adhesion and results in forming dental plaque, caries and other periodontal disease (Zero, 2004)

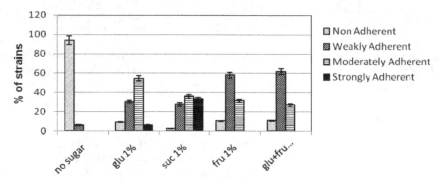

Fig. 3. The effect of different substrates in the adherence potential of streptococcal isolates. All isolates were classified into four groups. Data are expressed as means and standard deviations of triplicate experiments (Tahmourespour et al., 2010)

The ability of mutans Streptococci to adhere to teeth surfaces is vital for the progression of the disease. The bacterial adhesion mechanism is mediated by synthesis of both extracellular enzymes, glucosyltransferase (GTF) and fructosyltransferase (FTF). These extracellular enzymes identified in *Streptococcus mutans* are responsible for the synthesis of extracellular polysacharides such as glucans and fructans. These polymers are fundamental factors in dental biofilm formation. a-(1-3) - and a-(1-6)-linked glucan polymers through the concerted action of three secreted GTFs are encoded by the genes *gtfB*, *gtfC* and *gtfD*. In vitro studies have indicated that *gtfB* and *gtfC* are essential for the sucrose-dependent attachment of S. *mutans* cells to hard surfaces but *gtfD* is dispensable. The glucan polymers are involved in the colonization of cariogenic Streptococci and therefore have become a potential target for protection against dental caries.

The comparison between the mRNA level of *gtfB* in planktonic, biofilm and unattached cells of S. *mutans* by real time RT PCR also showed that, the level of *gtfB* gene expression in the biofilm condition was significantly higher than the planktonic condition (Fig4).

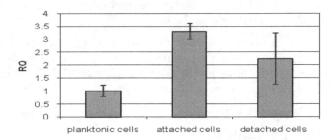

Fig. 4. The comparison of *gtfB* gene expression level in different condition (planktonic cells in the absence of sucrose, attached cells in the present of 1% sucrose and unattached or detached cells from biofilm in the presence of 1% sucrose) (Tahmourespour et al., 2010).

So, despite the fact that, the relationship between sugar consumption and caries is so strong; sugar consumption restriction still has an important role in prevention of caries going along with other new strategies.

4. Probiotics

In general, a probiotic, is a live microorganism which beneficially affects the host animal by improving its intestinal microbial balance. The concept of probiotic evolved from Elie Metchnikoff's ideas that the bacteria in fermented products could compete with microbes that are harmful to host and are hence injurious to health. The term probiotic, meaning "for life," is derived from the Greek language. It is the antonym of the term antibiotics, was introduced in 1965 by Lilly and Stillwell as substances produced by microorganisms which promote the growth of other microorganisms. Since then several definitions for probiotics have been proposed (Table 1).

Year with reference	Definition
1965 Lilly & Stillwell	Substances produced by microorganisms that promote the growth of other microorganisms
2001 Schrezemeir & de Vrese	A preparation of, or a product containing, viable, defined microorganisms in sufficient numbers, which alter the microflora (by implantation or colonization) in a compartment of the host and as such exert beneficial health effects in this host
2001 WHO/FAO report	Live microorganisms that, when administered in adequate amounts, confer a health benefit on the host
International Life Science Institute (ILSI) Europe	a live microbial food ingredient that, when ingested in sufficient quantities, exerts health benefits on the consumer

Table 1. Some definitions of probiotic bacteria.

The idea in the beneficial effects of probiotics is based on the knowledge that the intestinal flora can protect humans against infection and interruption of this flora can enhance susceptibility to infection. The most important sources of probiotics for humans are the bacteria in yogurt and fermented milk products.

The valuable effects of probiotics may be mediated by direct antagonistic effect against specific groups of organisms, resulting in a decrease in numbers or by an effect on their metabolism or by stimulation of immunity (Ouwehand et al.,2001; Teugheles et al., 2008; Millette et al., 2008; Tahmourespour & Kermanshahi, 2011).

Probiotics have been suggested to have the following properties and functions:

- adherence to host epithelial tissue,
- acid resistance and bile tolerance,
- elimination of pathogens or reduction in pathogenic adherence,
- production of acids, hydrogen peroxide and bacteriocins antagonistic to pathogen growth,
- safety, non-pathogenic and non-carcinogenic, and
- Improvement of intestinal microflora (Kaur *et al.* 2002; Ouwehand *et al.* 2002).

Lactic Acid Bacteria or LAB, as the main probiotic species, are thought to be safe that have been ingested from foods without any problems for many years and are known as GRAS (Generally Recognized As Safe) bacteria that are important for animal health(Saito, 2004). The proposed mechanisms of the actions of probiotics are summarized in Fig. 5.

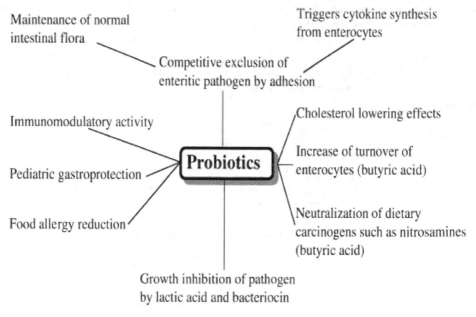

Fig. 5. Mechanisms of the actions of probiotics (Saito, 2004).

Promising probiotic strains include members of the genera Lactobacillus, Bifidobacterium and Enterococcus. The most commonly used probiotics mainly come from two genera Lactobacillus and Bifidobacterium (table2).

lactobacillus species	Bifidobacterium species	others
L. acidophilus	B bifidum lanimalisl	Bacillus cereus
L. rhamnosus	B. longum	Clostridium butyricum
L. gasseri	B. breve	Escherichia coli
L. casei	B. infantis	Proprionibacterium freundendsreichii
L. reuteri	B. lactis	Saccheromyces boulardii
L. bulgaricus	B. adolescentis	Enterococcus faecalis
L. plantarum		Streptococcus thermophilus
L. johnsonii		
L. lactis		

Table 2. The most commonly used probiotics.

4.1 Oral microbiota as a source of probiotics

The oral cavity is a complex habitat of a great diversity of microbial species.

Recently, it has been estimated that over 1000 bacterial species are present in it. The most commonly used probiotic bacterial strains belong to the genera Lactobacillus and Bifidobacteria. So, there is of special interest to realize whether such microbes naturally inhabit the oral cavity. In the oral cavity, lactobacilli usually comprise 1% of the total cultivable bacteria; commonly isolated species include L .paracaseie, L.plantarum, L.rhamnosus, L.salivarius. Bifidobacterial species isolated from oral samples include B.bifidum, B.dentium and B.longum.

A promising finding was that lactobacilli population differed in healthy and individuals with periodontal disease. In another study it is observed that healthy persons are populated by L. gasseriand L. fermentum, whereas the predominant species in periodontitis patients was L. plantarum while the first two were undetectable (Koll Kalis et al., 2005). Observations also showed that microorganisms with probiotic properties may really exist and inhabit in the oral cavity. Though, the complexity of biofilm development and interspecies interactions require more detailed investigations in order to state true probiotic candidates with activity in the oral cavity (Stamatova & Meurman, 2009).

4.2 Probiotics and resistance to oral defense mechanisms

At first, ingested probiotics are exposed to saliva. During this first step of contact, survival and resistance to oral environmental factors are very important. Salivary proteins such as lysozyme, lactoferrine, salivary peroxidase, and secretory IgA can collectively affect viability or cell surface morphology of probiotic species. The adhesion and metabolic activity of them is then affected. Saliva role on microbial establishment can be contradictory. In one hand, saliva can inhibit colonization of probiotics (by growth inhibition, killing, or prevention of adherence to host tissues), and on the other hand, it can promote microbial colonization. It has been observed that, Lysozyme pretreatment could significantly reduce the adhesion of L. rhamnosus GG, L. rhamnosus Lc705 and L. casei Shirota. However, the adhesive properties of L. johnsonii La1 and B. lactis Bb12 remained unaffected. These results highlight the strain-specific response to proteolytic enzymes and this feature needs to be considered when selecting probiotics for the oral cavity.

Other studies have also shown that lysozyme pretreatment of lactobacilli can slightly increase their adhesiveness to saliva coated surfaces. Lysozyme pretreatment could not significantly reduce the viability of lactobacilli but cell surface alterations might have contributed to the increased adhesion. Further studies on the mechanism whereby lysozyme affects adhesion are necessitated (Stamatova & Meurman, 2009).

Another aspect in oral establishment of probiotics is saliva-mediated aggregation.This ability is related to cell adherence properties. The adhesion mechanisms of lactobacilli involve hydrophobicity and surface charge, as well as specific carbohydrate and/or proteinaceous components. Organisms able to co-aggregate with other bacteria may have superior advantages over non-coaggregating organisms which are easily removed from the oral cavity. Recently, results have shown that *L. salivarius* was not able to form a biofilm in monoculture (in a microplate model), whereas when the species was added simultaneously with the inoculum of other commensal oral microorganisms, it established itself irrespective of pH. Similar findings were observed with *L. plantarum* SA-1 and *L. rhamnosus* that failed to form substantial biofilms in mono-culture but biofilm mass increased when cocultured with *A. naeslundii* (Filoche et al., 2004).

4.3 Probiotics and oral health

Several authors have suggested that probiotic bacteria could also be beneficial to oral health. Species of Lactobacillus and Bifidobacteria may exert beneficial effects in the oral cavity by inhibiting cariogenic Streptococci and Candida spp (Bhardwaj, 2010).

The mechanisms of probiotic action in the oral cavity could be similar to those described for the intestine. The mechanisms by which probiotics exert their effects are largely unknown, but may involve modifying pH, antagonizing pathogens through production of antimicrobial compounds, competing for pathogen binding and receptor sites, stimulating immune modulatory cells and producing lactase. It is also showed that they have influence to the immune system through several molecular mechanisms (Bhushan & Chachra, 2010).

To have a beneficial effect in oral cavity, a probiotic should have a tendency to form a biofilm that acts as a protective lining for oral tissues against oral diseases. Probiotics strains have been shown to vary broadly in their adhesiveness to saliva-coated HA and so in biofilm formation ability. Among probiotics strains *L. rhamnosus* GG exhibited the maximum values of adhesion, comparable to those of the early tooth colonizer *S. sanguinis*. Dairy starter *L. bulgaricus* strains adhered poorly to sHA.

Probiotic bacteria adhesion to oral soft tissues is another aspect that promotes their health effect to the host. Cell adhesion is a complex process involving contact between the bacterial cell and interaction with surfaces. The epithelial lining of the oral cavity despite its function as a physical barrier, actively participates in immune response. It has been shown that probiotic bacteria can stimulate local immunity and modulate the inflammatory response. Lactobacilli as well as other gram positive bacteria express ligands for toll-like receptors (TLRs) which initiate immune responses enabling detection of both pathogens and indigenous microbiota by epithelial cells. Recognition of commensal bacteria by these receptors (TLRs) is necessary for homeostasis, epithelial cells protection from injury and repair stimulation (Stamatova & Meurman, 2009).

Production of antimicrobial substances
• Organic acids • Hydrogen peroxide • carbon peroxide, • diacetyl • Biosurfactants • Bacteriocins
Binding in Oral Cavity
• Compete with pathogens for adhesion sites • Involvement in metabolism of substrates   (competing with oral micro organisms for substrates available)
Immuno modulatory
• Stimulate non specific immunity • Modulate humoral and cellular immune response
Modify oral conditions
• Modification of oxidation reduction potential • Modulating pH

Table 3. Possible mechanisms of a probiotic in oral health

4.4 Probiotics and dental caries

From a view point, probiotics (lactobacilli) could hydrolyse proteins, stimulate growth of streptococci: the streptococci are acidogenic bacteria and produce low pH conditions in the oral environment (Robinson and Tamine, 1981). Also untreated caries cavities should also be questioned at this point. On the other hand, in recent studies, it was stated that probiotic might decrease the risk of the highest level of Streptococcus mutans (Ahola et al, 2002) or might increases salivary counts of lactobacilli while *S. mutans* levels were not modified (Montalto et al, 2004).

To have a beneficial effect in limiting or preventing dental caries, a probiotic must be able to adhere to dental surfaces and integrate into the bacterial communities making up the dental biofilm. Such a biofilm holds pathogens off oral tissues by filling a space which in future, could have served as a niche for pathogens, and it should also compete with and antagonize the cariogenic bacteria and thus prevent their proliferation (Caglar et al., 2005; Sheikh et al., 2011). According to our researches, it is cleared that the presence of Lactobacillus Sp. Such as *L. acidophilus DSM 20079, L. fermentum ATCC 9338* and *L.rhamnosus ATCC 7469* can cause reduction in the adherence of Streptococcal strains that it is probably related to interaction between bacteria. The mutans streptococci adherence reduction was significantly stronger in the case of *L. acidophilus* and *L. rhamnosus* while in the other study showed that *L. fermentum* reduced the adherence of non mutans Streptococci more than mutans Streptococci (figure 6).

In general, Inoculation of probiotic strain before Streptoccocal isolates to in vitro system showed more effect on adherence reduction (about 25% reduction in adherence) with significant difference (Pvalue< 0.05) especially in the case of *L. rhamnosus*. It is thought that adhesion reduction is likely due to bacterial interactions and colonization of adhesion sites with probiotic strain before the presence of streptococci. Also, the probiotic strains were able to modify the proportion of the oral species within the biofilm (Tahmourespour & Kermanshahi, 2011).

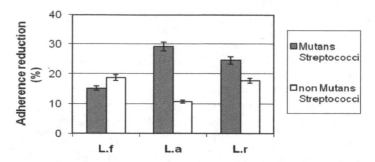

Fig. 6. The percentage of streptococcal adherence reduction in the presence of probiotic strains

Nikawa et al. (2004) also reported that consumption of yoghurt containing lactobacillus reuteri (L. reuteri) over a period of 2 weeks reduced the concentration of S. mutans in the saliva by up to 80%. Comparable results were obtained by incorporating probiotics into chewing gum or lozenges. Comelli et al (2002) reported that inoculation of dairy strains before adding the oral bacteria did not increase their colonization. They also found that dairy strains and particularly L. lactis NCC2211 were able to modify the extent of oral species within the biofilm and also able to reduce cariogenic bacteria levels. They suggest that the reduction of these strains can be explained either by competition for adhesion sites or growth factors. Miller et al., in their study about the effect of microbial interaction on In Vitro plaque formation by Streptococcus mutans found that microbial interaction may have the potential to affect the amount and type of plaque formed, depending upon the kinds of organisms involved. They also reported that the addition of the lactobacilli to cultures of S. sanguis resulted in more inhibition of plaque formation when compared with pure cultures of S. sanguis. A 34% inhibition of plaque formation was observed when L. casei interacted with S. mutans NCTC 10449. Furthermore Simark-Mattsson et al. (2007) have shown the interference capacities of lactobacilli against strains of Streptococcus mutans and Streptococcus sobrinus. Meurman (2005) showed the inhibitory activity of Lactobacillus rhamnosus GG against Streptococcus mutans in low pH and it can be useful for preventing the cariogenic effects of oral streptococci. In vivo studies have also confirmed the effects of probiotic bacteria consumption on decreasing the risk of dental caries and mutans Streptococcus counts. Nase et al., (2001) reported long term consumption of milk containing the probiotic Lactobacillus rhamnosus CG strain reduced caries in kindergarten children. In one of the earlier studies, Marquis et al, demonstrated a potential probiotic approach for reducing dental caries by using oral Streptococci that are able to metabolize arginine or urea to ammonia. Cagler et al have showed a reduced S. mutans level in patients receiving fluid or tablet probiotic forms. In another study by Cagler et al a significantly reduced level was observed for S.mutans not for Lactobacillus in an ice-cream containing Bifidobacterium lactis (Caglar et al., 2005; Kargul et al., 2003). Lactobacilli have been used to deliver vaccine components for active immunization in vivo. In this way, the vectors, with the ability of the streptococcal antigen I/II (*S. mutans* adhesion molecules) recognition were constructed and expressed in a strain of Lactobacilli. After the administration of such Lactobacilli to a rat model of dental caries development, *S. mutans* counts and caries scores were reduced obviously (Kruger et al., 2002). The above studies also suggest that consumption of products containing probiotic Lactobacilli or Bifidobacteria could reduce the number of mutans Streptococci in saliva. Oral probiotics may help fight tooth decay, since acid production from sugar is detrimental to teeth, care must be taken not to select strains with high fermentation capacity.

However, according to the researches, it is cleared that, there are some attractive vehicles for probiotic intake such as using fermented dairy products containing probiotic bacteria (milk, cheese, yogurt and ice cream) and also chewing gum, candies, tablets and water containing probiotics.

4.5 Probiotics-derived biosurfactant

Lactobacilli, as a probiotic (because of it`s known probiotic potential and it`s acid resistance and bile salt`s tolerance), are believed to interfere with pathogens by different mechanisms (table 3) and one of their mechanisms is biosurfactant production.

As it is mentioned before, lactobacilli have been recognized for their antimicrobial activity and ability to interfere with the adhesion of pathogens on epithelial cells and for their anti-biofilm production on catheter devices and voice prostheses. The mechanisms of this interfering have been demonstrated to include, among others, the release of biosurfactants. Biosurfactants, a structurally diverse group of surface active molecules synthesized by microorganisms, have recently attracted attentions in biotechnology for industrial and medical applications. Because the reason, they had several advantages on synthetic surfactants, such as low toxicity, inherent good biodegradability and ecological acceptability. Biosurfactants include unique amphipathic properties derived from their complex structures, which include a hydrophilic moiety and a hydrophobic portion (Vater et al. 2002). The use of biosurfactants from probiotic bacteria as antimicrobial and/or anti-adhesive agents has been studied before and their ability to inhibit adhesion of various micro organisms isolated from explanted voice prostheses has been demonstrated (Rodrigues et al. 2004). Biosurfactants adsorption to a surface modifies its hydrophobicity, interfering in the microbial adhesion and desorption processes; so, the release of biosurfactants by probiotic bacteria in vivo can be considered as a defence weapon against other colonizing strains (van Hoogmoed et al., 2004; Rodrigues et al., 2006). Consequently, previous adsorption of biosurfactants can be used as a preventive strategy to delay the onset of pathogenic biofilm growth, reducing the use of synthetic drugs and chemicals.

In a study, we showed that the biosurfactant derived from probiotic bacteria (*L.acidophilus, L. fermentum* and *L. rhamnosus*) could reduce the adhesion of *S. mutans* to the surfaces (fig 7) (Glass slide or Polystyrene micro titer plates). They also could make streptococcal chains shorter.

Other researchers demonstrated that, the biosurfactants from *L. acidophilus* RC14 and *L. fermentum* B54 could interfere in the adhesion and biofilm formation of the *S. mutans*. Also, it is reported that, the release of biosurfactant from *S. mitis BMS* could interfere in the adhesion of the cariogenic *S. mutans* to glass in the presence and absence of a salivary conditioning film. Others also confirmed that biosurfactants had inhibitory effect on bacterial adhesion and also biofilm formation. However; the precise mechanisms of such effects have not yet been explained. It seems to be highly dependent on biosurfactant type and the properties of the target bacteria. The simplest way to explain biosurfactant antiadhesion and antibiofilm activities would be their direct antimicrobial action. However, the antimicrobial activity of biosurfactants has not been observed in all cases (Tahmourespour et al., 2011 & vater et al., 2002). Thus, it is reported that the way in which surfactants influenced bacterial surface interactions appeared to be more closely related to the changes in surface tension and bacterial cell-wall charge. These factors are very important in overcoming the initial electrostatic repulsion barrier between the microorganism cell surface and its substrate. Surfactants may affect both cell-to-cell and cell-to-surface interactions. Their results support the idea that lactobacilli-derived agents remarkably have an effect on these interactions.

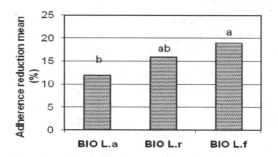

Fig. 7. The mean of adherence reduction percentage of mutans streptococci in presence of biosurfactants derived from *L. acidophilus*, *L. rhamnosus* and *L.fermentum* (Unpublished data).

As it is clear, colonization of the teeth by mutans streptococci has been associated with the etiology and pathogenesis of dental caries in humans. The ability of these organisms, particularly *Streptococcus mutans*, to synthesize extracellular glucans from sucrose using glucosyltransferases (Gtfs) is a major virulence factor of this bacterium.

The Gtfs secreted by *S. mutans* (particularly GtfB and GtfC) provide specific binding sites for either bacterial colonization of the tooth surface or attachment of bacteria to each other, modulating the formation of tightly adherent biofilms, the precursor of dental caries (Koo et al. 2010; Murata et al. 2010). However, the ability of *S. mutans* to adhere to the tooth surface is vital for the initiation and progression of dental caries. α-(1-3)- and α-(1-6)-linked glucan polymers are encoded by the genes gtfB, gtfC, and gtfD. In vitro studies have indicated that gtfB and gtfC are essential for the sucrose-dependent attachment of *S. mutans* cells to hard surfaces, but gtfD is dispensable (Yoshida et al. 2005). Therefore, these genes have become a potential target for protection against dental caries.

The effect of *L. fermentum* and *L. acidophilus* biosurfactant on gtfB and gtfC gene expression levels was also investigated in our other studies. The expression of these genes and the production of insoluble extracellular glucans mediate the attachment of *S. mutans* not only to surfaces but also to other active types of bacteria that are favorable to the organisms for the persistent colonization of tooth surfaces. Additionally, gtf genes are known virulence factors associated with the pathogenesis of dental caries and a high content of insoluble glucans in dental plaque, which is related to an elevated risk of biofilm cariogenicity in humans. Several environmental factors can influence the expression and activity of the gtf enzymes. The existence of various enzymes in the process of carbohydrate metabolism and transport, glucan synthesis and secretion and degradation in the oral streptococci, in addition to factors that involve Post-translational modifications of the gtf enzymes, have traditionally complicated the understanding of regulatory studies (Wen et al. 2010).

Our results (figure 8 & 9) suggest that either the *L .fermentum* or *L. acidophilus* derived biosurfactants themselves or a putative signaling molecule in the extract down-regulated the expression level of genes that play an important role in the process of *S. mutans* attachment and biofilm formation. In addition to down regulating gtfB and gtfC (genes involved in insoluble glucan production), it may also have an effect on converting gtf activity from producing insoluble glucans to water-soluble glucans, hence accounting for reduced *S. mutans* biofilm adherence, and this should be studied in the future.

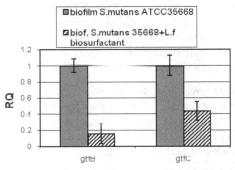

Fig. 8. The effect of *L.fermentum.*-derived biosurfactant on gtfB/C in immobilized biofilm of *S. mutans ATCC 35668;* The mRNA expression levels were calibrated relative to the control group (in the absence of biosurfactant)(Tahmourespour et al.,2011, Biofouling) .

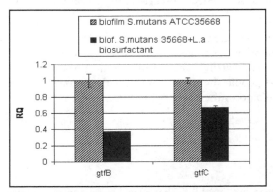

Fig. 9. The effect of *L.acidophilus*-derived biosurfactant on gtfB/C in immobilized biofilm of *S. mutans ATCC 35668;* The mRNA expression levels were calibrated relative to the control group (in the absence of biosurfactant) (Tahmourespour et al.,2011, Brazillian J of Microbiology).

Other studies have focused on the production and gene regulation of virulence factors, such as gtfs, which play an important role in biofilm formation by *S. mutans*, for controlling dental caries (Tamwsada and Kawabata 2004; Huang et al. 2008). The ability of *S. mutans* to produce extracellular polysaccharides from dietary carbohydrates has been demonstrated to significantly enhance its cariogenicity. Thus, the less extracellular polysaccharide produced, the lower the cariogenicity of *S. mutans*. Also it is demonstrated that chemical surfactants exerted different effects on the synthesis of glucosyltransferases in *S. mutans*; Tween 80 sig nificantly increased the level of gtfs, while Triton X-100 decreased gtf levels. So, It is proposed that the secondary metabolite of the probiotic bacteria (*L.fermentum and L.acidophilus*) decreases the expression level of gtf genes and therefore may be useful for the control of *S. mutans* and possibly other species.

4.6 Safty aspects of probiotics

Although probiotics can affect most important caries pathogens, lactobacilli may correlate with caries development. Some strains of *Lactobacillus* spp., together with *S. mutans*, play a key role in development of dental caries. The production of organic acids from dietary carbohydrates is also a main factor in dental caries progression. If lactobacilli taken orally are able to adhere or temporarily establish themselves in the oral environment, their metabolism and acid production should not support caries induction. Studies addressing sugar fermentation has shown a strain dependent

pH drop and the decrease was the fastest with glucose for all tested strains, thus highlighting the acidogenic potential of probiotics. The diversity of *in vitro* results does not allow clear conclusions about which probiotics may add benefit to the oral cavity. More large scale, multicenter clinical investigations are required to support the true effectiveness of probiotics in the prevention of oral and dental diseases.

It has been also observed that caries free subjects are colonized by lactobacilli that possess a significantly increased potential to suppress the growth of mutans streptococci compared with caries active or arrested subjects (Stamatova & Meurman, 2009). Finally, it can be concluded that the lactobacilli effect on caries prevention seems favorable when probiotic strains are well selected.

Furthure more, it should be mentioned that, orally lactobacillus species are well tolerated by about every one. Flatulence or gas is the most common side effect of Lactobacilli supplementation. It is usually very mild and goes away after 2 or 4 days. Immunocompromised people should be careful with the probiotics use as there have been reports of entering the blood stream (sepsis) in these individuals.

Bifidobacteria, is not associated with any side effects. It can occasionally cause mild diarrhea in children.

5. Future directions

According to the researches, probiotic bacteria have been characterized for different oral health purposes, including caries, periodontal diseases, and halitosis.

Genetically modified microbes including probiotics can take a new dimension to the concept of probiotics. Their main aim is the reduction of harmful effects of pathogenic strains naturally colonizing the oral cavity. The modified strain could then be used to replace the original pathogen. They also could be used to increase the properties of a potentially beneficial strain. In field of oral immunology, probiotics are being used as passive local immunization vehicles against dental caries. Bacteriophages, have also been detected in oral pathogens, such as *Actinobacillus Actinomycetemcomitans* (Sheikh et al., 2011).

The selection of the best probiotic for oral health and investigation the effect of other probiotic's metabolites on virulence genes and other traits of *S. mutans* are also issues that calls for further studies. It is possible that the administration way of probiotics might positively affect the effects observed as related to mutans streptococci reduction. So, further studies regarding the selection of best way for probiotic administration are necessitated.

Furthermore, the dosage of probiotic administration in each indication should be defined. Probiotics should be administered carefully and cautiously, and only on the basis of strong scientific evidence. Such evidence should direct the cautious, deliberate addition of clinically proven probiotics to commonly consumed food products to allow consumers to conveniently benefit from these organisms. Finally, safety issues are very important with any kind of bacteriotherapy.

Consequently, future studies should be conducted to investigate if phage therapy might be applied for oral and dental diseases in the same way as has been attempted for systemic infections.

6. Conclusion

Adhesion reduction can be an effective way on decreasing cariogenic potential of oral streptococci and all of the evidence has shown that probiotic bacteria such as Lactobacillus spp. can affect the oral ecology. In general, the above promising results suggest a potentially beneficial application of probiotics for the prevention of dental caries. These data also suggest that biosurfactant treatment can provide an option for controlling biofilm development and also influence the adhesive ability of bacterial pathogens

7. Acknowledgment

The author would like to thanks Dr. Ahmad Ali ForoughiAbari, the chancellor of Islamic Azad University Khorasgan (Isfahan), branch and Dr Mehran Hoodaji for their supports and Biotechnology Research Center of this University.

8. References

Ahola AJ., Yli-Knuuttila H. & Suomalainen T. (2002). Short term consumption of probiotic-containing cheese and its effect on dental caries risk factors. *Arch Oral Biol*, 47: 799–804.

Anderson MH. & Shi W. (2006). A probiotic approach to caries management. *Ped Dent*, 28 (2): 151-153.

Bhardwaj SB. (2010). Probiotics and oral health: an update. *Int J Contemporary Dent*, 1 (3): 116-119.

Bhushan J. & Chachra S. (2010). Probiotics-their role in prevention of dental caries. *J Oral Health Com Dent*, 4 (3): 78-82.

Bowen WH. (2002). Do we need to be concerned about dental caries in the coming millennium? *Crit Rev Oral Biol Med*, 13: 126-131.

Brown TA. Ahn SJ. Frank RN. Chen YY. Lemos JA. & Burne RA. (2005). A hypothetical protein of *Streptococcus mutans* is critical for biofilm formation. *Infect Immun*, 73(5): 3147-5.

Caglar E. Kargul B. & Tanbogaet I. (2005). Bacteriotherapy and probiotics role on oral health. *Oral Dis*, 11:1-7.

Carounanidy U. & Sathyanarayanan R. (2010). Dental caries: A complete changeover, PART III: Changeover in the treatment decisions and treatments. *J Conserv Dent*, 13: 209-17.

Comelli EM. Guggenheim B. Stingele F. & Nesser J. (2002). Selection of dairy bacterial strains as probiotics for oral health. *Eur j Oral sci*, 110: 218-224.

Cury JA. Rebelo MA. Del Bel Cury AA. Derbyshire MT. & Tabchoury CP. (2000). Biochemical composition and cariogenicity of dental plaque formed in the presence of sucrose or glucose and fructose. *Caries Res*, 34: 491-49.

Donlan RM. & Costerton JW. (2002). Biofilms: survival mechanisms of clinically relevant microorganisms. *Clin Microbiol Rev*, 15(2):167-93.

Filoche SK. Anderson SA. & Sissons CH. (2004). Biofilm growth of Lactobacillus species is promoted by Actinomyces species and *Streptococcus mutans*. *Oral Microbiol Immunol*,19:322-326.

Huang MJ. Meng L. Fan M. Hu P. & Bian Zh. (2008). Effect of biofilm formation on virulence factor *secretion via the general secretory pathway in Streptococcus mutans*. *Arch* Oral Biol, 53:1179-1185.

Kargul B. Caglar E. & Tanbogaet I. (2003). History of water fluoridation. *J Clin Pediatr Dent*,; 27 213-217.

Kaur IP. Chopra K. & Saini A. (2002). Probiotics: potential pharmaceutical applications. *Eur J Pharma Sci*, 15, 1–9.

Kõll-Klais P. Mändar R. Leibur E. Marcotte H. Hammarström L. & Mikelsaar M. (2005). Oral lactobacilli in chronic periodontitis and periodontal health: Species composition and antimicrobial activity. *Oral Microbiol Immunol*, 20:354-361.

Koo H. Xiao J. Klein MI. & Jeon JG. (2010). Exopolysaccharides produced by *Streptococcus mutans* glucosyltransferases modulate the establishment of microcolonies within multispecies biofilms. *J Bacteriol*, 192:3024–3032.

Kruger C. Hu YZ. Pan Q. Marcotte H. Hultberg A. & Delwar D. (2002). In situ delivery of passive immunity by lactobacilli producing single-chain antibodies. *Nature Biotech*, 20:702-6.

Leme AFP. Koo H. Bellato CM. Bedi G. & Cury JA. (2006). The role of sucrose in cariogenic Dental biofilm formation–New insight. *J Dent Res*, 85(10): 878-887.

Lilly DM. & Stillwell RH.(1965). Probiotics: growth-promoting factors produced by micro organisms. *Science*, 147: 747–8.

Loo CY. Mitrakul K. Voss IB. Hughes CV. & Ganeshkumar N. (2003). Involvement of an Inducible Fructose Phosphotransferase Operon in *Streptococcus gordonii* Biofilm Formation. *J Bacteriol*, 185: 6241-6254.

Marsh PD. (2005). Dental plaque: biological significance of a biofilm and community lifestyle. *J Clin Periodontol*, 32(supplement 6):7-15.

Meurman JH. (2005). Probiotics: do they have a role in oral medicine and dentistry. *Eur J Oral Sci*, 113:185-196.

Miller CH. & Kleinman JL. Effect of microbial interactions on in vitro plaque formation by *S.mutans*. *J Den Res*, 974.53(2): 427-434.

Millette M. Luquet FM. Ruiz MT. & Lacroix M. (2008). Characterization of probiotic properties of Lactobacillus strains. *Dairy Sci Technol*, 88 (6): 695-705.

Murata RM. Branco-de-Almeida EM. Franco R. Yatsuda MH. dos Santos SM. de-Alencarc H. Koo X. & Rosalen PL. (2010). Inhibition of *Streptococcus mutans* biofilm accumulation and development of dental caries in vivo by 7-epiclusianone and fluoride. *Biofouling*, 26:865–872.

Näse L. Hatakka K. Savilahti E. Saxelin M. Pönkä A. Poussa T. Korpela R. & Meurman J. (2001). Effect of long-term consumption of a probiotic bacterium, *Lactobacillus rhamnosus* GG. In milk on dental caries and caries risk in children. *Caries Res*, 35: 412-420.

Natcher WH. (2001). Diagnosis and Management of Dental Caries through out Life. *NIH Consensus Statement*, 18(1) 1-30.

Nikawa H. Makihira S. Fukushima H. Nishimura H. Ozaki K. Ishida K. (2004). *Lactobacillus reuteri* in bovine milk fermented decreases the oral carriage of mutans streptococci. *Int J Food Microbiol*, 95: 219-23.

Ouwehand AC. Salminen S. & Isolauri E. (2002). Probiotics: an overview of beneficial effects. *Antonie Van Leeuwenhoek*, 82: 279–289.

Pecharki GD. Cury JA. Paes Leme AF. Tabchoury CP. Del Bel Cury AA. Rosalen PL. (2005). Effect of sucrose containing iron (II) on dental biofilm and enamel demineralization in situ. *Caries Res*, 39: 123-129.

Ribeiro CC. Tabchoury CP. Del Bel Cury AA. Tenuta LM. Rosalen PL. & Cury JA. (2005). Effect of starch on the cariogenic potential of sucrose. *Br J Nutr* 94: 44-50.

Robinson RK. & Tamine AY. (1981). Microbiology of fermented milks. In: Robinson RK, ed. *Dairy microbiology*. Applied Science Publishers: Barking, UK, pp. 245-278.

Rodrigues L. Banat IM. Teixeira J. & Oliveira R. (2006). Biosurfactants: potential applications in medicine. *J Antimicrob Chemother*, 57:609–618.

Rodrigues L. Mei HC. Teixeira J. & Oliveira R. (2004). Influence of Biosurfactants from Probiotic Bacteria on Formation of Biofilms on Voice Prostheses. *Appl Environ microbial*, 70(7): 4408-10.

Saito T. (2004). Selection of useful probiotic lactic acid bacteria from the *Lactobacillus acidophilus* group and their applications to functional foods. *Animal Sci J*, 75, 1–13.

Schrezenmeir J. & de Vrese M. (2001). Probiotics, prebiotics, and synbiotics- approaching a definition. *Am J Clin Nutr*, 73: 361S-364S.

Sheikh S. Pallagatti S. Kalucha A. & Kaur H. (2011). Probiotics. Going on the natural way. *J Clin Exp Dent*, 3(2):e150-4.

Simark-Mattsson C. Emilson C G. Hakansson EG. Jacobsson C. Roos K. & Holm S. (2007). Lactobacillus-mediated interference of mutans streptococci in caries-free vs. caries-active subjects. *Eur J Oral Sci*, 115 (4): 308-314.

Stamatova I. & Meurman JH. (2009). Probiotics: Health benefits in the mouth. *Am J Dent*, 22:329-338.

Tahmourespour A. Kermanshahi RK. Salehi R. & Ghasemipero N. (2010). Biofilm formation potential of oral streptococci in related to some carbohydrate substrates. *Afr J Microbiol Res*, 4:1051-1056.

Tahmourespour A. & Kermanshahi RK. (2011). The effect of a probiotic strain (*Lactobacillus acidophilus*) on the plaque formation of oral Streptococci. *Bos J Basic Med Sci*, 11 (1): 4-7.

Tahmourespour A. Salehi R. Kermanshahi RK. & Eslami G. (2011). The anti-biofouling effect of *Lactobacillus fermentum*-derived biosurfactant against *Streptococcus mutans*. *Biofouling*, 27: 4, 385 – 392.

Tahmourespour A, Salehi R, Kermanshahi RK. (2011).Lactobacillus acidophilus-derived biosurfactant effect on gtfB and gtfC expression level in Streptococcus mutans biofilm cells. Brazil J Microbiol 42:330-339.

Tamwsada M. & Kawabata S. (2004). Synergistic effects of streptococcal glucosyltransferase on adhesive biofilm formation. *J Dent Res*, 83:874-879.

Teughels W. Essche M. & Sliepen I. (2008). Probiotics and oral health care. *Periodontol 2000*, 48: 111-147.

Thomas JG. Lindsay A. & Nakaishi BS. (2006). Managing the complexity of a dynamic Biofilm. *JADA,* 137(11 supplement):10S-15S.

Touger-Decker R. & Van Loveren C. (2003). Sugars and dental caries. (suppl): *Am J Clin Nutr*, 78: 881S-92S.

Van Hoogmoed CG. Van der Mei HC. & Busscher HJ. (2004). The influence of biosurfactants released by *S. mitis* BMS on the adhesion of pioneer strains and cariogenic bacteria. *Biofouling,* 20:261-267.

Vater J.Kablits B. Wild Ch. Franke P. Mehta N. & Cameotra SS. (2002). Matrix-assisted laser desorption ionization –time of flight mass spectrometry of lipopeptide biosurfactants in whole cells and culture filtrates of Bacillus subtilis C-1 isolated from petroleum sludge. *Appl Environ Microbiol,* 68:6210–6219.

Wen ZT. Yates D. Ahn SJ. & Burne RA. (2010). Biofilm formation and virulence expression by *Streptococcus mutans* are altered when grown in dual-species model. *BMC Microbiol* , 10:111-120.

Yoshida A. Ansai T. Takehara T. & Kuramitsu HK. (2005). LuxS-based signaling affects *Streptococcus mutans* biofilm formation. *Appl Environ Microbiol*, 71:2372-2380.

Zero DT. (2004). Sugars – The Arch Criminal. *Caries Res*, 38: 277-285. DOI: 10.1159/000077767

Part 2

Medical Treatment of Caries

6

Filling Materials for the Caries

Cafer Türkmen*

Marmara University, Dentistry Faculty, Depertment of Restorative Dentistry, Istanbul, Turkey

1. Introduction

Caries is a dynamic process in which mineral is removed during times of high acid production by bacterial plaque (demineralization) and replaced during periods of neutral pH (remineralization). Remineralization is the process by which mineral is deposited into tooth structure from salivary calcium and phosphate during periods of neutral pH. The remineralization process is facilitated by fluoride and can arrest carious demineralization by the formation of a hard outer surface [16].

Dentinal caries is similar to enamel caries, except that dentin demineralization begins at a higher pH (6.4 compared to 5.5) and proceeds about twice as rapidly since dentin has only half the mineral content. Low fluoride levels are insufficient to initiate dentin remineralization but are adequate to facilitate enamel remineralization. In enamel, at fluoride levels around 3 parts per million (ppm), the balance of mineral uptake and loss is shifted from net demineralization to net remineralization. Because dentin composes most root structure and because root surface caries lesions require significantly greater amounts of fluoride than enamel caries lesions to promote remineralization, restorative materials that release fluoride are often recommended for root surfaces [1]. Root caries appears as a softening and/or cavitation in the root surface with no initial involvement of the adjacent enamel. These lesions generally begin at or slightly occlusal to the free gingival margin but can extend into the gingival sulcus and/or undermine the coronal enamel as the caries progresses. Lesions also begin at the margins of restorations that have their cervical interfaces on root structure [19].

Traditional caries management has consisted of the detection of carious lesions followed by immediate restoration. In other words, caries was managed primarily by restorative dentistry. However, when the dentist takes the bur in hand, an irreversible process begins. Placing a restoration does not guarantee a sound future for the tooth; on the contrary, it may be the start of a restorative cycle in which the restoration will be replaced several times. The decision to initiate invasive treatment should be preceded by a number of questions: Is caries present and if so, how far does it extend? I a restoration required, or could the process be arrested by preventive treatment? Sometimes the decision to restore may be based on questionable diagnostic criteria.

---

*Corresponding Author

A different treatment strategy is recommended, based on a proper diagnosis of caries, taking into account the dynamics of the caries process. The activity of caries should be determined, and causative factors should be evaluated. Caries risk should be assessed before treatment is considered, and treatment should include preventive regimens to arrest the caries process by redressing the imbalance between demineralization and remineralization.

The treatment goal in caries management should be to prevent new lesions from forming and to detect lesions sufficiently early in the process so that they can be treated and arrested by nonoperative means. Such management requires skill and is time-consuming and worthy of appropriate payment. If these attempts have failed, high-quality restorative dentistry will be required to restore the integrity of the tooth surface [81].

The first popular fluoride-releasing tooth-colored restorative material was silicate cement. Although this material had no bonding properties and did not survive well in the oral environment, recurrent caries lesions associated with silicate cement restorations were rare. This anticaries effect was eventually associated with fluoride-releasing materials have the goal of inhibiting recurrent caries, especially in patients at high risk for developing new lesions.

Fluoride-releasing materials may be classified into four categories (1. Resin composites, 2. Compomers, 3. Resin-modified glass ionomers, and 4. Conventional glass ionomers based on similarities in physical, mechanical, and setting properties. Fluoride-releasing resin composites are on one end of the continuum and conventional glass ionomers on the other. Compomers appear near the resin composite end, and resin-modified glass ionomers are positioned nearer to the conventional glass ionomers [16].

The introduction of adhesive restorative materials has allowed dentists to make smaller preparations, which has led to preservation of hard dental tissues and, along with declining disease prevalence, has allowed elimination of G.V. Black's principle of "extension for prevention." Maximum tooth structure is preserved. However, this approach, sometimes described as a "dynamic treatment concept," cannot prevent repeated treatment procedures and the occurrence of iatrogenic damage [3]. Resin composites have better mechanical properties, no inherent adhesive properties, greater thermal expansion coefficients, and better wear resistance compared with other materials in the continuum, but they have the least fluoride release. Glass ionomers have inherent adhesive properties, release comparatively high amounts of fluoride, and have thermal expansion coefficients similar to tooth structure, but their mechanical properties and wear resistance are poor. Resin-modified glass ionomers contain elements of glass ionomers and light-cured resins. These materials have properties similar to glass ionomers and, like glass ionomers, should not be used for restorations in occlusal load-bearing areas. Although compomers are blends of resin composite and glass ionomer, they incorporate more resin than resin modified glass ionomers, and their physical and mechanical properties are more closely related to fluoride-releasing resin composites. Compomers require a bonding system and acid etching of tooth structure to achieve a clinically usable bond. They release more fluoride than resin composites but less than glass ionomers and are more abrasion resistant than conventional or resin-modified glass ionomers.

The early glass-ionomer restorative materials, called glass-ionomer cements, were rough, had less than optimum esthetic qualities, and had to be protected from hydration and dehydration with a varnish or light-cured resin, applied to the surface immediately after placement. Finishing was delayed for 24 hours with the earlier materials; this delay was later shortened, through modification of the material, to 7 minutes. The unmodified glass-ionomer materials are rarely used today [16].

Several mechanisms have been suggested for the anticaries effects of fluoride. These include the formation of fluorapatite, which is more acid resistant than hytdroxyapatite, the enhancement of remineralization, interference of ionic bonding during pellicle and plaque formation, and the inhibition of microbial growth and metabolism. Fluoride relased from restorative materials can inhibit caries through all these mechanisms, although it seems likely that enhancement of remineralization is the most important mechanism in the adult. Although the recurrent caries inhibition effects of fluoride-releasing materials are evident, their clinical effectiveness has been questioned based on the durability of the material. Even in primary teeth, these materials should be used selectively, and the time that the material will be expected to survive (how long the tooth will remain in the oral cavity) should be evaluated against its wear effectiveness [52].

For treating carious lesions, especially in the patient with high caries risk, resin-modified glass ionomers and fluoride-releasing resin composites have the greatest potential for success. Resin-modified glass ionomers are recommended as the esthetic restorative materials of choice in the Class 5 situation for patients with high caries risk, especially those with diminished salivary flow, due to their high fluoride release and fluoride recharge capability [16].

As materials continue to proliferate, it becomes increasingly difficult to choose the appropriate material for a particular clinical situation. Fluoride-releasing materials are no exception, and clinicians need guidelines to select and use these materials. There is modest but growing evidence from clinical trials that fluoride-releasing materials, especially glass ionomers, reduce the occurrence of recurrent caries. There is also evidence of a dose-response relationship between fluoride release and decreasing caries. While higher fluoride-releasing materials have greater caries protecting effects, these materials are not panaceas. The physical limitations of glass ionomers and compomers and their poor wear resistance contribute markedly to restoration failure. Evidence suggests that resin-modified glass-ionomer materials may provide an improved combination of physical integrity and caries inhibition [16].

The surfaces are important because all restorative dental materials meet and interact with tooth structure at a surface. Also, all dental surfaces interact with intraoral constituents such as saliva and bacteria. Changing a material's surface properties can mitigate the extent of that interaction. The type of interaction between two materials at an interface is defined as the energy of interaction, and this is conveniently measured for a liquid interacting with a solid under a standard set of conditions as the contact angle (θ). The contact angle is the angle a drop of liquid makes with the surface on which it rests (Fig. 1A). This angle is the result of an equilibrium between the surface tensions of the liquid-gas interface (Υ_{LG}), solid-gas interface (Υ_{SG}), and solid liquid interface (Υ_{SL}). These relationships can be expressed as an equation, as shown in fig. 1A. If the energy difference of the two materials in contact is large, then they will have a large contact angle. If the energy difference is very small, then the contact angle will be low and the liquid will appear to wet the solid by spreading. Wetting is a qualitative description of the contact angle. Good wetting, or spreading, represents a low contact angle. Partial (poor) wetting describes a contact angle approaching 90 degrees. Non wetting is a contact angle approaching 180 degrees (see fig. 1B).

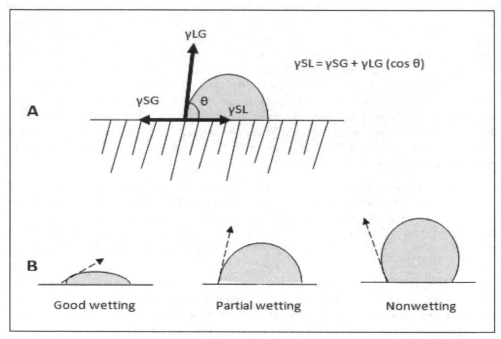

Fig. 1. Interfacial interactions of materials. A) Interaction quantified as contact angle (see formula). B) Interaction described in terms of good wetting (spreading), partial (poor) wetting, or nonwetting.

It is very important that film formers such as varnishes, liners, cements, and bonding agents have good wetting on tooth preparation surfaces on which these materials may be placed, so that they adapt to the microscopic interstices of the surfaces. However, in other instances, poor wetting may be an advantage. For example, experimental posterior composites have been formulated to have high contact angles to retard water and/or bacterial interactions. In most cases, wetting can be anticipated on the basis of the hydrophilicity (water-loving) or hydrophobicity (water-hating) of materials. Hydrophilic surfaces are not wet well by hydrophobic liquids [7].

Teeth also can be restored using indirect restorations are fabricated outside of the mouth. Most indirect restorations are made on a replica of the prepared tooth in a dental laboratory by a trained technician. Tooth-colored indirect systems include laboratory-processed composites or ceramics such as porcelain fired on refractory dies or hot pressed glasses. In addition, at least one chairside computer-aided design/computer-assisted manufacturing (CAD/CAM) system is currently available and is used to fabricate ceramic restorations [73].

This chapter reviews the glass-ionomer cements, compomers, and direct composite restorative materials (also dentin bonding agents) and their composition, classification, and clinical application and performance after removing caries.

2. Glass-ionomer cements

The original glass-ionomer cements (GICs), which are governed ISO 9917.1-2007 are water-based materials which set by an acid-base reaction between a polyalkenoic acid and a fluroaluminosilicate glass [86] and have been one of the most widely researched dental materials since their introduction in the 1970s. Since these were brittle materials, attempts were made to enhance the physical properties by the addition of either metal particles (silver or gold), by a fusion process resulting in a 'cermet' (ceramic-metal), or amalgam alloy particles by a simple addition ('admix'). An important characteristic of glass-ionomer is its ability to bond to tooth structure, one mechanism being that of a hydrogen bond between the carboxyl group of the polyacid and the camcium in the tooth structure. It has also been shown that there is a micromechanical penetration of the GI into the tooth. They have a coefficient of thermal expansion similar to the tooth, which may help reduce microleakage and therefore postoperative sensitivity and can be bulk-filled and finished faster than a composite. The newer generations of glass ionomer materials are faster setting and no longer sensitive to hydration or desiccation during setting. One main advantage of glass ionomer materials is their chemical bonding ability to tooth structure, making them more resistant to leaks. Compared with resin system bonding, glass ionomer bonding is more degeneration-resistant and does not breakup, unlike the hydrolytic degradation of the hybrid layer of the resin system. Further modification of water-based ('conventional') GICs took place in the early 1990s by the addition of water-soluble resin, to produce the 'resin-modified' GICs. The purpose of adding resin was to enhance the physical properties and to reduce the sensivity to water balance of the conventional GICs. The first of the 'resin-modified' GICs (RM-GICs) was Virtabond (3M Dental Products, St Paul, Minnesota, USA), now called Vitrebond (3M/Espe Dental). Other names for RM-GIC which have been used include 'resin-ionomers', 'resinomers', 'hybrid ionomers' and 'light-cured glass ionomers' [17, 79, 80, 84].

2.1 Setting reactions

After mixing powder and liquid, the acid etches the gllas which reslts in a release of calcium, aluminium, sodium and fluoride ions into solution. This is an acid-base reaction where the water serves as the medium for the reaction. The metal ions react with the carboxyl (COO) groups to form a polyacid salt, which becomes the cement matrix, and the surface of the glass becomes a silica hydrogel. The unreacted cores of the glass particles remain as a filler [79, 84].

Although the clinical set is completed within a few minutes, a continuing 'maturation' phase occurs over subsequent months. This is predominantly due to the slow reaction of the aluminium ions [45] and is the cause of the set material's sensitivity to water balance. The set material needs to be protected from salivary contamination for several hours, otherwise the surface becomes weak and opaque, and from water loss for several months, otherwise the material shrinks and cracks and may debond [45, 79].

The RM-GICs also undergo an acid:base reaction (which is a pre-requisite for any material to be described as a glass-ionomer cement). However, there is an additional resin polymerization phase. Depending on the product, the resin polymerization may be self-cure, light-cure or both. On mixing powder and liquid, the acid:base reaction, and if present, the self-cure resin polymerization reaction, begin and setting commences. Restorative RM-GICs (in contrast to luting RM-GICs) undergo photopolymerization on exposure to light, resulting in clinical set. However, the acid:base reaction continues, albeit much more slowly. Although the set material can be contoured and polished under water spray immediately following polymerization, delayed polishing has been recommended [88]. However, dehydration remains a potential problem. All GICs show an increase in translucency at seven days compared to that at placement, resulting in an aesthetic improvement [45, 79].

2.2 Classification

The most practical classification of the GICs is on their clinical usage [45, 87]. Type I GICs are the luting cements, characterized by low film thickness and rapid set; when available as an RM-GIC, the photopolymerization reaction will be absent. Type II GICs are restorative cements, with sub-types 1 and 2. Type II-1 GICs are aesthetic cements (available in both conventional and resin-modified presentations) and Type II-2 GICs are 'reinforced' (however, despite their description, are not necessarily stronger than Type II-1 products). However, they are more wear-resistant. Type III GICs are the lining cements and fissure sealants, characterized by low viscosity and rapid set.

In the mid- to late-1990s, high powder:liquid ratio conventional GICs were introduced, alternatively termed 'packable' or 'high viscosity' GICs [62]. These products (e.g., Ketac Molar, 3M/Espe, Seefeld, Bavaria, Germany; Chemflex, Dentsply, York, Pennsylvania, USA; Fuji IX and Fuji IX GP, GC International) are promoted principally for small cavities in deciduous teeth, temporary restorations, liner/base applications, and in the 'Atraumatic Restorative Treatment' (ART) technique [26, 79]. The most recently accepted uses of GICs have been as a liner and base under deep composite restorations, which was described in 1984 [38] and has been referred to as the *sandwich technique*, Deep cervical lesions and proximal boxes of class II cavities whose gingival floor is on root surfaces are areas where there is increased diameter of dentinal tubules that will affect the bond strength because of increased chances of hydrolytic degradation (The 'open sandwich' technique, also known as the 'cervical lining'). Because of their chemical bonding capabilities, glass ionomer adhere to these surface better then dental adhesive-bonding agents. Based on evidence-based dentistry protocols, the recommendation is to treat the surfaces with a polyacrylic acid conditioner, which is rinsed before glass ionomers are applied. This weak acid modifies the smear layer by leaving the smear plugs behind, improving the seal and eliminating postoperative sensitivity. A new self-conditioner for resin-modified glass ionomers, recently developed by Fuji (GC America, IL, USA), does not require rinsing before applying the glass ionomer material [9]. Both Fuji II and Fuji IX (GC America, IL, USA) have unique automix dispensing capsules, simplifying placement of these materials. Resin-modified ionomers, such as Fuji II LC, are routinely used as liners at 1 mm or less, and a material such as Fuji IX or Riva (SDI, Bensenville, IL, USA) is preferred for larger areas of dentin replacement.

Based on abundant evidence, conventional and metal-modified glass ionomers are not recommended in class 2 restorations in both primary and permanent molars. To compensate for this, RM-GICs were developed to produce better mechanical properties than the conventional ones. The resin hydroxyethyl methacrylate (HEMA) or bis-glycerol methacrylate was added to the liquid. The resin modification of these cements allowed the base curing reaction to be supplemented by a light or chemical curing process, allowing for a command set. The obvious advantages were better fracture toughness, increased tensile strength, and a decrease in desiccation and hydration problems [20]. The limiting factors were the setting shrinkage, which was found to be greater than with conventional cements, and the limited depth of cure with more opaque lining cements [5]. The mean age of these failed glass ionomer restorations at replacement in permanent teeth in general practice was found to be 5.5 years for patients older than 30 years [43]. Secondary caries, bulk fracture (1.4%–14%), and marginal fracture (from poor anatomic form) constituted the main reasons for failure. In developing countries, highly viscous glass ionomer materials have became popular in atraumatic restorative treatment techniques for class 1 restorations in posterior teeth. In class 2 restorations, these high viscous glass ionomers are still considered satisfactory after 3 years of clinical service, despite large percentages of failed restorations. However, a recently concluded retrospective study showed that the failure of class 2 restorations with these materials rose to 60% at 72 months. It was hypothesized that caries-like loss of material was seen on radiographs and that the presence of proximal contacts promoted disintegration of these materials [66, 80].

2.3 Bonding mechanism

The bonding mechanism of the GICs to dental hard tissues is very complex, and may be different for RM-GICs compared to conventional GICs. Simplistically, an ionic bond occurs between the carboxyl (COO^-) ions in the cement acid and the calcium (Ca^{++}) ions in enamel and dentine.

When freshly mixed conventional GIC is placed on enamel or dentine, dissolution of any smear layer occurs but demineralization is minimal since the tooth hydroxyapatite buffers the acid, and polyalkenoic is quite weak [83]. Phosphate ions (negatively charged) and calcium ions (positively charged) are displaced from the hydroxyapatite, and are absorbed into the unset cement. This results in an intermediate layer between the 'pure' GIC and the 'pure' hydroxyapatite; the so called 'ion-exchange' layer [45]. Problems of specimen preparation of a water-based material have hindered investigation of this layer, although better techniques are now becoming available [49].

The ion-exchange layer appears to consist of calcium and phosphate ions from the GIC, and aluminium, silicic, fluoride and calcium and/or strontium ions (depending on glass composition) from the GIC [67]. The thickness of the ion-exchange layer appears to be in the order of a few micrometres, and merges into the GIC on one side and into the enamel/dentine on the other. Unfortunately there is some confusion in the literature [24, 31, 49, 76] regarding the ion-exchange layer. Other terms have been proposed such as 'zone of interaction', 'interdiffusion zone', 'hybrid layer', 'interphase', and 'intermediate layer'. In particular, the notation 'hybrid layer' causes confusion with the 'hybrid layer' formed between resin composite and dentine (see below). The term 'ion-exchange layer' should be used, since it accurately describes its nature. It has been shown that this layer is resistant to acid and base treatment, and has thus also been referred to as the 'acid-base resistant layer' [79].

Measurement of the bond strength of GIC to enamel and dentine is complicated by the brittle nature of the GIC. Laboratory bond strength tests invariably result in cohesive failure of the GIC, rather than failure within the ion exchange layer. Consequently, the true strength of the ion-exchange layer is not known; values in the range 3-10 MPa are commonly reported, i.e., approximately the cohesive strength of GIC [76, 79].

2.4 Fluoride release

The release of fluoride ions is one of the notable characteristics of GICs. It is present originally as a flux in the manufacture of the glass, and is released from the glass particles on mixing with the polyalkenoic acid. The presence of fluoride also has benefits in increasing translucency and strength and improving handling properties [29]. The mechanism of release is complex and not fully understood. However, it is maximum in the first few days and decreases rapidly to a lower level over weeks, and maintains a low level over months. It has also been shown that GIC can be 'recharged' with fluoride, resulting in a subsequent short-term boost in release. Most of the fluoride is released as sodium fluoride, which is not critical to the cement matrix, and thus does not result in weakening or disintegration of the set cement. Resin-modified GICs show similar dynamics of fluoride release, although for both types of material the dynamics of release and the amounts released depend on the particular material and the experimental design [79, 89].

2.5 Biological properties

Several metallic ions are released from GIC, as well as fluoride. The highest release occurs from the unset material, and as described above, most research has been done on fluoride. Hydroxethylmethacrylate (HEMA) is released from RM-GICs and can diffuse through dentine in laboratory studies. Since HEMA can induce allergic and toxic responses, the clinical relevance of its release requires more investigation [70]. Nevertheless, to date there is no evidence that HEMA in dental materials is responsible for any local or systematic adverse effects.

Glass-ionomer cement has been shown to have an antimicrobial effect in several studies, and greater than that shown by other materials such as amalgam and resin composite. However, again it is difficult to do more than generalize, as the results depend on the experimental method, the bacteria used and the product tested [70]. There are several theories regarding the antibacterial activity. Most workers propose that fluoride is responsible, possibly acting synergistically with pH. However, other released agents have been cited as possible antibacterials, including zinc [77] and polyalkenoic acid [68], acting alone or synergistically with pH and fluoride [79].

2.6 Clinical performance

One of the principal benefits of GICs is their adhesion to the dental hard tissues, and this has been confirmed in non-undercut non-carious cervical lesions (NCCLs) where dentine is the main substrate. However, because of the low fracture toughness of GICs (including RM-GICs), they are recommended principally for non-stress-bearing areas, e.g., carious and non-carious cervical lesions and approximal anterior lesions. Nevertheless, the high powder:liquid ratio materials may be useful in the restoration of small cavities in deciduous teeth. Clinical studies on RM-GICs are less extensive because of their more recent introduction [6, 13]. However, the results are mixed with respect to both brand comparisons and comparisons with polyacid-modified resin composites. One presentation of an RM-GIC is in a low powder:liquid ratio form (Fuji Bond LC; GC International), and is used in a similar way to a dentine bonding agent. Excellent five-year results have been obtained for the retention by this material of resin composite in non-carious cervical lesions [78].

Evidence is accumulating that GIC may have an important role in minimum intervention dentistry. Modern concepts of operative dentistry propose that only the 'infected' dentine should be removed, leaving the 'affected' dentine which has the potential to remineralize. Recent evidence suggests that such remineralization may be potentiated by GIC [3], and this has special relevance in the ART technique [79].

3. Compomers (Polyacid-modified resin composites)

Polyacid-modified composite resins, known trivially as compomers, are a group of aesthetic materials for the restoration of teeth damaged by dental caries. They were introduced to the profession in the early 1990s [40], and were presented as a new class of dental material designed to combine the aesthetics of traditional composite resins with the fluoride release and adhesion of glass-ionomer cements. The trivial name was devised from the names of these two "parent" materials, the "comp" coming from composite, and "omer" from ionomer [60]. The term *polyacid-modified composite resin* was originally proposed for these materials in 1994 [39] and has been widely adopted both by manufacturers and researchers since that time. However, it has been criticised on the grounds that it ". . .may over-emphasize a structural characteristic of no or little consequence" [60]. This is a somewhat strange criticism, since to formulate these materials, manufacturers have modified them specifically by the introduction of acid functional macro-monomers. They are, therefore, without question "polyacid modified". Whether this modification confers clinical benefits, or indeed whether these materials can usefully be considered to be distinctive materials is more debateable. The conclusion of Ruse is that ". . . They are, after all, just another dental composite", but this seems to the present author to be somewhat extreme, and there is considerable evidence that compomers possess characteristic properties, and are therefore distinct from conventional composite resins [50, 55, 60, 85].

3.1 Composition and setting

As has already been stated, compomers resemble traditional composite resins in that their setting reaction is an addition polymerization. It is usually light-initiated, and the initiator is camphorquinone with amine accelerator, and as such is sensitive to blue light at 470 nm [40]. There is, however, at least one brand, designed for use as luting cement, Dyract Cem, that is a two-paste system. Cure is brought about as a result of mixing the two pastes, each of which contains a component of the free radical initiator system. The set material, though, does not differ in any fundamental way from those compomers that cure photochemically.

A key feature of compomers is that they contain no water and the majority of components are the same as for composite resins. Typically these are bulky macro-monomers, such as bisglycidyl ether dimethacrylate (bisGMA) or its derivatives and/or urethane dimethacrylate, which are blended with viscosity-reducing diluents, such as triethylene glycol dimethacrylate (TEGDMA). These polymer systems are filled with non-reactive inorganic powders, such as quartz or a silicate glass, for example $SrAlFSiO_4$. These powders are coated with a silane to promote bonding between the filler and the matrix in the set material. In addition, compomers contain additional monomers that differ from those in conventional composites, which contain acidic functional groups. The most widely used monomer of this type is so-called TCB, which is a di-ester of 2-hydroxyethyl methacrylate with butane tetracarboxylic acid [23]. This acid-functional monomer is very much a minor component and compomers also contain some reactive glass powder of the type used in glass-ionomer cements [25, 50].

Despite the presence of these additional components, compomers are similar to composite resins in that they are fundamentally hydrophobic, though less so than conventional composite resins. They set by a polymerization reaction, and only once set do the minority hydrophilic constituents draw in a limited amount of water to promote a secondary neutralization reaction [23]. They lack the ability to bond to tooth tissues, so require bespoke bonding agents of the type used with conventional composite resins, and their fluoride release levels are significantly lower than those of glass-ionomer cements. Such low levels of fluoride release have been shown to compromise the degree of protection afforded by these materials in *in vitro* experiments using an artificial caries medium [41].

3.2 Effect of water uptake

A distinctive feature of compomers is that, following the initial polymerization reaction, they take up small amounts of moisture *in situ*, and this triggers an acid–base reaction between the reactive glass filler and the acid groups of the functional monomer [51, 60]. Among other features, this process causes fluoride to be released from the glass filler to the matrix, from where it can readily be released into the mouth, and act as an anticariogenic agent [41]. Polymerization is associated with contraction and the development of measurable stresses, and it may be that the sorption of water plays some part in reducing these stresses *in vivo* [25, 50].

The role of the reactive glass in the water uptake process has been considered in one report [1]. A conventional composite resin formulation was used as the matrix phase, with filler being either an unreactive glass, Raysorb T-4000, or the ionomer glass G338, whose composition and properties have been described extensively in the literature. In each case, the glass was used both with and without a coating of silane coupling agent (Y-methacryloxy propyl trimethoxysilane). The results show that silanation reduced the water uptakefor both of the glasses and also improved the strength. However, incorporating G338 rather than Raysorb T-4000 gave an inferior material since it took up more water and was of lower strength. Previous studies of water sorption by composite resins have shown that the water accumulates around the filler particles [69], so that one conclusion of the study is that G338 is more hydrophilic than Raysorb T-4000. This suggests that it provides part of the driving force for water uptake by compomers, and also that it is responsible for a decline in their overall mechanical properties relative to conventional composite resins.

Compomers are designed to absorb water, and are able to up of the order of 2–3.5% by mass of water on soaking. This water uptake has been shown to be accompanied by neutralization of the carboxylic acid groups, as shown by changes in bands at 1705 and 1555 cm−1. The former band arises from the presence of carboxylic acid groups within the material, and gradually reduces in intensity on exposure to water. By contrast the latter band arises from the presence of carboxylate salts, and shows a corresponding increase in intensity with time. Neutralization has been shown to be controlled by rate of water diffusion and is therefore fairly slow. Although compomers are designed to take up water in order to promote a later neutralization, these processes have been shown to have an adverse effect on many of their mechanical properties [50].

3.3 Fluoride release

Compomers are designed to release fluoride in clinically beneficial amounts. Fluoride is present in the reactive glass filler, and becomes available for release following reaction of this glass with the acid functional groups, triggered by moisture uptake. In addition, commercial compomers contain fluoride compounds such as strontium fluoride or ytterbium fluoride, which are capable of releasing free fluoride ion under clinical conditions, and augment the relatively low level of release that occurs from the polysalt species that develops. Fluoride release occurs to enhanced extents in acidic conditions, and in lactate buffer has been shown to be diffusion-based [64].

The conventional way of determining fluoride release is to employ an ion-selective electrode, and to treat the sample solution with an equal volume of the decomplexing TISAB (total ionic strength adjustment buffer). This liberates fluoride from any potential complexes, and enables to full amount of fluoride to be determined [50].

The authors speculated that the complexation was caused by the elevated levels of aluminium released under acidic conditions. As an example, for Compoglass F, aluminium concentration rose from 4.68 ppm in water to 104ppm in lactic acid solution. Aluminium is known to form complexes of the type AlF_2^+ and AlF^{2+} [2] and these have been widely assumed to occur, for example in glass-ionomer cements. However, an alternative suggestion has been made by Billington et al. [8], who have suggested that complexation as monofluorophosphate is also a possibility, and they note that phosphorus levels released by glass-ionomer cements are also typically elevated under acidic conditions. This is also possible for compomers, as their glass filler components are similar to those used in glass-ionomers, and they, too, show elevated phosphorus release under acidic conditions [25, 50].

3.4 Clinical performance

Right from the time they were first launched, compomers have shown acceptable clinical performance in a variety of clinical applications. However, wear characteristics of early materials were poor and there were concerns about their durability. Despite this, the early results were promising, and more recently, results with newer formulations have also been good.

Compomers are designed for the same sort of clinical applications as conventional composites. These include Class II and Class V cavities, as fissure sealants, and as bonding agents for the retention of orthodontic bands. Their fluoride release, however, is seen as a useful feature for use in paedodontics, and certain brands have been produced that are specifically aimed at children [25, 50].

Compomers have been widely used in Class V restorations. For example, the compomers Dyract AP, Compoglass F and F2000 were evaluated for use in this application over a 2-year period [37]. This study concluded that, after this time, all three materials showed an acceptable level of clinical performance.

Colour stability has been found to be somewhat of a problem with compomers in a few studies. This is not entirely surprising, given that they are designed to take up water, which is likely to alter appearance through a change in refractive index, and also to carry with it coloured chemical species (stains) from certain foodstuffs such as coffee and red wine. In a 3-year study of Class V restorations of Dyract, Demirci et al. [21] found that all Ryge criteria were good, except those relating to colour change, i.e. colour stability and marginal discoloration. In both of these there were significant changes [21].

Compomers have been used as fissure sealants [28], and a clinical study examined the teeth of children aged between 7 and 10 years sealed by the compomer Dyract Seal. Sealed teeth were examined post-operatively at 3, 6, 12 and 24 months, and were also evaluated by the Ryge criteria. In general Dyract Seal behaved as well as a conventional composite resin sealant, except on the criterion of marginal integrity, showing that this material was acceptable for its clinical application, at least of the 24 months period of the study [28].

Compomers have also been used for Class I [56] and Class II restorations. In the Class I study, they were used in composite laminate restorations, and were shown to perform as well as conventional composite resins [56]. In the Class II study, they were studied over 7 years in children aged between 3.6 and 14.9 years. Again performance was indistinguishable from that of conventional composite resins.

Lastly, compomers have been employed as cements for orthodontic bands and there have been a number of full studies of compomers in this application [34]. Results have been generally extremely good for compomers, except in the realms of taste, as determined by the patient, and in which compomers scored less well than glass-ionomers. Thus, compomers have been shown to have acceptable performance as materials for use in orthodontic band retention, though the final choice of cementing agent could be left to patients. If they found the taste of the compomer particularly objectionable, a resin-modified glass-ionomer could be used equally effectively instead [50].

Overall, the major conclusion from these clinical results is that compomers perform well, and are suited to their suggested uses in dental restoration. The reduction in strength due to water uptake does not seem to be important clinically and these materials are suited to use in vivo.

4. Dentine Bonding Agents (DBAs)

The concept of bonding a restorative material to the dentine surface is by no means a new idea. Even at the time of Buonocore using phosphoric acid to bond to enamel, the idea of bonding to dentine was considered. However, due to limitations of materials and knowledge of the structure and nature of dentine the dream remained just that until the late '70s. In fact Buonocore did try to introduce a dentine adhesive but was unsuccessful [15]. The earliest bonding agent which showed some success was introduced by Fusayama [27]. At the same time Bowen [12] in the USA started investigating new formulations of resins that were more water tolerant as well as methods of treating the dentine with oxalates to gain adhesion. The concern of many clinicians at that time was the potential damage phosphoric acid was going to cause the dental pulp if dentine was etched [79]. The first work to investigate the mechanism of bonding to the dentine was by Nakabayashi [47]. His paper of 1982 has now become one of the classic papers to first identify a layer between the resin and dentine substrate referred to as 'hybrid' dentine, in that it was the organic components of the dentine that had been permeated by resin (Fig. 2). The term 'hybrid layer' has now become synonymous with bonding of resins to etched dentine. There has been a tremendous amount of research done on the hybrid layer, its structure, formation and how it can be improved. Without a hybrid layer a bond will not be formed to the dentine. Therefore, it is essential for some modification to be made to the dentine surface so a mechanical interlocking of resin around dentinal collagen can occur. This layer has also been referred to as the 'resin-dentine interdiffusion zone' [79].

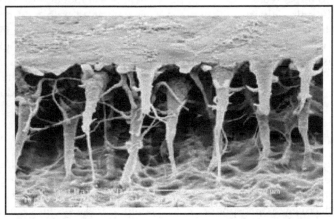

Fig. 2. Bonded specimen in which the dentine (mineral and protein) has been removed. The infiltration of resin into the acid-etched dentine can be seen with an associated permeation of resin throughout the dentine tubular network and its lateral branches.

4.1 Classification

Dentine bonding agents have gone through many changes over the last 10 years. This has led some people to refer to the changes as 'generations' of material, implying that there has been some chronological development. This is a falsehood — for example, the first 'self-etching' type material was introduced by Coltène (Altstätatten, Switzerland) as 'ART Bond'. Therefore, it is more logical to classify materials by the number of steps needed to complete the bonding process.

4.1.1 'Three-step' or 'Conventional' systems

This group represents those materials that have separate etching, priming and adhesive steps. It just so happens that this group of materials is also the oldest. However, they are still widely used and have been shown to provide reliable bonding. The greatest problem with this group would seem to be that three distinct steps are needed, which gives rise to possible problems through contamination of the bonded surface prior to placement of the resin composite filling material; in other words, they are more technique sensitive [47, 79].

4.1.2 'Two-step' systems

This group has two subgroups; the first includes those systems that have a separate etch and have combined the priming and bonding steps. These systems are often referred to as 'Single-bottle' systems. In general, the problems experienced with the Conventional Systems still exist with the Single-bottle systems. Although one step has been eliminated, the great problem is ensuring good infiltration of the priming-bond into the demineralized dentine. The other subgroups combine the etching and priming steps together and are referred to as 'Self-etching primers'. These systems also have not been without their problems. The major concern has been their ability to etch the enamel to a great enough extent to ensure a good seal. This seems to be overcome now [42]. The problem of technique sensitivity also seems to have been significantly reduced with these systems compared with the Conventional and Single-bottle systems. This is attributed to the fact that the self-etching priming agent does not have to be washed off the dentine, therefore eliminating the need to maintain the dentine in a moist state. The method of demineralization of these materials is by the use of an acidic resin that etches and infiltrates the dentine simultaneously. The dentine is an excellent buffer, so the acidity of the self-etching primer is rapidly reduced and after polymerization is neutralized [32].

4.1.3 'One-bottle' or 'All-in-one' systems

This fourth group is the simplest of all the DBAs. They combine all steps into one process. Their mode of demineralization is identical to that of the self-etching priming materials, but the bonding resin is also incorporated. These systems also have the problem of not etching the enamel as effectively as phosphoric acid. In addition these systems are the newest and have no long-term clinical data to demonstrate their effectiveness, although early studies are showing some variability in the success of these materials [14].

4.2 Bonding mechanism

As already mentioned, the mechanism of bonding of resin-based DBAs is via a hybrid layer. This is a micromechanical interlocking of resin around dentinal collagen fibrils that have been exposed by demineralization. The interlocking occurs by the diffusion of the resins in the primer and bonding resin. The formation and structure of the hybrid layer has been extensively studied, and has also been referred to as the resin-impregnated layer, the resin-dentine interdiffusion zone. The thickness of the hybrid layer ranges from less than 1μm for the all-in-one systems to up to 5μm for the conventional systems. The strength of the bond is not dependent on the thickness of the hybrid layer, as the self-etching priming materials have shown bond strengths greater than many other systems but exhibit a thin hybrid layer. Sugizaki [72] showed that the etching, washing and drying process caused the dentine to collapse due to the loss of the supporting hydroxyapatite. Further work showed that this collapse of the collagen was an impediment to the successful diffusion of the resin to the base of the region of demineralization. To overcome this problem, Kanca [33] introduced the 'wet bonding technique' which left the demineralized collagen fibres supported by residual water after washing. This allowed the priming solution to diffuse throughout the collagen fibre network more successfully. However, when it comes to clinical practice, it is very difficult to find the correct balance of residual moisture. Sano *et al.* [65] showed in their work on nanoleakage that most resin-based DBAs allowed the ingress of silver nitrate along the base of the hybrid layer. However, the clinical significance of this is unclear. It may be a pathway for fluid to affect collagen not coated by resin, and the outcome may be degradation of the bond over time. However, the degree of nanoleakage is very much material dependent rather than system dependent, meaning that there are conventional systems and self-etching priming systems that show small amounts of nanoleakage whereas others show more. For the self-etching systems, these are able to solubilize the smear layer and demineralize the underlying dentine, forming a quite thin hybrid layer [25, 35, 36, 79].

4.3 Bonding substrate

Dentine is quite a variable tissue. Within the tooth itself the dentine approaching the dentino-enamel junction is more highly mineralized and the area occupied by the tubules is less than that of dentine adjacent to the pulp. In addition to this, dentine should be considered as a dynamic tissue that changes due to ageing, in response to caries and restoration placement. Most changes relate to occlusion of tubules and also an increase in the mineralization of the dentine. The implication of this is that the dentine becomes slightly more difficult to etch and exposure of collagen fibrils can also be reduced, hence there is a potential for the bond to be somewhat tenuous. This is particularly the case for the highly sclerosed dentine of non-carious cervical lesions (NCCLs). Laboratory studies indicate that the hybrid layer of the dentine surface of NCCLs is thinner than that of normal dentine [29, 63]. In addition, it seems that some bonding systems do not adhere as well to this surface and show a slightly decreased bond strength [25, 35, 79].

A considerable amount of work has also been done looking at the variation of the bond to caries-affected dentine. Some of the early studies used artificial caries like lesions. However, this does not reproduce the situation that occurs in the oral cavity since caries is a process of demineralization and remineralization associated with the damage of the supporting collagen matrix [48, 53]. The increased thickness of the hybrid layer is mainly because the dentine is already partially demineralized from the caries and the action of the acid etch is therefore somewhat greater. This provides a clear basis for not etching for longer than that recommended by the manufacturer. In addition, the water content of caries-affected dentine is believed to be greater than normal dentine. This too will also have an effect on the ability of the resins to penetrate to the full depth of the demineralized dentine. In the case of caries-affected dentine treated with chemo-mechanical caries removal solutions, there appear to be no adverse effects on the bond with a DBA [79].

However, the bond to radicular and pulp chamber dentine does seem to vary quite a lot depending on the DBA used. This perhaps provides a strong case for being careful with the selection of a DBA for these regions of the tooth. It is believed that it may be necessary to use different DBAs for different regions of the tooth, or a system needs to be selected where it has been shown to provide a reliable bond to all parts of the tooth. Another alternative is the use of GIC restorative materials when then is a deep cavity on the radicular surface of a tooth, as it is known that a reliable bond can be achieved and moisture control is not such a problem [25, 35, 79].

4.4 Clinical studies

There has been a considerable amount of work done to evaluate the success or otherwise of DBAs in clinical studies. However, one of the great problems has been that many of the DBAs have been considerably changed or a new material introduced by the time these studies are completed or published. Many of the studies have also been performed on NCCL, which means the outcomes cannot really be applied to restorations in other parts of the mouth because NCCL dentine is usually sclerosed and therefore different from that of an intracoronal cavity. However, these outcomes will provide some indication as to whether the DBA is able to achieve a durable bond under very harsh conditions. Since the early materials were introduced, the retention rates of the DBAs to sclerosed cervical dentine have steadily improved to extent that retention rates are little different from GICs [79].

With regard to clinical studies on posterior teeth restored with a DBA, there is still little evidence available. It would seem though, that clinical studies of resin composite restorations are showing evidence that when placed in the correct manner and the patient has a low caries rate, restoration survival is approaching that of amalgam [30].

When it comes to the use of DBAs, it is important to follow the manufacturers' directions carefully. Overetching can create a situation where there will potentially be a region of poorly or uninfiltrated dentine. This zone may be susceptible to acid or enzyme attack from oral bacteria, hence leading to bond failure [82].

In the case of the self-etching priming materials, this is not believed to be a problem. However, the converse problem may occur: as mentioned, the dentine or smear layer may neutralize the etching primer if the primer has a relatively high pH. The anecdotal evidence would seem to indicate that gentle agitation of these solutions may assist with the etching. However, there are no research data to support this [35, 79].

5. Direct composite restorative materials

A generalized definition of a composite is a multiphase material that exhibits the properties of both phases where the phases are complimentary, resulting in a material with enhanced properties. The first tooth-colored composite was silicate cement, which was introduced in 1870s. This composite formulation was based on alumino-fluro-silicate glasses and phosphoric acid. The dispersed phase was residual glass particles, and the matrix phase was the aluminum phosphate salt formed from the partial acid dissolution of the glass particles; however, these were brittle, required mechanical retention, and had an average longevity of only a few years. of only a few years. The first polymeric tooth-colored composite used in dentistry was based on poly (methylmethacrylate). This material was developed in the 1940s, and consisted of a poly (methylmethacrylate) powder, methyl methacrylate monomer, benzoyl peroxide, and n,n-dimethlyparatoluidine. These materials could be classified as composites, because upon mixing, the polymer powder formed a dispersed phase and the monomer polymerized to form the continuous phase. The polymerization was initiated at room temperature, using the redox initiator combination of benzoyl peroxide and n,ndimethlyparatoluidine. Although these materials were initially esthetic, they were plagued with a variety of problems, including poor color stability, high polymerization shrinkage, a lack of bonding to tooth structure, and a large coefficient of thermal expansion (CTE). The first polymer matrix composite incorporating silica fillers was introduced in the 1950s. These composites had improved mechanical properties and good esthetics; they did not bond to tooth structure, and still exhibited significant polymerization shrinkage [10, 46, 55, 58].

One way to address the polymerization shrinkage problem is to use high molecular weight monomers. In 1962 Bowen [11], while at the National Bureau of Standards, synthesized an acrylated epoxy using glycidylmethacrylate and Bisphenol A epoxy for use as a matrix for dental composite. The resulting monomer, called Bis-GMA or Bowen's resin, possessed the viscosity of honey, and therefore limited the amount of filler particles that could be incorporated. Subsequent experiments incorporated triethylene glycol dimethacrylate (TEGDMA) as a diluent to reduce the viscosity. This monomer combination worked well, and has become one of the most widely used matrix monomer combinations for dental composites to date. The structures of Bis-GMA and TEGDMA are shown in Figs. 3 and 4, respectively.

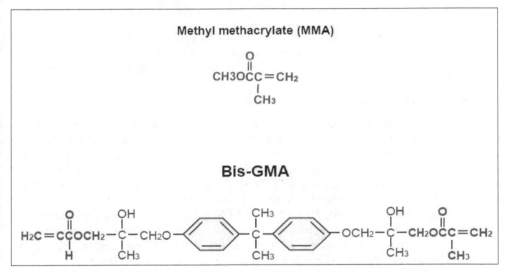

Fig. 3. The chemical structure of Bis-GMA, a resin invented by Ray Bowen. It also is referred to as Bowen's resin.

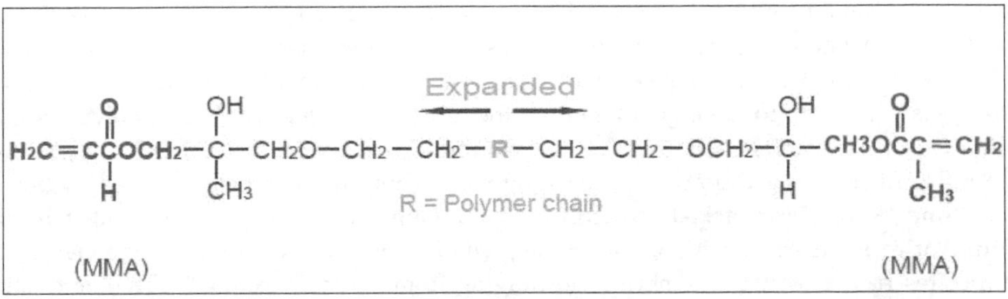

Fig. 4. TEGDMA. The chemical structure of triethyleneglycol dimethacrylate (TEGDMA, which is also abbreviated TEDMA and TEGMA). The structure of methyl methacrylate (MMA) is shown for comparison.

Both of these monomers contain two reactive double bonds, and when polymerized, form covalent bonds between the polymer chains known as cross-links. Cross-linking improved the properties of the matrix phase, and the composite produced had improved mechanical and physical properties. Additional composite formulations have been prepared using various diluent monomers such as methyl methacrylate (MMA) and ethylene glycol dimethacrylate (EGDMA), and an additional high molecular weight monomer based on a urethane dimethacrylate (UDMA). The chemical structure for UDMA is illustrated in Fig. 5 [10, 25, 46, 55, 58, 75].

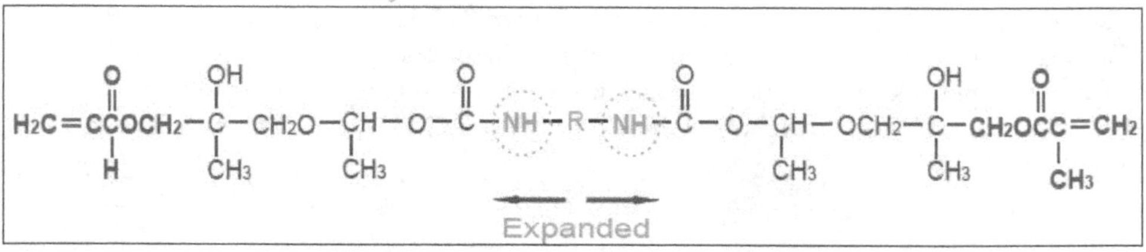

Fig. 5. Urethane dimethacrylate. The chemical structure of popular difunctional urethane resins. R = a number of carbon compounds that can be used to lengthen or alter the properties of the monomer. Nitrogen in the form of NH–R–NH is the urethane component.

5.1 Composite resin chemistry

To reduce polymerization shrinkage and increase mechanical and physical properties requires the use of high molecular weight monomers that have the ability to cross-link. The high molecular weight reduces the volume change during polymerization. Cross-linking forms covalent bonds between the polymer chains, resulting in a dramatic increase in modulus and reduction in solubility [57]. Bowen's resin is the reaction product between Bisphenol A and glycidyl dimethacrylate. A lower molecular weight monomer such triethylene glycol dimethacrylate (TEGDMA) or EDMA is added to reduce the viscosity and allow increased filler loadings to be used. These monomers are also multifunctional and increase the number of cross-linking reactions during setting of resin matrix. These lower viscosity monomers may comprise 10% to 50% of a composite's composition.

One of the most significant problems with current monomers used for direct composite restorative materials is the shrinkage that occurs during polymerization. Currently, all commercial dental composites are based on vinyl monomers polymerized using free radical initiators. Conversion of these monomers results in a decrease in distance between the molecules, from a Van der Waals gap to the distance of a covalent bond. Although this distance is very small for a single monomer, the distance change over a long polymer chain is significant. Inclusion of filler reduces the volume of resin and its volume change, but the amount of filler incorporation is approaching the maximum theoretical packing fraction of 74 volume % for close-packed structures. The amount of shrinkage is controlled by the volume of resin, its composition, and the degree of conversion. Current commercial dental composites have a volumetric shrinkage ranging from 1.6 to 8 volume%. The contraction stress developed at the margin of the restoration can be sufficient to overcome the bond strength of the bonding system, resulting in a contraction gap. The contraction gap can lead to microleakage and all its associated problems (eg, secondary caries and pain) [55, 57].

One approach to reduce polymerization shrinkage and contraction stress is through the development of low-shrinkage or expanding monomer systems. These resin systems are based on ring-opening polymerization reactions that do not shrink to the extent of conventional vinyl polymerization resins. Monomers based on spiro-ortho carbonate have been prepared and evaluated in composite formulations. Although the composites formulated using these monomers did show less polymerization shrinkage, the property improvements were only incremental, and probably not significant enough to be realized clinically [10, 25, 55, 57].

One problem that has not been addressed is the large difference between the Coefficient of Thermal Expansion (CTE) of resin composites and tooth structure. The CTE of tooth structure ranges from 9 to 11 ppm/_C, compared with 28 to 50 ppm/_C for dental composite restoratives [4]. The differential expansion and contraction of composites cause additional stress at the margin of the restoration that contributes to fatigue failure of the bond between the composite and tooth structure. Currently the only way to lower the CTE of composites is to increase the filler loading.

5.2 Composite fillers

The reinforcing phase in direct dental restoratives is based on glass or ceramic particles. Incorporation of these inorganic particles imparts improved strength and wear properties, decreased CTE, and reduced polymerization shrinkage. In addition, incorporation of heavy metals into the filler provides radiopacity. The initial composite fillers were limited in size because of the limited ability to grind and sieve quartz, glass, borosilicate, or ceramic particles. The particle size range was from 0.1 to 100 mm. Smaller particles have been prepared through hydrolysis or precipitation to produce what is termed fumed or pyrolitic silica. The particle sizes obtained from this process range from 0.06 to 0.1 mm 6.

The most recent process to form particles is through sol-gel chemistry, which uses silicate precursors that are polymerized to form particles ranging from nm to mm dimensions. This sol-gel process can be used to form almost mono dispersed particle sizes, which can be a significant advantage because different particle sizes can be produced and blended to optimize the packing efficiency and filler loading of the composite. In addition, the ability to produce submicron size particles allows the production of nanocomposites in which the particles approach the size of the polymer matrix molecules. Theoretically, nanocomposites have the potential to exhibit excellent mechanical and physical properties at higher filler loadings [25, 55, 80].

5.3 Curing of dental composites

The majority of current dental composites are cured using visible light ranging from 450 to 475 nm. Light sources include quartz halogen, laser, plasma arc, and most recently, light emitting diodes (LED). The minimum energy required for adequate curing is 300 mW/cm^2. Newer lights have incorporated curing modes that step or ramp up the light intensity with time. These modes were added in an attempt to control the polymerization shrinkage and reduce the polymerization contraction stress. Although these lights have shown some promise, the clinical effectiveness of these controlled polymerization techniques is unknown. All of the lights used for curing composite increase the temperature of the composite to varying extents, which can actually increase the degree of conversion; however, high-intensity light sources may cause sufficient temperature increases to result in damage to the pulp [7, 25, 55].

5.4 Composite classification: properties and applications

Composites generally are classified with respect to the components, amounts, properties of their filler or matrix phases, or by their handling properties. The most common classification method is based on filler content (weight or volume percent), filler particle size, and method of filler addition. Composites also could be defined on the basis of the matrix composition (BIS-GMA or UDMA) or polymerization method (self-curing, ultraviolet light-curing, visible light-curing, dual curing, or staged curing), but these do not communicate as much information about the properties. One of the most often used classification systems is based upon filler particle sizes. That system is extended here to include the particle size by order of magnitude, acknowledging mixed ranges of particle sizes, and distinguishing procured composite pieces as special filler. Composite filler particles are called *macrofillers* in the range of 10 to 100 μm, *midifillers* from 1 to 10 μm, *minifillers* from 0.1 to 1 μm, and *microfillers* 0.01 to 0.1 μm. Very large individual filler particles, called *megafillers*, also have been used in special circumstances. New ultrasmall fillers are being used that are from 0.005 to 0.01 μm in diameter and are called *nanofillers*. Accordingly, composites are classified by particle size as *megafill, macrofill, midifill, minifill, microfill,* and *nanofill*. Composites with mixed ranges of particle sizes are called hybrids, and the largest particle size range is used to define the hybrid type (e.g., minifill hybrid) because microfillers are normally the second part of the mixture. If the composite simply consists of filler and uncured matrix material, it is classified as homogeneous. If it includes procured composite or other unusual filler, it is called heterogeneous. If it includes novel filler modifications in addition to conventional fillers, then it is called modified, such as fiber-modified homogeneous. Another consequence of advances in the control of filler particle size, particle size distribution, particle morphology, and monomer technology has been the introduction of composites with specific handling characteristics. These include *flowable composites* and *packable composites*. *Flowable composites* are a class of low-viscosity materials that possess particle sizes and particles size distrubutions similar to those of hybrid composites, but with reduced filler content, which allows the increased amount of resin to decrease the viscosity of the mixture. *Packable composites*, also referred to as *condensable composites*, were developed in a direct effort to produce a composite with handling characteristics similar to amalgam, thus the moniker of "packable" or "condensable". These "amalgam alternatives" are intended primarily for Class I and Class II restorations. For posterior composite restorations, it is also possible to place one or two large glass inserts (0.5-to 2-mm particles) into composites at points of occlusal contact or high wear. These pieces of glass are referred to as *inserts* (or *megafillers*). Although they have demonstrated improved wear resistance to contact area wear, the techniques are more complicated and do not totally eliminate contact frea area wear. Furthermore, the bonding of the composite to the insert is questionable [7, 16, 55].

5.4.1 Microfilled composites

Microfilled composites were introduced to the market from the late 1970s to the early 1980s. Microfilled composites were developed to provide the dental profession with a material that possessed outstanding polishability and esthetics. These composites incorporate particles ranging from 0.04 μm to 0.4 μm. The early versions of microfilled resins were limited in the amount of filler that could be incorporated, because of the high surface area-to-volume ratio of the filler that caused large viscosity increases in the formulation. These composites only contained 35 to 67 weight % and 20 to 59 volume % glass fillers. One way to increase the volume of small particles is through the use of prepolymerized particles. In this process, submicron-sized particles are mixed with monomers such a Bis-GMA and TEGDMA at elevated temperatures. The mixture is then cured at elevated temperature and pressure, using benzoyl peroxide as an initiator. After polymerization, the material is chilled and ground to form particles having a size range of 1 to 200 μm. The prepolymerized particles allow higher filler loadings to be obtained with smaller particles; however, the prepolymerized particles cannot be bonded to the matrix phase using silane coupling agents. Interfacial bonding requires diffusion of the matrix monomers into the particles, with subsequent polymerization to provide micromechanical interlocks. Some investigators have suggested that the lack of interfacial bonding in these systems may contribute to failure [55, 57, 59].

Therefore microfilled composites have a lower elastic modulus and lower fracture strength than materials that contain higher concentrations of filler. The prepolymerized particles allow the filler content to be maximized and polymerization shrinkage to be minimized, however, while making these composites highly polishable and possessing the ability to maintain a smooth surface during clinical wear. Because of these properties, microfilled composite resins are indicated for Class V restorations, non–stress-bearing Class III restorations, and small Class I restorations. They are also indicated for direct composite resin veneers if the patient does not demonstrate any parafunctional habits, such as bruxism. Because of their lower fracture strength and potential for marginal breakdown, microfills are generally contraindicated for posterior load bearing restorations such as Class II and large Class I restorations [55, 71].

5.4.2 Hybrid composites

The majority of resin composites in clinical use today are categorized in the general term of "hybrid composites." This broad category includes traditional hybrids, micro-, and nanohybrids. The "hybrid" moniker implies a resin composite blend containing submicron inorganic filler particles (.04 μm) and small particles (1 μm–4 μm). The combination of various sizes of filler particles corresponds to an improvement in physical properties as well as acceptable levels of polishability. These improvements in wear resistance and fracture strength, along with good polishability, make hybrids the material of choice for Class III and Class IV restorations. In addition, practitioners have used these traditional hybrids in posterior load-bearing surfaces such as Class I and Class II restorations because of their improved strength and wear resistance.

Recent improvements in filler technology by manufacturers have allowed blends of both submicron particles (0.04 μm) and small particles (0.1 μm–1.0 μm) to be incorporated into a composite formulation. These materials are classified as micro-hybrid composites. The mixture of smaller particles distinguishes microhybrids from traditional hybrids and allows for a finer polish, along with improved handling. The desirable combination of strength and surface smoothness offers the clinician flexibility for use in posterior stress-bearing areas as well as anterior esthetic areas. Although microhybrids offer superior strength, their polishability is not better than a traditional microfilled composite resin. The trend in the newer microhybrid materials is to maximize filler loading and minimize filler size. The latest version of microfilled hybrids has used nanofiller technology to formulate what have been referred to as nanohybrid composite resins. Nanohybrids contain nanometer-sized filler particles (.005–.01 microns) throughout the resin matrix, in combination with a more conventional type filler technology. Nanohybrids may be classified as the first truly universal composite resin with handling properties and polishability of a microfilled composite, and the strength and wear resistance of a traditional hybrid. These nanohybrids can be used in any situation similar to the microhybrids, with possibly a slight improvement in polishability because of the smaller particle size [55, 74].

5.4.3 Packable composites

Packable or condensable composites were developed to provide a composite that handled more like amalgam. This marketing ploy by dental product manufacturers was an attempt to increase the use of composites by older dentists who were not trained in their use in dental school, and younger dentists who were looking for a more user-friendly material. Packable composites have a higher viscosity and are less "sticky" than other composite restoratives. The viscosity increase is obtained through changes in the particle size distribution and incorporation of fibers [81]. These composites were introduced to the market as amalgam substitutes, as practitioners searched for the ideal esthetic material with handling properties similar to amalgam. Another desire was to find a material that would establish adequate proximal contacts more easily than traditional hybrid composites. Claims of improved handling properties and better adaptation to the matrix band in Class II restorations have piqued the interest of many clinicians. The dental professions have referred to these materials as "packable composites" instead of "condensable," because of their greater viscosity and decreased stickiness compared with conventional hybrid composites. When initially placed, these materials were more viscous than traditional hybrid composites; however, after placement the viscosity decreased as the temperature of the material equilibrated with the temperature of the oral cavity. Although the "packable composites" showed improved handling properties for restoring Class I and II preparations, they have not fully solved the problem of achieving adequate interproximal contacts. Because packable composites do not have substantially better mechanical properties than hybrid composites, they would not be expected to perform better clinically [86]. In addition, because of the development of improved placement instruments and matrix systems to achieve better interproximal contacts, the need for packable or condensable materials has decreased, resulting in a decreased market share. In summary, the mechanical properties of the packable composites are not significantly better than other hybrid formulations, and there have not been sufficient long-term clinical studies to determine how these materials will perform long-term in the oral cavity. Their use as a direct dental restorative may be limited [18, 55, 57].

5.5 Clinical survive probability of composites

Composites are monitored in clinical studies by using United States Public Health Service (USPHS) categories [61] of interest: color matching, interfacial staining, secondary caries, anatomic form (wear), and marginal integrity [7].

Changes in restorative treatment patterns, the introduction of new and improved restorative materials and techniques, effective preventive programs, enhanced dental care, and growing interest in caries-free teeth have greatly influenced the longevity of dental restorations; however, failure of restorations is a major problem in a practice treating primarily permanent teeth. Studies show that 60% of all operative work done is attributed to the replacement of restorations [44]. Composites have improved since their introduction, and their survival rates are improving. Clinical studies to evaluate the latest composite technologies have not been published; therefore most of the survival data are on older composite compositions.

In the 1970s, degradation or wear was considered the main reason for failure of composite restorations. Improvements in filler technology and formulation of composite materials have resulted in new reasons for replacement. Twenty years later, studies revealed secondary caries to be the new cause of failure. The main factors responsible for the change in reasons for replacement include improved clinical technique based on more adequate teaching of posterior composites at dental schools, and on gained experience through trial and error of clinicians in practice [55]. Advancements in composite properties and adhesive technology also contributed to these changes.

In comparison of survival probability between amalgam and composite, a time period involving 3, 4, 5, and 7 years was considered [54]. In permanent teeth, the following values were measured: 3 year, 97.2% (amalgam) to 90% (composite); 4 year, 96.6% (amalgam) to 85.6% (composite); 5 year, 95.4% (amalgam) to 78.2% (composite); and 7 year, 94.5% (amalgam) to 67.4% (composite).

In summary, longevity of composite restorations depends upon factors involving the materials, the patient, and the dentist. The request for these esthetic, tooth-colored restorations will continue to increase, and patients must be educated about the expected life of these restorations as well as their advantages and disadvantages, so they can make an informed decision on a treatment option.

6. References

[1] Adusei, G.O.; Deb, S. & Nicholson, J.W. (2004). The role of the ionomer glass component in polyacid-modified composite resin dental restorative materials. *Journal of Material Science & Material Medicine*, Vol. 15, pp. 751-754.

[2] Akitt, J.W.; Greenwood, N.N. & Lester, G.D. (1971). Nuclear magnetic resonance and Raman studies of aluminium complexes formed in aqueous solutions of aluminium salts containing phosphoric acids and fluoride ions. *Journal of Chemical Social Association*, Vol. 14, pp. 2450-2457.

[3] Alves, J.B. & Brandao, P.R. (2002). Atraumatic restorative treatment: Clinical, ultrastructural and chemical analysis. *Caries Research*, Vol. 36, pp. 430-436.

[4] Anusavice, K.J. & Brantley, W.A. (2003). Physical properties of dental materials. In: *Phillip's science of dental materials*, (11th edn). Anusavice, K.J. (Ed.). pp. 41-71, WB Saunders, Phalladelphia.

[5] Atin, T.; Buchalla, W., Keilbassa, A.M., et al. (1995). Curing shrinkage and volumetric changes of resin-modified glass ionomer restorative materials. *Dental Materials*, Vol. 11, pp.359–362.

[6] Azzopardi, A.; Bartlett, D.W., Watson, T.F. & Sherriff, M. (2001). The measurement and prevention of erosion and abrasion. *Journal of Dentistry*, Vol. 29, pp. 395-400.

[7] Bayne, S.C.; Thompson, J.Y. & Taylor, D.F. (2002). Dental materials, In: *Sturdevant's art & science of operative dentistry*, (4th Edn). Roberson, T.M.; Heymann, H.O. & Swift, E.J. (Eds), pp. 135-233, Mosby Inc., A Harcourt Health Sciences Company, ISBN: 0-323-01087-3, St. Louis, Missouri, USA.

[8] Billington, R.W.; Williams, J.A., Dorban, A. & Pearson G.J. (2004). Glass ionomer cement: Evidence pointing to fluorine release in the form of monofluorophosphate in addition to fluoride ion. *Biomaterials*, Vol. 25, pp. 3399-3402.

[9] Bishara, S.; Ostby, A. Lafoon J. et al. (2007). A self-conditioner for resin-modified glass ionomers in bonding orthodontic brackets. *Angle Orthodontics*, Vol. 77, pp. 711-715.

[10] Bowen, R.J. (1958). Synthesis of a silica-resin filling material progress report (abstract). *Journal of Dental Research*, Vol. 27, p. 90.

[11] Bowen, R.J. (1962). Dental filling material comprising vinyl silane treated fused silica and a binder consisting of the reaction product of bisphenol and glycidyl acrylate. *US Patent*, pp. 306-319.

[12] Bowen, R.L. & Cobb, E.N. (1983). A method for bonding to dentin and enamel. *Journal of American Dental Association*, Vol. 107, pp. 734-736.

[13] Brackett, M.G.; Dib, A., Brackett, W.W., Estrada, B.E. & Reyes, A.A. (2002). One year clinical performance of a resin-modified glass ionomer anda resin composite restorative material in unprepared Class V restorations. *Operative Dentistry*, Vol. 27, pp. 112-116.

[14] Brackett, W.W.; Covey, D.A. & St Germain, H.A. Jr. (2002). One-year clinical performance of a self-etching adhesive in class V resin composites cured by two methods. *Operative Dentistry*, Vol. 27, pp. 218-222.

[15] Brudevold, F.; Buonocore, M. & Wileman, W. (1956). A report on a resin composition capable of bonding to human dentin surfaces. *Journal of Dental Research*, Vol. 35, pp. 846-851.

[16] Burgess, J.O. (2001). Fluoride-releasing materials, In: *Fundamentals of operative dentistry: A contemporary approach*, (2nd Edn). Summitt, J.B.; Robbins, J.W. & Schwartz, R.S. (Eds), pp. 377-385, Quintessence Publishing Co. Inc., ISBN: 0-86715-382-2, Illinois, USA.

[17] Chalmers, J.M. (2006). Minimal intervention dentistry: Part 2. Strategies for addressing restorative challenges in older patients. *Journal of Canadian Dental Association*, Vol. 72, pp. 435-440.

[18] Cobb, D.S.; MacGregor, K.M., Vargas, M.A., et al. (2000). The physical properties of packable and conventional posterior resin-based composites: A comparison. *Journal of American Dental Association*, Vol. 131, pp. 1610-1615.

[19] Cochran, M.A. & Matis, B.A. (2001). Diagnosis and treatment of root caries, In: *Fundamentals of operative dentistry: A contemporary approach*, (2nd Edn). Summitt, J.B.; Robbins, J.W. & Schwartz, R.S. (Eds), pp. 365-376, Quintessence Publishing Co. Inc., ISBN: 0-86715-382-2, Illinois, USA.

[20] Davidson, C. (2006). Advances in glass-ionomer cements. *Journal of Applied Oral Science*, Vol. 14, pp. 3-9.

[21] Demirci, M.; Ersev, H., Topçubaşı, M. & Uçok, M. (2005). Clinical evaluation of a polyacid-modified resin composite in class V carious lesions: 3-year results. *Dental Materials Journal*, Vol. 24, pp. 321-327.

[22] Eliades, G. (1999). Chemical and biological properties of glass-ionomer cements. In: *Advances in glass ionomer*. Davidson, C.L. & Mjör, I.A. (eds). Pp. 67-84, Quintessence, Chicago.

[23] Eliades, G.; Kakaboura, A. & Palaghias G. (1998). Acid base reaction and fluoride release profiles in visible light-cured polyacid modified composite resin restorations. *Dental Materials*, Vol. 14, pp. 57-63.

[24] Ferrari, M. & Davidson, C.L. (1997). Interdiffusion of a traditional glass ionomer cement into conditioned dentin. *American Journal of Dentistry*, Vol. 10, pp. 295-297.

[25] Ford, H. (2002). Resins. In: *Tooth colored restoratives: Principles and techniques*, (9th Edn). Albers, H.F. (Ed.). pp. 111-156. BC Decker Inc., ISBN: 1-55009-155-7, Hamilton, London. 45

[26] Frencken, J.E.; Pilot, T., Songpaisan, Y. & Phantumvanit, P. (1996). Atraumatic restorative treatment (ART): Rationale, technique and development. *Journal of Public Health Dentistry*, Vol. 56, pp. 135-140.

[27] Fusayama, T.; Nakamura, M., Kurosaki, N. & Iwaku, M. (1979). Non-pressure adhesion of a new adhesive restorative resin. *Journal of Dental Research*, Vol. 58, pp. 1364-1370.

[28] Gungor, H.C.; Altay, N. & Alpar, R. (2004). Clinical evaluation of a polyacid-modified resin composite-based fissure sealant: two-year results. *Operative Dentistry*, Vol. 29, pp. 254-260.

[29] Harnirattisai, C.; Inokoshi, C. Shimada, Y. & Hosoda H. (1993). Adhesive interface between resin and etched dentin of cervical erosion/abrasion lesions. *Operative Dentistry*, Vol. 18, pp. 138-143.

[30] Hickel, R. & Mmanhart, J. (2001). Longevity of restorations in posterior teeth and reasons for failure. *Journal of Adhesive Dentistry*, Vol. 3, pp. 45-64.

[31] Hosoya, Y. & Garcia-Godoy, F. (1998). Bonding mechanism of Ketac-molar Aplicap and Fuji IX GP to enamel and dentin. *American Journal of Dentistry*, Vol. 11, pp. 235-239.

[32] Hume, W.R. (1994). Influence of dentine on the pulpward release of eugenol or acids from restorative materials. *Journal of Oral Rehabilitation*, Vol. 21, pp. 469-473.

[33] Kanca, J. (1992). Resin bonding to wet substrate. I. Bonding to dentin. *Quintessence International*, Vol. 23, pp. 39-41.

[34] Knox, J.; Chye, K.Y. & Durning, P. (2004). An ex vivo evaluation of resin-modified glass polyalkenoates and polyacid-modified composite resins as orthodontic band cements. *Journal of Orthodontics*, Vol. 31, pp. 323-328.

[35] Landuyt, K.L.V.; Snauwaert, J., Munck, J.D. et al. (2007). Systematic review of the chemical composition of contemporary dental adhesives. *Biomaterials*, Vol. 28, pp. 3757-3785.

[36] Li H.; Burrow, M.F. & Tyas, M.J. (2000). Nanoleakage patterns of four dentin bonding systems. *Dental Materials*, Vol. 16, pp. 48-56.

[37] Luo, Y.; Lo, E.C.M., Fang, D.T.S., Smales, R.J. & Wei, S.H.Y. (2002). Clinical evaluation of Dyract AP restorative in permanent molars: 2 year results. *American Journal of Dentistry*, Vol. 15, pp. 403-406.

[38] McLean, J.W. & Gasser, O. (1985). Glass-cermet cements. *Quintessence International*, Vol. 16, pp. 333-343.

[39] McLean, J.W.; Nicholson, J.W. & Wilson, A.D. (1994). Proposed nomenclature for glass-ionomer dental cements and related materials. *Quintessence International*, Vol. 25, pp. 587–589.

[40] Meyer, J-M.; Cattani-Lorente, M.A. & Dupuis, V. (1998). Compomers: Between glass-ionomer cements and composites. *Biomaterials*, Vol. 19, pp. 529–39.

[41] Millar, B.J.; Abiden, F. & Nicholson, J.W. (1998). In vitro caries inhibition by polyacid-modified composite resins ("compomers"). *Journal of Dentistry*, Vol. 26, pp. 133-136.

[42] Miyazaki, S.; Iwasaki, K., Onose, H. & Moore, B.K. (2001). Enamel and dentin bond strengths of single application bonding systems. *American Journal of Dentistry*, Vol. 14, pp. 361-366.

[43] Mjör, I.; Dahl, J., Moorhead, J.E., et al. (2000). Age of restorations at replacement in permanent teeth in general dental practice. *Acta Odontologica Scandinavia*, Vol. 58, pp. 97–101.

[44] Mjör, I.A. (1989). Amalgam and composite resin restorations: Longevity and reasons for replacement. In: *Quality of evaluation of dental restorations*. Anusavice, K. (Ed.), pp. 61-80, Quintessence Publishing Corp, Inc., Chicago.

[45] Mount, G.J. (2002). *An atlas of glass-ionomer cements. A clinician's guide*, (3rd Edn). pp. 10-45.Martin Dunitz Ltd, London. 12

[46] Murchison, D.F.; Roeters, J., Vargas, M.A., et al. (2006). Direct anterior restorations. In: *Fundamentals of operative dentistry: A contemporary approach*, (3rd Edn). Summitt, J.B.; Robbins, J.W. & Schwartz, R.S. (Eds), pp. 261-288, Quintessence Publishing Co. Inc., ISBN: 0-86715-382-2, Illinois, USA.

[47] Nakabayashi, N.; Kojima, K. & Masuhara, E. (1982). The promotion of adhesion by the infiltration of monomers into tooth substrates. *Journal of Biomedicine & Material Research*, Vol. 16, pp. 265-273.

[48] Nakajima, M.; Ogata, M., Harada, N., Tagami, J. & Pashley, D.H. (2000). Bond strengths of self-etching primer adhesives to in vitro demineralized dentin following mineralizing treatment. *Journal of Adhesive Dentistry*, Vol. 2, pp. 29-38.

[49] Ngo, H.; Mount, G.J. & Peters, M.C. (1997). A study of glass-ionomer cement and its interface with enamel and dentin using a low temperature, high resolution scanning electron microscope technique. *Quintessence International*, Vol. 28, pp. 63-69.

[50] Nicholson, J.W. (2007). Polyacid-modified composite resins ("compomers") and their use in clinical dentistry. *Dental Materials*, Vol. 23, pp. 615-622.

[51] Nicholson, J.W. & McKenzie, M.A. (1999). The properties of polymerizable luting cements. *Journal of Oral Rehabilitation*, Vol. 26, pp. 767-774.

[52] Niessen, L.C. & Gibson, G. (1997). Oral health for a lifetime: Preventive strategies for the older adult. *Quintessence International*, Vol. 28, pp. 626-630.

[53] Perdigao, J. & Swift, E.J. (1994). Analysis of dental adhesive systems using scanning electron microscopy. *International Dental Journal*, Vol. 44, pp. 349-359.

[54] Pounder, B.; Gregory, W.A. & Powers, J.M. (1987). Bond strengths of repaired composite resins. *Operative Dentistry*, Vol. 12, pp. 127-131.

[55] Puckett, A.D.; Fitchie, J.G., Kirk, P.C. & Gamblin, J. (2007). Direct composite restorative materials. *The Dental Clinics of North America*, Vol. 51, pp. 659-675.

[56] Qvist, V.; Laurberg, L., Poulsen, A. & Teglers, P.T. (2004). Class II restorations in primary teeth: 7-year study on three resin-modified glass ionomer cements and a compomer. *European Journal of Oral Science*, Vol. 112, pp. 188-196.

[57] Rawls, H.R. & Upshaw, J.E. (2003). Restorative resins. In: *Phillip's science of dental materials*, (11th edn). Anusavice, K.J. (Ed.). pp. 399-441, WB Saunders, Philladelphia.

[58] Roberson, T.M.; Heymann, H.O. & Ritter A.V. (2002). Introduction to composite restorations. In: *Sturdevant's art & science of operative dentistry*, (4th Edn). Roberson, T.M.; Heymann, H.O. & Swift, E.J. (Eds), pp. 471-500, Mosby Inc., A Harcourt Health Sciences Company, ISBN: 0-323-01087-3, St. Louis, Missouri, USA.

[59] Roulet, J.F. (1987). Polymer constructions used in restorative dentistry. In: *Degradation of dental polymers*, pp. 3-59, Karger, New York.

[60] Ruse, N.D. (1999). What is a compomer? *Journal of Canadian Dental Association*, Vol. 65, pp. 500-504. 39

[61] Ryge, G. (1980). Clinical criteria. *International Dental Journal*, Vol. 30, pp. 347-358.

[62] Saito, S.; Tosaki, S. & Hirota, K. (1999). Characteristics of glass ionomer cements. In: *Advances in glass-ionomer cements*. Davidson, C.L. & Mjör, I.A. (eds). Quintessence, Chicago.

[63] Sakoolnamarka, R.; Burrow, M.F. & Tyas, M.J. (2002). Micromorphological study of resin-dentin interface of non-carious cervical lesions. *Operative Dentistry*, Vol. 27, pp. 493-499.

[64] Sales, D.; Sae-Lee, D., Matsuya, S. & Ana, I.D. (2003). Short-term fluoride and cations release from polyacid-modified composites in distilled water and an acidic lactate buffer. *Biomaterials*, Vol. 21, pp. 1687-1696.

[65] Sano, H.; Takatsu, T. Ciucchi, B. et al. (1995). Nanoleakage: Leakage within the hybrid layer. *Operative Dentistry*, Vol. 20, pp. 18-25.

[66] Scholtanus, J. & Huysmans, M. (2007). Clinical failure of class-II restorations of a highly viscous glass-ionomer material over a 6-year period: a retrospective study. *Journal of Dentistry*, Vol. 35, pp. 156-162.

[67] Sennou, H.E.; Lebugle, A.A. & Gregoire, G.L. (1999). X-ray photoelectron spectroscopy study of the dentin-glass ionomer cement interface. *Dental Materials*, Vol. 15, pp. 229-237.

[68] Seppa, L.; Fors, H. & Ogaard, B. (1993). The effect of fluoride application on fluoride release and the antibacterial action of glass ionomers. *Journal of Dental Research*, Vol. 72, pp. 1310-1314.

[69] Sideridou, I.; Achilias, D.S., Spyroudi, C. & Karabela, M. (2004). Water sorption characteristics of light-cured dental resins and composites based on Bis-EMA/PCDMA. *Biomaterials*, Vol. 25, pp. 367-76.

[70] Sidhu, S.K. & Schmalz, G. (2001). The biocompatibility of glass-ionomer cement materials. A status report for the American Journal of Dentistry. *American Journal of Dentistry*, Vol. 14, pp. 387-396.

[71] Stansbury, J.W. (1992). Synthesis and evaluation of new oxaspiro monomers for double ring-opening polymerization. *Journal of Dental Research*, Vol. 71, pp. 1408-1412.

[72] Sugizaki, J. (1991). The effect of various primers on the dentin adhesion of resin composite. *Japanese Journal of Conservative Dentistry*, Vol. 34, pp. 228-265.

[73] Swift JR, E.J.; Sturdevant, J.R. & Ritter, A.V. (2002). Classes I and II indirect tooth-colored restorations, In: *Sturdevant's art & science of operative dentistry*, (4th Edn).

Roberson, T.M.; Heymann, H.O. & Swift, E.J. (Eds), pp. 571-589, Mosby Inc., A Harcourt Health Sciences Company, ISBN: 0-323-01087-3, St. Louis, Missouri, USA.

[74] Swift, E.J. (2005). Nanocomposites. *Journal of Esthetic Restorative Dentistry*, Vol. 17, pp. 3-4.

[75] Taira, M.; Suzaki, H., Wakasa, K. et al. (1990). Preparation of pure silica-glass filler for dental composites by the sol-gel process. *Journal of British Ceramics Transactions*, Vol. 89, pp. 203-207.

[76] Tay, F.R.; Smales, R.J., Ngo, H., Wei, S.H. & Pashley, D.H. (2001). Effect of different conditioning protocols on adhesion of a GIC to dentin. *Journal of Adhesive Dentistry*, Vol. 3, pp. 153-167.

[77] Tobias, R.S. (1988). Antibacterial properties of dental restorative materials: A review. *International Endodontic Journal*, Vol. 21, pp. 155-160.

[78] Tyas, M.J. & Burrow, M.F. (2002) Clinical evaluation of a resin modified glass ionomer adhesive system: Results at five years. *Operative dentistry*, Vol. 27, pp. 438-441. 36

[79] Tyas, M.J. & Burrow, M.F. (2004). Adhesive restorative materials: A review. *Australian Dental Journal*, Vol. 49, pp. 112-121. 8

[80] Vaderhobli, R.M. (2011). Advances in dental materials. *Dental Clinic of North America*, *Vol*. 55, pp. 619-625. 9

[81] Van Amerongen, JP.; Van Loveren, C. & Kidd, E.A.M. (2001). Caries management: Diagnosis and treatment strategies, In: *Fundamentals of operative dentistry: A contemporary approach*, (2nd Edn). Summitt, J.B.; Robbins, J.W. & Schwartz, R.S. (Eds), pp. 70-90, Quintessence Publishing Co. Inc., ISBN: 0-86715-382-2, Illinois, USA.

[82] Wang, Y. & Spencer, P. (2003). Hybridization efficiency of the adhesive/dentin interface with wet bonding. *Journal of Dental Research*, Vol. 82, pp. 141-145.

[83] Watson, T. (1999). Bonding of glass-ionomer cements to tooth structure. In: *Advances in glass-ionomer cements*. Davidson CL, Mjör IA, (eds). pp. 121-136, Quintessence Chicago.

[84] Weiner, R. (2011). Liners and bases in general dentistry. *Australian Dental Journal*, Vol. 56, pp. 11-22.

[85] Wiegand, A.; Buchalla, W. & Attin, T. (2007). Review on fluoride-releasing restorative materials- Fluoride release and uptake characteristics, antibacterial activity and influence on caries formation. *Dental Materials*, Vol. 23, pp. 343-362.

[86] Wilson, A.D. & Kent, B.E. (1972). A new translucent cement for dentistry. The glass-ionomer cement. *Journal of Applied Chemical Biotechnique*, Vol. 132, pp. 133-135.

[87] Wilson, A.D. & McLean, J.W. (1988). *Glass-ionomer cement*. pp. 15-65, Quintessence, Chicago.

[88] Yap, A.U.; Sau, C.W. & Lye, K.W. (1998). Effects of finishing/polishing time on surface characteristics of tooth-coloured restoratives. *Journal of Oral Rehabilitation*, Vol. 25, pp. 456-461.

[89] Yap, A.U.: Khor, E. & Foo, S.H. (1999). Fluoride release and antibacterial properties of new-generation tooth-colored restoratives. *Operative Dentistry*, Vol. 24, pp. 297-305.

7

White-Spot Lesions in Orthodontics: Incidence and Prevention

Airton O. Arruda, Scott M. Behnan and Amy Richter
University of Michigan,
USA

1. Introduction

The most common negative effect of orthodontic treatment with fixed appliances is the development of incipient carious lesions around brackets. The objectives of this chapter are to present some of the results of two studies aiming: 1) to evaluate patients treated with comprehensive orthodontics to determine the incidence of new carious lesions during treatment; and 2) to investigate the potential of ACP-containing resin cement and other treatments (fluoride varnish, resin sealer, MI Paste) to prevent incipient carious lesions on bracketed teeth. In the first study, 350 orthodontic patients were selected randomly. The pre- and post-treatment photographs of the patients were examined to determine lesion development. The labial surface of each tooth was scored with a standardized system based on the *International Caries Determination and Assessment System II*. The independent variables were collected by chart abstraction. In the second study, 100 extracted human premolars were allocated randomly to five groups (N = 20). Brackets were bonded with ACP-cement (Aegis-Ortho), Transbond

XT (Control), Transbond XT followed by application of fluoride varnish (Vanish), resin sealer (Pro-seal) and CPP-ACP paste (MI Paste). All teeth were pH cycled for 15 days in demineralization solution and artificial saliva. The extent of demineralization in each group was assessed using Quantified Light-induced Fluorescence (QLF) and Confocal Laser Scanning Microscopy (CLSM). The incidence of patients who developed at least one new white-spot lesion during treatment was 73%. Treatment length was associated significantly with new white-spot lesion development. The independent variables of gender, age and extraction/non-extraction were not associated with lesion development. Fluorescence loss and lesion depth measurements demonstrated that the Pro-seal and Vanish groups had the least amount of demineralization. The control group showed the most demineralization. Although the MI Paste and Aegis-Ortho groups experienced less demineralization than controls, neither was significant statistically. Only the Pro-seal and Vanish groups had significantly smaller lesions than the control group for both QLF and CLSM. Thus, the development of new lesions appeared to be related to treatment duration and, to a lesser degree, to initial oral hygiene score. Light-cured filled sealer (Pro-seal) and the fluoride varnish (Vanish) have the potential to prevent enamel demineralization adjacent to orthodontic brackets exposed to cariogenic conditions.

2. White-spot lesions

One of the most common negative side effects of orthodontic treatment with fixed appliances is the development of incipient caries lesions around brackets and bands, particularly in cases with poor oral hygiene (Fig. 1). Caries lesions typically form around the bracket interface, usually near the gingival margin (Gorelick *et al.*, 1982). Certain bacterial groups such as mutans streoptococci and lactobacilli ferment sugars to create an acidic environment that over time might lead to the development of dental caries. Since orthodontic appliances make plaque removal more difficult, patients are more susceptible to carious lesions. The irregular surfaces of brackets, bands, wires, and other attachments also limit naturally occurring self-cleaning mechanisms, such as movement of the oral musculature and saliva (Rosenbloom and Tinanoff, 1991).

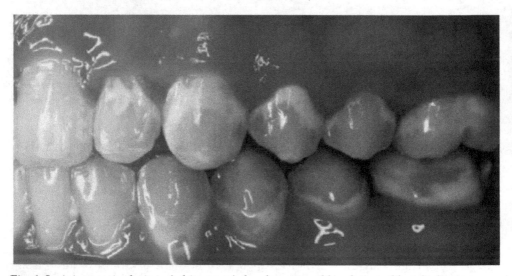

Fig. 1. Incipient caries lesions (white spots) develop around brackets and bands due to poor oral hygiene

Incipient lesions are characterized by their opacity, mineral loss, and decrease of fluorescence radiance when compared to healthy enamel surfaces. Many incipient enamel lesions have a white appearance due to an optical phenomenon caused by mineral loss in the surface and sub-surface that alters the refractive index and increases the scattering of light in the affected area, all resulting in greater visual enamel opacity.

Studies have shown that white spot lesions can take only one month to develop (Øgaard *et al.*, 1988; O'Reilly and Featherstone, 1987; Gorton and Featherstone, 2003). A clinical study reported the prevalence at 50% (Gorelick *et al.*, 1982), while recent investigations put the incidence of white spot lesions in the orthodontic populations studied at 73-95% (Richter *et al.*, 2009; Lovrov *et al*, 2007). Orthodontists and patients will notice these lesions after removal of the fixed appliances, especially since the white spots tend to form in the maxillary esthetic zone (Gorelick *et al.*, 1982; Banks and Richmond, 1994). While some studies have reported a decrease in the display of white spot lesions over time post-orthodontic treatment, these unesthetic spots tend to remain unless they are resolved with more aggressive treatment, such as minimally invasive or even full restorative dentistry (Øgaard, 1989; Årtun and Thylstrup, 1989).

3. Measures to counteract this problem

3.1 Oral hygiene

The first line of defense against the development of incipient caries lesions has traditionally been patient education, with a special emphasis on optimal oral hygiene. The advocacy organization for orthodontists in the United States known as the American Association of Orthodontists (AAO) has developed patient manuals and a website to provide recommendations for patients undergoing orthodontic treatment (AAO, 2009). Specifically, the website suggests extra time for toothbrushing, specialized tips to get in between the braces, floss threaders, oral irrigators, and over-the-counter mouthrinses. Additionally, the AAO sponsored informed consent form emphasizes the need for excellent oral hygiene and routine visits to the general dentist (AAO, 2005). It also warns that inadequate oral hygiene could result in caries, discolored teeth, and periodontal disease. Finally, the form explains that the aforementioned problems may be aggravated if the patient has not had the benefit of fluoridated water. In many cases, patient education will also include an emphasis on proper diet with reduced intake of sugars. Despite these efforts by the orthodontist and staff members, many patients will still be non-compliant with oral hygiene instructions. Unfortunately, most orthodontists have a limited background in the behavioral basis of compliance (Mehra et al., 1998). Thus, patient non-compliance presents a unique challenge to orthodontic practices.

3.2 Fluoride during orthodontic treatment (rinses, etc)

In addition to reinforced oral hygiene instructions, orthodontists have turned to various products and preventive measures to reduce this problem. Dental professionals have employed fluoride for years to prevent caries and remineralize enamel in patients. A systematic review found a reduced level of caries and adolescents who have regular supervised rinsing with a fluoride mouthwash (Marinho, 2004). Daily fluoride rinses have shown promising results, and a significant reduction in enamel lesions can be achieved during orthodontic therapy through the daily use of a 10 mL neutral 0.05% sodium fluoride rinse. However, typical patient compliance rates with this protocol have been relatively low (Geiger et al., 1992).

3.3 Fluoride varnish

Preventive measures that do not require patient compliance would seem to make more sense for the typical orthodontic patient population of adolescents. For some patients, professional fluoride varnish application by orthodontic auxiliaries at routine appointments can in part address this compliance issue (Vivaldi-Rodrigues et al., 2006). On the other hand, each application requires over five minutes of chair-time, and whether or not today's high efficiency/high volume orthodontic practice will devote the time and resources to apply this protocol is debatable. Generally however, fluoride varnishes have a proven track record in caries reduction when applied properly. Vanish (3M/Omni) is a very popular 5% NaF white varnish used for prevention of dental caries. The manufacturer advertises the ease of use, lack of an unesthetic yellow color found in other varnishes, enhanced flow characteristics, and its fluoride delivery of 22,600 ppm. Its name comes from an alleged ability to disappear after application. Data gathered by the manufacturer declare greater fluoride release over a 48-hour period in comparison to other fluoride products. To date, Vanish in particular has not been tested in any of the *in-vitro* or *in-vivo* trials in the literature.

3.4 Resin sealer

Just as sealants have been shown to prevent caries in molars with deep fissures, resin-based sealers have been applied on facial surfaces of bracketed teeth to prevent enamel caries. In addition to the increased chair-time for this procedure, earlier generations of resin sealers have been found to have very low wear resistance. Previous studies have proven that most of the chemically cured sealants (Zachrisson *et al.*, 1979) do not effectively seal smooth enamel surfaces, because of oxygen inhibition of polymerization when the sealant is in contact with the air in a thin layer. Instead, only "islands" of cured sealant remain where resin pooling occurs. Even light-cured sealants (Banks and Richmond, 1994) that were unfilled or lightly filled could not provide any more protection than the chemically cured sealants. A more recent developed product Pro-seal (Reliance, Itasca, IL) has been marketed as a sealer that is more resistant to toothbrush abrasion than earlier generations, since it is a highly filled resin. In patients with poor oral hygiene, Pro-seal can be added before bracket bonding or after bonding. Additionally, the manufacturer claims that Pro-seal releases fluoride, which further enhances its anticariogenic properties.

3.5 ACP/CPP-ACP

Recently, there has been increased interest and development in calcium phosphate-based remineralization technology (Reynolds and del Rio, 1984; Rosen *et al.*, 1984). One of the newest modalities in preventive dentistry is the introduction of amorphous calcium phosphate (ACP) into methacrylate composites, gum, pastes, and other dental products. Casein is the predominant phosphoprotein in bovine milk and accounts for almost 80 percent of its total protein, primarily as calcium phosphate stabilized micellular complexes (Aimutis, 2004). Several laboratory and animal experiments have investigated the low cariogenic potential and the possible cario-static activity of dairy products (milk, casein, caseinates and cheeses). The use of casein as an anticariogenic additive to food, toothpaste or drinking water has not been implemented because of its adverse organoleptic properties and the large amount required for efficacy (Reynolds, 1998).

Casein phosphopeptide (CPP) contains the cluster sequence of -Ser (P)-Ser (P)-Ser (P)-Glu-Glu from casein (Iijima *et al.*, 2004). CPP does not have the limitations of casein, has the potential for specific anticariogenic activity, and is at least 10 times greater on a weight basis than it is for casein (so not as much is needed for it to be effective). CPP can remarkably stabilize calcium phosphate (which usually is highly insoluble) in a state-forming CPP-amorphous calcium phosphate (ACP) complex. There is no conclusive evidence that ACP is an integral mineral component in hard tissues. Its advocates theorize that it likely plays a special role as a precursor to bioapatite and as a transient phase in biomineralization. In solutions, ACP is converted readily to stable crystalline phases such as octacalcium phosphate or apatitic products (Mathew and Takagi, 2001). Reynolds and colleagues have proposed that under acidic conditions, localized CPP-ACP buffers the free calcium and phosphate ions, substantially increasing the level of calcium phosphate in plaque and, therefore, maintaining a state of supersaturation that inhibits enamel demineralization and enhances remineralization (Reynolds et al., 1999). Rose conducted a laboratory experiment in which he showed that CPP-ACP binds well to dental plaque, providing a large calcium reservoir that may inhibit demineralization and assist in subsequent remineralization (Rose, 2000).

This technology has entered the orthodontic marketplace in two different forms: resin bracket bonding cement containing ACP and topical paste containing the CPP-ACP complex. Aegis-Ortho, an ACP-including resin bonding cement, has been marketed by Bosworth (Skokie, IL) as a substitute for ordinary bracket bonding cement, with the added benefit of caries prevention. The manufacturer claims that the acidic challenge (pH at or below 5.8) to the surrounding bracket area will trigger the release of calcium and phosphate from the cement, and a supersaturated calcium phosphate matrix will not only inhibit demineralization, but also remineralize the enamel. ACP-filled composite resins have been shown to recover 71% of the lost mineral content of demineralized teeth (Skrtic et al., 1996).

A similar chemical process is manifested with MI paste (GC America, Alsip, IL). Instead of residing in the resin cement, the casein phosphopeptide-amorphous calcium phosphate (CPP-ACP) is applied topically in the mouth to affected areas. The manufacturer implicates this product not only lesion prevention (applied twice daily after brushing throughout orthodontic treatment), but also claims the patient can expect the complete reversal of such lesions after three months use post-debonding. Additionally, the manufacturer has recommended MI paste for dental patients with xerostomia, dental sensitivity, gastric reflux, fluorosis, exposed root surfaces, and as an adjunct to tooth bleaching.

4. Current level of evidence

4.1 Fluoride varnish

A myriad of in-vivo and in-vitro studies have been carried out to study the efficacy of preventive measures against white spot lesion formation during orthodontic treatment. Fluoride varnish has by far the strongest evidence base. The potential of fluoride varnish has been evaluated in-vitro (Adriens et al., 1990; van der Linden and Dermaut, 1998; Todd et al., 1999; Demito et al., 2004) as well as in-vivo (Vivaldi-Rodrigues et al., 2006; Øgaard et al., 2001). Generally, investigations carried out in-vitro indicate a moderate to strong beneficial effect of the tested varnishes on enamel demineralization. Two in-vivo studies have emerged. In a split-mouth prospective study, there was 44.3% less demineralization noted for teeth that had been treated every 12 weeks with fluoride varnish during orthodontic treatment (Vivaldi-Rodrigues et al., 2006). In a double-blinded randomized placebo-controlled trial, Stecksén-Blicks et al. reported that although fluoride varnish did not totally prevent white spot lesion formation, the incidence was significantly reduced in the fluoride varnish group. In addition to differences in study design, the frequency of fluoride application also varied among the studies. Stecksén et al. applied the fluoride varnish at six week intervals, the typical appointment interval for most orthodontic patients.

4.2 Resin sealer

After less successful earlier sealers, findings about the application of a filled-resin sealer (Pro-seal) have been published in the literature. One *in-vitro* study using an acid challenge found that demineralization was significantly less with Pro-seal treatment, compared to an untreated enamel surface (Hu and Featherstone, 2005). In fact, the demineralization levels established by microhardness profiles showed that the Pro-seal group had 98% less demineralization than the control group. This study also featured a group of teeth treated with fluoride varnish. While both the Pro-seal and fluoride varnish had significantly less demineralization than the control group, the sealer had significantly less demineralization than the varnish. Furthermore, the study also found that Pro-seal can stand up to acid challenge and toothbrush abrasion in a laboratory environment. These outcomes were corroborated by another *in-vitro* study, that also found that the filled-resin sealer (Pro-seal) provided significantly more protection than either fluoride varnish or an unfilled resin sealer, with a 92% reduction in lesion depth compared with the controls using polarized light microscopy (Buren *et al.*, 2008). In looking at its supposed fluoride release, one study found that Pro-seal released fluoride ions in a sustained way – with significantly decreasing amounts over a 17-week period, though this release was measured to be sub-ppm (Soliman *et al.*, 2006). Despite some favorable results with *in-vitro* models, no *in-vivo* trials with Pro-seal have been published in the literature.

4.3 Amorphous calcium phosphate (ACP)

4.3.1 CPP-ACP paste

Due to the early stages of this technology, published independent research on the ACP products like MI Paste is limited. Generally, the studies on caries prevention with CPP-ACP consist of *in-situ* caries models with gums, mouthrinses, or lozenges (Iijima *et al.*, 2004; Reynolds *et al.*, 2003). In addition, the vast majority of these studies were carried out by the same group that first isolated CPP-ACP at the University of Melbourne, Australia. For example, using topical applications of CPP-ACP via sugar-free chewing gum and mouthrinse, Reynolds et al. showed that CPP-ACP incorporated into dental plaque can significantly increase the levels of plaque calcium and phosphate ions (Reynolds *et al.*, 2003). Conversely, an *in-vitro* study carried out by an American group found that while fluoride 5000 ppm paste had a statistically significant protective effect against demineralization on enamel sections, MI Paste had no effect (Pulido *et al.*, 2008).There are two published studies that examine the role of CPP-ACP paste in orthodontics. In an *in-vitro* study that assessed the demineralization around bonded molar tubes on extracted third molars, a mild decrease in demineralization was found with the application of CPP-ACP (Sudjalim *et al.*, 2007). On the other hand, the authors of this very article recommended combining CPP-ACP with a fluoride gel to enhance the treatment effect. For the most part, clinicians loyal to the CPP-ACP protocol apply it without a fluoride gel, and the brochures by the manufacturer make no mention of additional rinses or gels. Andersson et al. conducted an *in-vivo* post-orthodontic treatment study, in which they compared the remineralization capabilities of 0.05% Sodium Fluoride mouthwash and the application of Topacal (CPP-ACP topical cream) on patients with white spot lesions. The study found significant remineralization with both protocols, and found no significant differences between the groups over time.

Still, the authors pointed out that the remineralization that occurred with CPP-ACP treatment was generally more esthetic than with the fluoride rinse.

4.3.2 ACP-containing bonding cement

As for ACP bonding cement products like Aegis-Ortho, there are currently no published comparative studies on its ability to prevent white spot lesions in the peer-reviewed literature. Two reports detail the questionable bond strength of ACP-containing cement. In spite of its potential benefits, frequent bond failures with ACP-cement have been reported. An *in-vitro* study with an earlier generation of Aegis-Ortho showed that orthodontic brackets bonded to teeth with an ACP-containing composite material failed at significantly lower forces than brackets bonded to teeth with a conventional resin-based composite orthodontic cement (Dunn, 2007). Another *in-vitro* study found that brackets bonded with the conventional Transbond XT had more than two times the shear bond strength in comparison to brackets bonded with Aegis-Ortho cement (Foster *et al.*, 2008). In evaluating the current evidence base for ACP and its various products, the number of published *in-vitro* and *in-vivo* trials is clearly underwhelming. In a 2008 systematic literature review published in the Journal of the American Dental Association (JADA), the authors concluded that there is insufficient clinical trial evidence to make a recommendation regarding the long-term effectiveness of casein derivatives, specifically CPP-ACP, in preventing caries *in-vivo* (Azarpazhooh and Limeback, 2008).

5. Summary of evidence

Of all the treatments for incipient caries lesions during orthodontic treatment, agents with fluoride including varnish have the highest level of evidence. Multiple laboratory and clinical studies have demonstrated its efficacy. Highly-filled resin sealers like Pro-seal are relatively new, although the results from a few *in vitro* studies have demonstrated impressive results. On the other hand, a clinical study on its demineralization prevention has not yet surfaced. At this juncture, the evidence level for ACP products like CPP-ACP paste or ACP resin bonding cement is low. There is a clear need for more independent research of casein derivatives like CPP-ACP to make conclusions about its efficacy in caries prevention.

6. Clinical status quo

In terms of the clinical status quo for prevention of incipient caries lesions during orthodontic treatment, one has to first reference the AAO sponsored informed consent form, in which there is an emphasis on excellent oral hygiene, regular visits to the general dentist, and access to fluoridated water (AAO, 2009). In looking at practice trends, a recent survey by the Journal of Clinical Orthodontics does provide some information about the usage of some of the preventive measures previously outlined (Keim *et al.*, 2008). Despite its proven efficacy, only 9.3% of orthodontists deliver fluoride varnish to their patients. The article also mentions that only 7.4% of orthodontists employ the fluoride-releasing glass ionomer adhesive for bracket bonding, which is understandable given its questionable physical properties. There were no data in the article detailing the usage of ACP products or resin sealers. In any event, the fact that more than half of orthodontic patients develop incipient caries lesions (Gorelick *et al.*, 1982; Richter *et al.*, 2009) and that only 9.3% of orthodontists give their patients fluoride varnish (Keim *et al.*, 2008), raises questions about emphasis of preventive care in today's orthodontic practice.

7. Need for investigation

Due to high caries incidence, low patient compliance, and low usage of fluoride varnish by orthodontists, there appears to be a need for a better treatment modality for patients undergoing orthodontic treatment. Regardless of the exact prevalence rate for white spot lesion development, most dental professionals would agree that it is currently far too high. While adjuncts to treatment such as fluoride rinse can potentially reduce the incidence of white spot lesions, the required compliance of high caries-risk patients is dubious. Equally troublesome, available non-compliant and proven treatments like professionally applied fluoride varnish have failed to catch the attention of practicing orthodontists. The resin sealer (Pro-seal) seems to address the patient compliance issue, but if orthodontists have neither the time nor the interest to deliver fluoride varnish, their likelihood of investing the resources and chair time to etch and light cure Pro-seal on twenty teeth is probably low. Aegis-Ortho bracket cement containing ACP seems to address all these issues. It does not require patient compliance, and it does not require any additional chair time in the office, since time allotted for orthodontic bracket bonding is already a part of the treatment plan. In spite of some reports, which document a low bond strength of its earlier generations, if ameliorated, this product holds immense potential for preventive care during orthodontic treatment. First however, there is a need to test and document the preventive properties of ACP-containing bracket cement with *in-vitro* studies.

8. Methods to assess demineralization

With a heightened interest in evidenced-based dentistry, the dental research community has over the years employed various modes of technology to quantify extent of enamel demineralization. The ideal method of assessment should be simple, noninvasive, reproducible, and precise. The following is brief description of four commonly employed techniques (TMR, PLM, QLF, and CLSM).

8.1 Microradiography

Transverse Microradiography (TMR) or contact-microradiography is one of the most widely accepted methods used to assess demineralization and remineralization in dental hard tissues in *in-situ* and *in-vitro* studies. It is a highly sensitive method to measure the morphology of and the change in mineral content of enamel and dentin samples (Arends and Ten Bosch, 1992). In TMR the tooth sample to be investigated is cut into thin slices (about 80 μm and 200 μm for dentine samples). A microradiographic image is made on high resolution film by X-ray exposure of the sections together with a calibration stepwedge. The microradiogram is digitized by a video camera or photomultiplier. The mineral can be automatically calculated from the gray levels of the images of section and stepwedge using a custom-made software. In examining the reliability of TMR, Exterkate et al. found that repeated microradiographs of the same thin enamel sections resulted in a negligible spread in mineral loss among them (Exterkate *et al.*, 1993). Such reliability and the more recent application of computer imaging make microradiography a standard method used in caries research for the assessment of lesion profiles.

8.2 Polarized light microscopy

Polarized light evaluations of enamel sections have been useful in describing the early caries lesion and alterations in structure upon further demineralization or remineralization. Generally, it provides information on absorption color and boundaries between minerals of differing refraction indices. Materials such as enamel act as beam splitters and divide light rays into two parts. Polarized Light microscopy (PLM) in turn exploits the interference of split light rays, as they are reunited along the same optical path to extract information about materials. Essentially, polarized light microscopy allows the visualization of areas with different porosities. The histologic features seen under a polarized light microscope allow the examiner to distinguish carious and non-carious enamel by their respective distribution of pores (Gwinnett, 1966). Polarized light examination of enamel specimens is a well-established procedure in which it is customary to view quinoline-imbibed sections orientated so that normal enamel is blue/green in color (Gilmour and Edmunds, 1998).

8.3. Quantitative light-induced fluorescence

Quantitative Light-induced Fluorescence (QLF) is one method of assessing levels of enamel demineralization. With QLF, real-time fluorescent images are captured into a computer and stored in an image database. Optional quantitative analysis tools enable the user to quantify parameters like mineral loss, lesion depth, lesion size, stain size and severity with high precision and repeatability. The QLF method is based on the auto-fluorescence of teeth. When teeth are illuminated with high intensity blue light they will start to emit light in the green part of the spectrum. When enamel demineralization takes place, minerals are replaced mainly by water from saliva, causing a decrease in the light path in the tooth substance. This results in less light absorption by enamel. Because fluorescence is a result of light absorption, the intensity of fluorescence decreases in demineralized regions of the enamel, which appear darker than sound tooth structures (de Josselin et al., 1995; al-Khateeb et al., 1998; Rousseau et al., 2002). Thus, the fluorescence of the dental tissue has a direct relation with the mineral content of the enamel. The effectiveness of QLF for measurement of enamel demineralization has been demonstrated in several studies. The use of QLF allows for quantitative analysis has been reported to be well correlated (0.73-0.83) with the degree of mineral loss from early enamel lesions in-vitro when measured by longitudinal microradiography. (Hafstrom-Bjorkman et al., 1992; Emami et al., 1996; Lagerweij et al., 1996). The use of QLF as a method of following caries development during orthodontic treatment has been suggested and encouraged by the results of several in-vitro studies. (Benson et al., 2003 and Pretty et al., 2003). Recent studies also indicate that QLF is suitable for in-vivo monitoring of mineral changes in incipient enamel lesions (Van der Veen et al., 2000 and Al Khateeb et al., 2002).

8.4 Confocal laser scanning ,icroscopy

Confocal Laser Scanning Microscopy (CLSM) is yet another method of assessing enamel demineralization. This technique accelerates and simplifies the measuring of mineral loss. The enamel specimens are sectioned in half, stained with fluorescent dye, and analyzed using a CLSM system (Fontana *et al.*, 1996). The major advantage of this method is that it enables quantitative analysis of thick samples without the problems of thin section preparation required for microradiography or polarized light microscopy. Essentially, CLSM allows a subsurface examination since the scattered, reflected, and fluorescent light from planes out of focus is eliminated – providing a subsurface image only from a thin layer upon which it is focused. This processed digital image can be used to determine surface features, area and volume analysis of given structures, and views of the total structure from any angle in three dimensions. In terms of efficacy, a statistically significant high correlation was found between mineral changes measured using microradiography and the changes in lesion parameters analyzed by confocal microscopy (González-Cabezas *et al.*, 1998)

With all the treatment modalities flooding the marketplace, the orthodontist might find it difficult to sort out what works best and why when oral hygiene deteriorates. The objectives of this chapter are to highlight the results of two recent studies that investigated:

1. The incidence of new WSLs before and after orthodontic treatment using photographic records; and
2. The potential of ACP-containing resin cement and other treatments (fluoride varnish, resin sealer, MI Paste) to prevent incipient caries lesions next to bracketed teeth.

9. Methods and materials: Part I

9.1 Selection of subjects

From a population of 2,296 patients treated in the graduate orthodontic clinic at the University of Michigan School of Dentistry (UMSD) between 1997 and 2004, 350 patient records were selected randomly using a random number sequence. Inclusion criteria for record selection consisted of patients who:

1. Underwent comprehensive orthodontic treatment utilizing full fixed appliances on labial tooth surfaces;
2. Had complete initial and final series of intraoral photographs; and
3. Had complete treatment log information within their chart.

9.2 Chart abstraction

Data collection from de-identified patient charts included gender and age at initiation of orthodontic treatment, and treatment variables such as extraction therapy and comprehensive treatment time. Comprehensive treatment time was defined as the period between initiation of full fixed appliance therapy and removal of all active fixed appliances. Initial oral hygiene score, frequency of oral hygiene discussion, oral hygiene instruction and fluoride application and/or rinse were recorded from progress notes in the chart.

9.3 Photography

Intraoral pre-treatment (initial) and post-treatment (final) photographs of each patient were taken as part of standard orthodontic recordkeeping procedures. All photographs, stored as 35 mm slides, were taken in the Clinical Photography Department at the UMSD by two professional photographers utilizing a standardized intraoral photography procedure.

Individual slides were scanned into digital format using a Nikon Slide Feeder SF-200 (S) and Super Coolscan 4000 ED scanner. Scanned images were enlarged 325% and imported into an individual Microsoft PowerPoint presentation for each patient.

9.4 Dental caries determination

Images were evaluated by trained investigators using a scoring system specifically adapted for use with photographed images (*International Caries Detection and Assessment System II*; Ismail, 2005). Visible labial surfaces examined included maxillary and mandibular central and lateral incisors, canines, first and second premolars, and first molars. The evaluators scored each visible labial tooth surface before and after orthodontic treatment. The scores were combined to determine the labial caries incidence for each patient. Teeth were examined and scored from first molar to first molar, maxilla and mandible (Fig. 2).

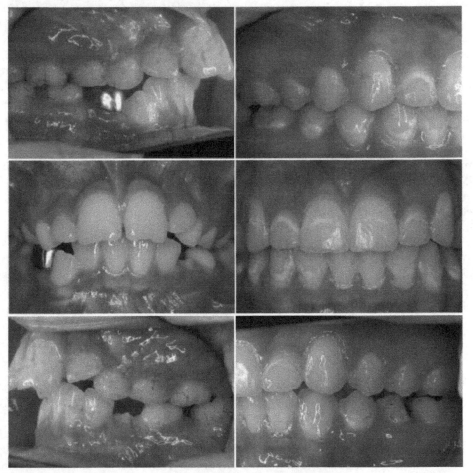

Fig. 2. Tooth labial surfaces were examined and scored from left first molar to right first molar, maxilla and mandible, before and after orthodontic treatment.

10. Results: Part I

The overall incidence of patients who developed at least one WSL during orthodontic treatment was 72.9% (N = 255; Table 1 and Fig. 3), while for newly developed cavitated lesions that were unrestored on the final record was 2.3%. Of the eight patients that developed cavitated lesions during orthodontic treatment, four (1.1%) developed one new cavitated lesion, three (0.9%) developed two new cavitated lesions and one (0.3%) developed four new cavitated lesions. Of the maximum 24 surfaces investigated per patient, on average 4.2 surfaces in each patient showed new WSL. The average of surfaces with new cavitations was only 0.04 and 0.05 with restorations. Even though infrequently, some early WSL regressed to sound (0.07 per patient). Demographic variables of gender and age at initiation of treatment were not related significantly to development of new decalcified or cavitated lesions. There was a significant relationship between increased treatment length and number of newly developed lesions (P = 0.03; Table 2). The mean number of labial surfaces per patient that developed new WSL was 3.01 for patients with a treatment length of less than 22 months. This increased to 5.28 teeth for patients with therapy longer than 33 months. The number of new cavitations, however, showed only a nonsignificant trend (P = 0.08) with increased treatment time. In addition, the number of newly developed lesions (both WSL and cavitations) showed no significant association with extraction or non-extraction treatment protocols (Table 3). Although no relationship was demonstrated between pretreatment oral hygiene scores and lesion development, the recorded number of oral hygiene discussions between provider and patient were associated significantly with development of both white-spot (P <0.0001) and cavitated (P = 0.0006) lesions. The mean number of new lesions for patients with whom oral hygiene discussions had never been noted in the chart was 3.08, while the mean number of decalcified lesions for patients who were given oral hygiene instruction on three or more occasions increased to 7.78. A similar increase was exhibited for the mean number of cavitated lesions for patients given three or more oral hygiene discussions (mean = 0.20) *vs.* those with whom oral hygiene was not discussed after initial instruction (mean = 0.01). Age group (P = 0.03), treatment length (P = 0.01) and number of oral hygiene discussions (P < 0.0001) were associated with development of WSL. There was a decrease in WSLs associated with increasing age group (regression coefficient = -0.59). An increase in WSLs was associated with both increased treatment time (regression coefficient = 0.07) and increased number of oral hygiene discussions (regression coefficient = 1.88).

11. Methods and materials: Part II

11.1 Sample preparation

One hundred human premolar teeth were collected from various oral surgery practices located in southeast Michigan. Only premolars presenting a healthy facial enamel surface were included. All teeth were assigned randomly to five equal groups of 20 teeth. One of the groups had brackets bonded with Aegis-Ortho resin cement while the remaining groups were bonded with Transbond XT. Of the four Transbond XT groups, one served as a control, another received Vanish (3M, Espe, MN) fluoride varnish, another received MI Paste and the final received a coat of Pro-seal as adjunctive treatments.

11.2 Demineralization protocol

Teeth were exposed to a pH cycling system to develop caries-like lesions. Each day teeth were incubated in demineralization solution (lactic acid and Carbopol [pH = 5.0], 50% saturated with hydroxyapatite) for eight hours, rinsed with de-ionized water and placed in artificial saliva for 30 minutes, followed by two seconds of brushing with a powerbrush (Sonicare, Philips) and fluoridated dentifrice (NaF, 1,100 ppm F), rinsed again and placed back in artificial saliva until next demineralization period (next day).

Number of teeth with newly developed WSL	Frequency of patients (N)	Percent of total patients	Cumulative frequency	Cumulative percent
0	95	27.1	95	27.1
1	57	16.3	152	43.4
2	48	13.7	200	57.1
3	18	5.1	218	62.2
4	21	6.0	239	68.3
5	18	5.1	257	73.4
6	21	2.3	265	75.7
7	11	3.1	276	78.9
8	10	2.8	286	81.7
9	9	2.6	295	84.3
10	6	1.7	301	86.0
11	5	1.4	306	87.4
12	8	2.3	314	89.7
13	6	1.7	320	91.4
14	5	1.4	325	92.9
15	7	2.0	332	94.9
16	5	1.4	337	96.3
17	4	1.1	341	97.4
18	4	1.1	345	98.6
19	1	0.3	346	98.9
20	2	0.6	348	99.4
21	1	0.3	349	99.7
22	1	0.3	350	100.0

Table 1. Incidence of white-spot lesions (WSLs)

Solutions were refreshed daily during the experimental period of 15 days. On day 15, all teeth were removed from the saliva solution, rinsed under tap water and stored in 100% humidity. To assess demineralization, Quantitative Light-induced Fluorescence (QLF) and Confocal Laser Scanning Microscopy (CLSM) were used. Both procedures were carried out at the Oral Health Research Institute (IU) in Indianapolis, IN.

Variable	Parameter estimate	Standard error	t-value	P-value
Sex	-0.73	0.55	-1.33	0.19
Age group	-0.59	0.28	-2.12	0.03*
Treatment length	0.07	0.02	2.76	0.01*
Initial oral hygiene score	-0.08	0.56	-0.14	0.89
Number of oral hygiene discussions	1.88	0.39	4.86	<0.00*

*= P- value significant at $P<0.005$.

Table 2. Multivariabile regression model.

Age	Trend, fewer new lesions as age increases
Treatment length	Trend, 0.08 new lesions per month of treatment
Oral hygiene	Counter-intuitive trend, number increases as number of discussions increased

Table 3. Inferential statistics. Adjusted R-square = 0.11. This model accounts for 11% of the variation inWSL development.

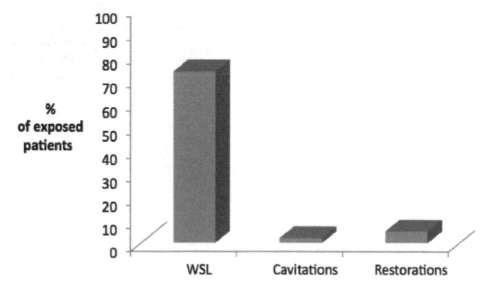

Fig. 3. Distribution of patients with at least one new lesion.

12. Results: Part II

Demineralization assessed by QLF is shown in Table 4. The Proseal group had the least amount of fluorescence loss followed by the Vanish group. Aegis-Ortho group, MI Paste group and the control group (Transbond) had the most fluorescence loss and were not different significantly. Demineralization assessed by CLSM is shown in Table 5. No detectable lesion depth was seen in any of the specimens of Pro-seal and Vanish groups. The greatest lesion depth was found in the control group (Transbond), but it was not different significantly from Aegis-Ortho and MI Paste.

Treatment Group	Mean ΔF	SD
TbXT + Pro-seal	-7.0	4.4
TbXT + Vanish	-19.7	3.5
* Aegis-Ortho	-22.9	3.7
* TbXt + MI Paste	-25.0	6.2
* Transbond XT (TbXT) – Control	-29.6	8.2

*Groups not different significantly ($P>0.05$). ΔF=fluoresce loss.

Table 4. Loss of fluorescence per group(N=20).

Treatment Group	Mean ΔF	SD
TbXT + Pro-seal	0.0	0.0
TbXT + Vanish	0.0	0.0
* Aegis-Ortho	15.9	7.4
* TbXt + MI Paste	16.4	15.8
* Transbond XT (TbXT) – Control	32.9	19.3

*Groups not different significantly ($P>0.05$). ΔF=lesion depth.

Table 5. Lesion depth for each group (N=20).

13. Discussion

The use of intraoral photographs for caries determination in orthodontic patients is a well-accepted method. Standardized photographs taken before and after appliance placement are available readily as a standard procedure in orthodontic care. Color photography as a means of recording prevalence of enamel opacity is a powerful method (Ellwood, 1993). Studies have shown that assessment of enamel demineralization from color images appears to be more reproducible than direct clinical observation utilizing only the naked eye (Benson et al., 1998). Moreover, photographic records provide an efficient means to capture the appearance of enamel and provide a permanent record at a given time point. It allows an examiner, therefore, to assess the caries experience of a patient blindly and randomly. Based on pre- and post-orthodontic treatment photographic patient records, this study showed a high incidence of new WSLs (72.9%) in patients treated with comprehensive orthodontics, while the incidence of new cavitated lesions in this population was 2.3%. Gender, age and oral hygiene at start of treatment were not associated with lesion development, while a significant association was evidenced with treatment duration. Patients in treatment for less than 22 months developed on average three WSLs, while patients in treatment for 33 months or longer developed on average more than five lesions. Linear regression analysis suggested that as the duration of fixed appliances increased one month, 0.08 new WSLs were developed. The *in vitro* study sought to test four different treatments, which comprise much of the currently available therapies to prevent WSLs. The four experimental groups differed in their application, chemistry and physical properties. The Aegis-Ortho cement serves as a replacement for a typical bracket bonding cement. This ACP-containing material supposedly reduces the incidence of enamel demineralization with the release of calcium and phosphate ions – not only to reduce demineralization, but also to promote the remineralization of enamel. The fluoride varnish group received the same bonding cement as the control plus an application of Vanish, a popular fluoride varnish used for caries prevention. Unlike fluoride rinses that require patient compliance, the delivery of Vanish takes place in the dental chair and could be applied at the monthly orthodontic appointment. The CPP-ACP group teeth received an adjunctive daily application of MI Paste, whose chemical mechanism of action resembles that of the ACP cement. Instead of having ACP just residing in the bracket cement, the preventive protocol for MI Paste demands a daily application and, thus, a certain degree of patient compliance. MI Paste is claimed to have the ability to prevent WSLs during orthodontic treatment. Teeth in the final group received a light cured filled sealant as adjunctive treatment. Though it claims to offer some fluoride release, Pro-seal at its core functions as a protective physical barrier against the acid attacks.

Compared with the control group, the Pro-seal group had a statistically significant difference in regard to both outcome measures (*i.e.*, lesion depth and fluorescence loss). The CLSM results indicated that there was no demineralization on any of the specimens in this group. Similarly, the QLF test demonstrated that teeth treated with Pro-seal had the least amount of fluorescence loss by far. The findings of this study confirmed that the Pro-seal functions as a protective barrier that is impermeable to the daily acid challenge. This impressive display of demineralization prevention under *in vitro* cariogenic conditions also has been observed in other studies (Hu and Featherstone, 2005; Buren *et al.*, 2008).

When interpreting the results of the current study, it is important to examine the experimental methods used. Obviously, the oral cavity of the typical teenager presents a much more dynamic and abrasive environment than those used in this *in vitro* study. However, it has been shown that Pro-seal sealant also displays physical properties when subjected to abrasion (Hu and Featherstone, 2005). Pro-seal prevented enamel demineralization convincingly and, thus, seems to be a reasonable treatment option that requires zero patient compliance.

The results from this study also indicated that teeth treated with the fluoride varnish had less enamel demineralization than the control and the ACP groups. Although it had a statistically significant difference in both lesion depth and fluorescence loss when compared to the control group, the difference was not nearly as dramatic in the QLF test. Currently, there are no other *in vitro* studies in the literature that examine fluoride varnish around orthodontic brackets with both CLSM and QLF.

In that there was zero demineralization measured with the CLSM but some degree of fluorescence loss found with the QLF raises questions. In spite having the specimens brushed daily, for the most part the fluoride varnish remained unexpectedly on the tooth surface throughout the experiment and had to be removed with a plastic scaler at the end of the experiment. Therefore, its mechanism of action must be considered. In addition to the anti-cariogenic properties of fluoride as rationale for use, the fluoride may not have been the only mechanism of action in this *in vitro* experiment in that the varnish formed a physical barrier to the acid challenge.

In this study, the Aegis-Ortho group and the MI Paste group showed less demineralization numerically than the control group for both the CLSM and QLF test, though neither had statistical significance. Thus, both Aegis-Ortho and MI Paste were not different from the control group. The similar numerical levels of effectiveness for Aegis-Ortho and MI Paste are not surprising, given their similar mode of action. In analyzing these two treatments, the obvious disadvantage for the MI Paste group is that it requires daily application, whereas the ACP in Aegis-Ortho simply resides in the bracket bonding cement.

While the results of this study help us better understand the prevention potential of these products, *in vitro* experimental conditions cannot encapsulate all the complexities of a living oral cariogenic environment.

The ultimate answer on efficacy of these products has to come from well-designed controlled clinical trials. An *in vivo* randomized controlled trial study that employs proven methods for clinical evaluation of incipient lesions around brackets and also includes the patient compliance factor would provide the highest level of evidence with respect to the preventive treatment modalities discussed.

14. Conclusions

The incidence of WSLs in patients treated with comprehensive orthodontics was very high, suggesting that any preventive therapy provided appeared to be ineffective. This widespread problem poses an alarming concern and warrants significant attention from both patients and providers that should result in greatly increased emphasis on effective caries prevention. Results from this study suggest that both the lightcured filled sealer (Proseal) and the fluoride varnish (Vanish) have the potential to prevent enamel demineralization next to orthodontic brackets exposed to cariogenic conditions.

15. References

Adriens ML, Dermaut LR, Verbeeck RM: The use of Fluor Protector, a fluoride varnish as a prevention method under orthodontic bands. Eur J Orthod 1990;12:316–9.

Aimutis WR. Bioactive properties of milk proteins with particular focus on anticariogenesis. J Nutr 2004;134:989–95.

Al-Khateeb S, Forsberg CM, de Josselin de Jong E, Angmar-Mansson B. A longitudinal laser fluorescence study of white spot lesions in orthodontic patients. Am J Orthod Dentofacial Orthop 1998;113:595–602.

Al-Khateeb S, Exterkate RA, de Josselin de Jong E, Angmar-Månsson B, ten Cate JM Light-induced fluorescence studies on dehydration of incipient enamel lesions. Caries Res. 2002 ;36:25-30.

American Association of Orthodontists [Internet] Missouri; AAO; [cited 2009 Jan 5]. Available from http://www.braces.org/knowmore/care/.

Andersson A, Sköld-Larsson K, Hallgren A, Petersson LG, Twetman S. Effect of a dental cream containing amorphous cream phosphate complexes on white spot lesion regression assessed by laser fluorescence. Oral Health Prev Dent. 2007;5:229-33.

Arends J, Ten Bosch JJ. Demineralization and remineralization evaluation techniques. J Dent Res 1992;71:924-8.

Årtun J, Thylstrup A. A 3-year clinical and SEM study of surface changes of carious enamel lesions after inactivation. Am J Orthod Dentofacial Orthop 1989;95:327-33.

Azarpazhooh A, Limeback H. Clinical efficacy of casein derivatives: A systematic review of the literature. J Am Dent Assoc 2008;139:915-924.

Banks PA, Richmond S. Enamel sealants: a clinical evaluation of their value

Benson PE, Pender N, Higham SM. Quantifying enamel demineralization from teeth with orthodontic brackets – a comparison of two methods. Part 1: repeatability and agreement. Eur J Orthod 2003;25:149-58.

Benson PE, Pender N, Higham SM. Quantifying enamel demineralization from teeth with orthodontic brackets – a comparison of two methods. Part 2: validity. Eur J Orthod 2003;25:159-65.

Buren JL, Staley RN, Wefel J, Qian F. Inhibition of enamel demineralization by an enamel sealant, Pro-seal: An *in vitro* study. Am J Orthod Dentofacial Orthop 2008;133:S88-S94.

de Josselin de Jong E, Sundstrom F, Westerling H, Tranaeus S, ten Bosch JJ, Angmar-Mansson B. A new method for *in-vivo* quantification of changes in initial enamel caries with laser fluorescence. Caries Res 1995;29:2-7.

Demito CF, Vivaldi-Rodrigues G, Ramos AL, Bowman SJ. The efficacy of a fluoride varnish in reducing enamel demineralization adjacent to orthodontic brackets: an *in-vitro* study. Orthod Craniofacial Res 2004;7:205-10.

Dunn W. Shear bond strength of an amorphous calcium phosphate – containing orthodontic resin cement. Am J Orthod Dentofacial Orthop 2007;131:243-7.

Emami Z, al-Khateeb S, de Josselin de Jong E, Sundstrom F, Trollsas K, Angmar-Mansson B. Mineral loss in incipient caries lesions quantified with laser fluorescence and longitudinal microradiography. A methodologic study. Acta Odontol Scand 1996;54:8-13.

Exterkate RAM, Damen JJM, ten Cate JM (1993). A single section model for enamel de- and remineralization studies. I. The effects of different Ca/P ratios in remineralization solutions. J Dent Res. 1993;72:1599-1603.

Fontana M, Dunipace AJ, Gregory RL, Noblitt TW, Li Y, Park KK, Stookey GK. An *in- vitro* microbial model for studying secondary caries formation. Caries Res 1996a;30:112-8.

Fontana M, Dunipace AJ, Noblitt TW, Fischer GM, Katz BP, Stookey GK. Measurement of enamel demineralization using microradiography and confocal microscopy. Caries Res 1996b;30:317-25.

Foster JA, Berzins DW, Bradley TG. Bond strength of an amorphous calcium phosphate-containing orthodontic adhesive. Angle Orthod. 2008;78:339-44.

Geiger AM, Gorelick L, Gwinnett AJ, Benson BJ. Reducing white spot lesions in orthodontic populations with fluoride rinsing. Am J Orthod Dentofacial Orthop 1992;101:403-7.

Gilmour AS, Edmunds DH. The polarized light microscopic appearance of caries-like lesions adjacent to restored cavities in the crowns and roots of extracted human teeth. J Oral Rehabil. 1998;25:929-39.

González-Cabezas C, Fontana M, Dunipace AJ, Li Y, Fischer GM, Proskin HM, Stookey GK. Measurement of enamel remineralization using microradiography and confocal microscopy. Caries Res 1998;32:385-92.

Gorelick L, Geiger AM, Gwinnett AJ. Incidence of white spot formation after bonding and banding. Am J Orthod Dentofacial Orthop 1982; 81:93-98.

Gorton J, Featherstone JDB. In vivo inhibition of demineralization around orthodontic brackets. Am J Orthod Dentofacial Orthop 2003; 123:10-14.

Gwinnett J. Normal Enamel II: Qualitative polarized light study. J. Dent. Res. 1966 45: 261-5.

Hafstrom-Bjorkman U, Sundstrom F, de Josselin de Jong E, Oliveby A, Angmar-Mansson B. Comparison of laser fluorescence and longitudinal microradiography for quantitative assessment of in-vitro enamel caries. Caries Res 1992;26:241-7.

Hu W, Featherstone JDB. Prevention of enamel demineralization: An in vitro study using light-cured filled sealant. Am J Orthod Dentofacial Orthop 2005;128:592-600.

Iijima Y, Cai F, Shen P, Walker G, Reynolds C, Reynolds EC. Acid resistance of enamel subsurface lesions remineralized by a sugar-free chewing gum containing casein phosphopeptide-amorphous calcium phosphate. Caries Res 2004;38:551-6.

Informed consent for the orthodontic patient: risks and limitations of orthodontic treatment. American Association of Orthodontists (2005).

Ismail A. Rationale and evidence for the International Caries Detection and Assessment System (ICDAS II). In: Stookey G, ed. Clinical Models Workshop: Remin-demin, Precavitation, Caries: Proceedings of the 7th Indiana Conference. Indianapolis: Indiana University School of Dentistry 2005:161-222.

Keim RG, Gottlieb EI, Nelson AH, Vogels DS 3rd. 2008 JCO study of orthodontic diagnosis and treatment procedures, Part 1: Results and trends. J Clin Orthod. 2008;42:625-40.

Lagerweij M, van der Veen M, Ando M, Lukantsova L, Stookey G. The validity and repeatability of three light-induced fluorescence systems: an in-vitro study. Caries Res 1999;33:220-6.

Lovrov S, Hertrich K, Hirschfelder U. Enamel Demineralization during Fixed Orthodontic Treatment - Incidence and Correlation to Various Oral-hygiene Parameters. J Orofac Orthop. 2007;68:353-63.

Marinho VCC, Higgins JPT, Logan S, Sheiham A. Fluoride mouthrinses for preventing dental caries in children and adolescents (Cochrane Review). In: The Cochrane Library, Issue 1, 2004. Chichester, UK: John Wiley & Sons.

Mathew M, Takagi S. Structures of biological minerals in dental research. J Res Natl Inst Stand Technol 2001;106:1035-44.

Mehra T, Nanda RS, Sinha PK. Orthodontists' assessment and management of patient compliance. Angle Orthod. 1998; 68:115-22.

Øgaard B, Rolla G, Arends J. Orthodontic appliances and enamel demineralization. Part 1. Lesion development. Am J Orthod Dentofacial Orthop 1988;94:68-73.

Øgaard B. Prevalence of white spot lesions in 19-year-olds: a study on untreated and orthodontically treated persons 5 years after treatment. Am J Orthod Dentofacial Orthod 1989;96:423-7.

Øgaard B, Larsson E, Henriksson T, Birkhed D, Bishara SE: Effects of a combined application of antimicrobial and fluoride varnishes in orthodontic patients. Am J Orthod Dentofacial Orthop 2001;120:28-35.

O'Reilly MM, Featherstone JDB. Demineralization and remineralization around orthodontic appliances: An in vivo study. Am J Orthod Dentofacial Orthop 1987;92:33-40.

Pretty IA, Pender N, Edgar WM, Higham SM. The in-vitro detection of early enamel de- and re-mineralization adjacent to bonded orthodontic cleats using quantitative light-induced fluorescence. Eur J Orthod 2003;25:217-23.

Pulido MT, Wefel JS, Hernandez MM, Denehy GE, Guzman-Armstrong S, Chalmers JM, Qian F. The inhibitory effect of MI paste, fluoride and a combination of both on the progression of artificial caries-like lesions in enamel. Oper Dent. 2008;33:550-5.

Reynolds EC, del Rio A. Effect of Casein and whey-protein solutions on caries experience and feeding patterns of the rat. Arch Oral Biol 1984;29:927-33.

Reynolds EC. Anticariogenic complexes of amorphous calcium phosphate stabilized by casein phosphopeptides: a review. Spec Care Dentist 1998;18:8-16

Reynolds EC, Black CL, Cai F, et al. Advances in enamel remineralization: anticariogenic casein phosphopeptide-amorphous calcium phosphate. J Clin Dent 1999;10:86-8

Reynolds EC, Cai F, Shen P, Walker GD. Retention in plaque and remineralization of enamel lesions by various forms of calcium in a mouthrinse or sugar-free chewing gun. J Dent Res 2003;82:206-11.

Richter AE, Arruda AO, Peters MC and Sohn W. Incidence of caries lesions for patients treated with comprehensive orthodontics. J Dent Res 88(Spec Iss A): Abstract Miami meeting, 2009.

Rose RK. Binding characteristics of Streptococcus mutans for calcium and casein phosphopeptide. Caries Res 2000;34:427-31.

Rosen S, Min DB, Harper DS, Harper WJ, Beck EX, Beck FM. Effect of cheese, with and without sucrose, on dental caries and recovery of Streptococcus mutans in rats. J Dent Res 1984;63:894-6.

Rosenbloom RG, Tinanoff N. Salivary Streptococcus mutans levels in patients before, during and after orthodontic treatment. Am J Orthod Dentofacial Orthop 1991;100:35-7.

Rousseau C, Vaidya S, Creanor SL, Hall AF, Girkin JM, Whitters CJ, et al. The effect of dentine on fluorescence measurements of enamel lesions in-vitro. Caries Res 2002;36:381-5.

Skrtic D, Hailer AW, Antonucci JM, Takagi S, Eanes ED. Quantitative assessment of the efficacy of amorphous calcium phosphate/methacrylate composites in remineralizing caries-like lesions artificially produced in bovine enamel. J Dent Res. 1996;75:1679-86.

Soliman MM, Bishara SE, Wefel J, Heilman J, Warren JJ. Fluoride release rate from an orthodontic sealant and its clinical implications. Angle Orthod. 2006;76:282-8

Stecksén-Blicks C, Renfors G, Oscarson ND, Bergstrand F, Twetman S. Caries-preventive effectiveness of a fluoride varnish: A randomized controlled trial in adolescents with fixed orthodontic appliances. Caries Res 2007;41:455-459.

Sudjalim TR, Woods MG, Manton DJ, Reynolds EC. Prevention of demineralization around orthodontic brackets in-vitro. Am J Orthod Dentofacial Orthop 2007;131:705.

Todd MA, Stanley RN, Kanellis MJ, Donly KJ, Wefel JS: Effect of a fluoride varnish on demineralization adjacent to orthodontic brackets. Am J Orthod Dentofacial Orthop 1999;116:159-67.

van der Linden RP, Dermaut LR: White spot formation under orthodontic bands cemented with glass ionomer with or without Fluor Protector. Eur J Orthod 1998;20: 219-24.

van der Veen MH, de Josselin de Jong E Application of quantitative light-induced fluorescence for assessing early caries lesions. Monogr Oral Sci. 2000;17:144-62.

Vivaldi-Rodrigues G, Demito CF, Bowman SJ, Ramos AL. The effectiveness of a fluoride varnish in preventing the development of white spot lesions. World J Orthod 2006;7:138-144.

Zachrisson BU, Heimgard E, Ruyter IE, Mjor IA. Problems with sealants for bracket bonding. Am J Orthod 1979;75:641-9.

8

Laser Technology for Caries Removal

Adriana Bona Matos, Cynthia Soares de Azevedo,
Patrícia Aparecida da Ana, Sergio Brossi Botta and Denise Maria Zezell
University of São Paulo, School of Dentistry and Nuclear and Energetic Research Institute,
Brazil

1. Introduction

Laser technology has been in the scope of dentistry community since Stern & Sognnaes (1964) studied laser application on dental hard tissues. Lasers have become an attractive instrument for many dental procedures including soft tissues surgery (Sperandio et al., 2011), decontamination (Benedicenti et al., 2008; Koba et al., 1998) and for assuring anti-inflammatory effects (Lang-Bicuto et al., 2008). In restorative dentistry, laser has been used successfully for cavity preparation (De Moor et al., 2010; Obeidi et al., 2009), caries prevention (Namour et al., 2011; Rechmann et al., 2011; Zezell et al., 2009), caries decontamination (Namour et al., 2011) and caries removal (Neves et al., 2011; White et al., 1993). For that, high intensity lasers are indicated, which are able to promote controlled temperature rise in a small and specific area of dental hard tissue (Ana et al., 2007). Depending on the temperature rise and the interaction of laser irradiation with dental tissues, it is possible to produce specific micro structural and/or mechanical changes related to a correct clinical application.

The use of lasers for cavity preparation and caries removal is based on the ablation mechanism, in which dental hard tissue can be removed by thermal and/or mechanical effect during laser irradiation (Seka et al., 1996). This mechanism relies on the type of tissue to be irradiated, as well as the characteristics of laser equipments. The knowledge of laser wavelength, laser emission, pulse duration, pulse energy, repetition rate, beam spot size, delivery method, laser beam characteristics (Ana et al., 2006), and optical properties of the tissue, such as the refractive index, the scattering coefficient (μ_s), the absorption coefficient (μ_a), and the scattering anisotropy (Featherstone, 2000a) are necessary to assure better clinical results without thermal or mechanical damages to the dental hard tissue.

For irradiation in dental hard tissues, the most frequent laser systems used are Nd:YAG λ = 1.064 µm), Argon (λ = 0.488 µm), Ho:YLF (λ = 2.065 µm), Ho:YAG (λ = 2.100 µm), Er:YAG (λ = 2.940 µm), Er,Cr:YSGG (λ = 2.780 µm), Diode (λ = 0.810 µm) and CO_2 (λ = 9.300 µm or 9.600 µm or 10.600 µm). With the exception of the argon laser, these lasers emit in infrared range of electromagnetic spectrum, and a good number of equipment operates at the free running mode, with pulse durations of microseconds (µs). Considering that laser wavelength must be absorbed by enamel and dentin to assure the efficient caries removal and cavity preparation (Seka et al., 1996), the most successful laser systems for this purpose are erbium and CO_2 (λ = 9.6 μm) lasers. However, the CO_2 (λ = 9.6 μm) systems are not commercially available for applications in dentistry.

Considering the advances in technology for the development of ultra short pulse lasers (USPLs) (Niemz, 1995; Strickland & Mourou, 1985), efforts have been implemented to understand their interaction with dental hard tissues and to determine safe and proper parameters to provide a future clinical application in dentistry (Altshuler et al., 1994; Freitas et al., 2010; Kruger et al., 1999; Lizarelli et al., 2008; Strassl et al., 2008). Due to the extremely short pulse length, these systems promote precise cutting and have a strong potential for obtaining well-defined cavities and controlled caries removal (Niemz, 2004; Serbin et al., 2002). Also, due to the use of low energies per pulse, it is possible to adjust parameters bellow the ablation threshold for sound tissue which, at the same time, can ablate and remove the carious tissue (Niemz, 2004; Strassl et al., 2008). In this way, the selective removal of carious tissue could be seen as a minimal intervention that does not depend on the professional experience, but essentially relies on the tissue chemistry (Serbin et al., 2002).

The operation of laser systems and interactions with dental hard tissues, the clinical diagnosis and the knowledge of the characteristics of the tissue to be irradiated are extremely important to assure a well-succeeded therapy. Professionals must evaluate the mineralization degree and chemical composition of the tissue to be removed, the extension and localization of caries, the activity degree of lesions and the interference of the irradiation on the restorative procedure.

In this chapter, focus will be given on the last developments concerning the use of high-intensity lasers in restorative dentistry, describing the different laser wavelengths, the mechanisms of interaction with dental hard tissue and the influence of pulse width on removing these tissues. Also, the effects of laser irradiation on carious tissues will be described, and the possibility of removing dental caries with laser irradiation will be discussed to help dentists to choose a suitable equipment and technique for improving their clinical practice.

2. Laser interaction with dental hard tissues

Depending on laser wavelength and tissue characteristics, laser irradiation can be absorbed, scattered, reflected or transmitted into dental tissues (Ana et al., 2006; Featherstone, 2000; Niemz, 2004; Seka et al., 1996). These effects must be well known by professionals to help them choose the best equipment for a specific clinical application and to avoid thermal and mechanical damages to the target and surrounding tissues. Depending on the clinical situation, dentists need different laser wavelengths and irradiation parameters to obtain distinct effects on the same tissue.

Considering the applications in restorative dentistry, the conventional high-intensity infrared lasers can be well-suited for caries removal (Neves et al., 2010; Tachibana et al., 2008; White et al., 1993), cavity preparation (De Moor & Delme, 2010; Moldes et al., 2009; Obeidi et al., 2009;) and tissue conditioning (Botta et al., 2009; Dundar & Gunzel, 2011). For that, continuous emission lasers or pulsed laser longer than 1 picosecond should be well absorbed by the main components of teeth, i.e., water and hydroxyapatite; to promote the desired thermal and mechanical effects on these tissues, in a process called *thermal ablation* due to a *thermomechanical* effect (Fried, 2000; Niemz, 1995; Seka et al., 1996). For shorter pulses, such as femtosecond laser pulses, the ablation occurs due to non-linear interactions with the tissue resulting in a plasma-mediated ablation.

The thermal ablation process that occurs in dental hard tissues is also known as explosive (water-mediated) tissue removal (Fried, 2000; Niemz, 1995; Seka et al., 1996). In a few words, this process can be explained as a result of the fast heating of the subsurface water confined by the hard tissue matrix, due to the higher interaction with infrared laser irradiation. The heating of these water molecules leads to an increase on molecular vibration and, consequently, an increase on subsurface pressures that can exceed the strength of the above tissue. Finally, it can be noted an "explosion" of tissue due to the material failure, resulting in the material removal. This process happens in temperatures below the melting point of dental hard tissues (around 1200°C) and varies according to the laser wavelength (e.g., Er:YAG reaches 300° C at the ablation threshold, while Er,Cr:YSGG reaches 800° C and CO_2 9.6 μm reaches 1000° C) ((Seka et al., 1996; Fried et al., 1996). This process has been studied for the past 30 years, with the intention of choosing the best laser wavelength and parameter to effectively promote tissue removal or selective caries removal with minimal thermal consequences (Stern & Sognnaes, 1964; White et al., 1993; Neves et al., 2010; Ana et al., 2007; Seka et al., 1996; Tachibana et al., 2008; Moldes et al., 2009; Botta et al., 2009; Dundar & Gunzel, 2011).

For understanding how laser irradiation can provide a more conservative treatment of caries lesions, the chemical composition of target tissue must be known by the professional. Human enamel is composed by 95% hydroxyapatite ($Ca_{10}(PO_4)_6(OH_2)$), 4% water and 1% collagen fibers (Gwinnett, 1992); as well as human dentine contains 70% hydroxyapatite, 20% collagen fibers and 10% water (Ziip & Bosch, 1993). Considering the differences in composition and the higher resonance of Er:YAG (λ = 2.94 μm) by water (λ = 3 μm), we can infer that Er:YAG laser can ablate dentin faster than enamel. The same rule is valid when comparing carious tissue with sound ones, taking into account that decayed tissues have a significant higher amount of water. In this way, in a clinical application, professionals can observe easier caries removal when compared to the removal of sound surrounding tissues, and this fact can influence the laser irradiation parameters that should be used for different application.

Dental enamel and dentin have a weak absorption in the visible (400–700 nm) and near-infrared (1064 nm) wavelength ranges; however, absorption bands of water and carbonated hydroxyapatite is found from 2.7 to 11 μm (Figure 1) (Ana et al., 2006; Fried 2000). The optical penetration of Nd:YAG on enamel is significantly high, indicating that the dentin irradiation with Nd:YAG laser can affect the pulp tissue in case of high energy densities, long exposure or in the absence of a photoabsorber (Boari et al., 2009). However, Nd:YAG laser can be indicated for removal of stained caries tissue, promoting a selective removal of caries lesion without pulpal damages due to the higher interaction of Nd:YAG by pigments (Seka et al., 1996), as it was demonstrated by a clinical trial performed by White *et al.* (1993).

Considering the use of Er,Cr:YSGG laser, literature evidences (Stock et al., 1997) that the 2.78 μm is strongly absorbed by the dental hard tissue since the optical absorption coefficient of enamel is about 7000 cm^{-1}. In this way, the optical penetration is a few micrometers smaller than the obtained by Er:YAG laser.

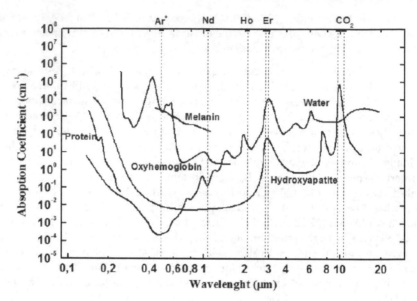

Fig. 1. Absorption coefficients for the main chromophores of biological tissues (Ana et al., 2006).

Since the approval of erbium lasers for dental hard tissues use by FDA in 90's, Er:YAG and Er,Cr:YSGG have been extensively studied for caries therapy. The literature present a number of advantages over the high-speed drills for the removal of caries, such as reduction of pain, noise, vibration (Fried, 2000; Niemz, 2004; Seka et al., 1996; White et al., 1993), the possibility of selective removal (Eberhard et al., 2005; Neves et al., 2010) and the changes in chemical composition of remaining tissue (Ana et al., 2006; Bachmann et al., 2009; Botta et al., 2011), leading to a tissue that is resistant to demineralization. That is why erbium lasers can be considered a clinical reality in dental offices.

3. The use of erbium lasers for caries therapy

The erbium lasers are solid-state lasers produced with different types of matrix crystals. Some of them, such as Er:YAG (λ = 2.94 μm), Er,Cr:YSGG (λ = 2.78 μm), Er:YLF (λ = 2.81 μm), Er:YAG (λ = 2.73 μm) and CTE:YAG (λ = 2.69 μm), were already studied for ablation of dental hard tissues (Altshuler et al., 1994). From all of them, the most popular and with commercially available equipments for dentistry are Er:YAG and Er,Cr:YSGG.

Comparing the absorption of Er:YAG with Er,Cr:YSGG lasers by dental hard tissues, it is possible to observe that Er:YAG have a strong interaction with OH- from water molecules contained in the teeth, while Er,Cr:YSGG is better absorbed by water and OH- contents of hydroxyapatite (Figure 2)(Ana et al., 2006). Due to this fact, Er:YAG promotes surface temperatures up to 300º C at the ablation threshold, and Er,Cr:YSGG reaches 800º C during ablation of enamel (Fried et al., 1996).

Although it have been tested some erbium lasers operating in the Q-switched mode (with pulse duration in the range of ns) (Fried, 2000), the commercially available erbium lasers operate in free running mode, with pulse duration of 150-400 μs. This pulse duration is shorter than the thermal relaxation time of dental hard tissues (< 1ms) (Niemz, 2004), which provide heat dissipation during ablation and avoid excessive heat transmission to the pulp, for instance. However, at higher energy per pulses, erbium lasers can induce thermal injuries to dental hard tissue, such as the presence of microcracks, melting or even carbonization. In this way, during the clinical application, it is essential to use the correct set up of laser parameters and the use of an adequate air-water spray to provide proper refrigeration and avoid these side effects. However, although the presence of a thin layer of water can increase the ablation process (Fried at al., 2002), an excessive water layer can decrease erbium interaction with dental hard tissues (Niemz, 2004); in this way, the use of saliva suction is recommended.

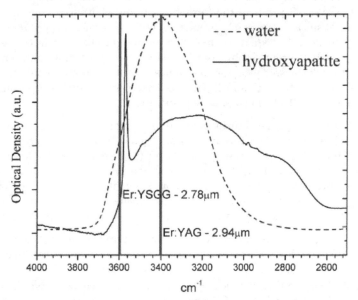

Fig. 2. Absorbance of water and hydroxyapatite and their relation with Er:YAG and Er,Cr:YSGG lasers (Ana et al., 2006).

Er:YAG lasers became popular for using in dental hard tissues at the end of 1980s, when researchers tested the Er:YAG for ablation of enamel, dentin and caries lesions on extracted teeth (Hibst & Keller, 1989). Since then, several studies have been performed to determine parameters and conditions for a safe and efficient application in daily practice for soft and hard tissue applications (Altshuler et al., 1994; De Moor & Delme, 2010; Eberhard et al., 2005; Fried et al., 1996, 2002; Hibst & Keller, 1989; Moldes et al., 2009; Neves et al., 2010; Stock et al., 1997; White et al., 1994). On the other hand, the popularity of Er,Cr:YSGG laser started later, since the first studies tested the possibility of ablation of dental hard tissues on early 90's. In vitro (Altshuler et al., 1994; Ana et al., 2007; Bachmann et al., 2009; Botta et al., 2011; Dundar & Guzel, 2011; Fried et al., 1996; Moldes et al., 2009; Obeidi et al., 2009; Stock et al., 1997; Tachibana et al., 2008) and in vivo (Yazici et al., 2010; Yilmaz et al., 2011) studies confirmed the feasibility of this wavelength for several applications on dental hard tissues, such as cavity preparation and caries removal.

During cavity preparation, the ablation of sound enamel by Er:YAG laser promotes cavities with rough enamel margins, with irregular and rugged walls, with depth that depends on the energy density and pulse width (Navarro et al., 2010). As well, it is reported the absence of smear layer, cracks, carbonization or melting if the adequate parameters and refrigeration were used (Botta et al., 2009). As Er:YAG, the enamel cavities produced by Er,Cr:YSGG laser irradiation present their floor with fissures and conical craters with sharp enamel projections and, in some areas, with the exposition of the enamel rods. The roughness of cavities is also dependent on the energy densities used (Ana et al., 2007; Olivi et al., 2010; Tachibana et al., 2008).

In sound dentin, due to the differences in composition and morphology, erbium lasers promote a higher removal of peritubular than the intertubular dentin. In this way, both Er:YAG and Er,Cr:YSGG promote the formation of rough surfaces with opened dentinal tubules, absence of smear layer, cracks or melting, with protrusion of peritubular dentin due to its less amount of water when compared to the intertubular dentin (Botta et al., 2009, 2011). The irregularities promoted by laser irradiation vary according to the energy density applied. Considering these facts, the differences in temperature rises at the ablation threshold promoted by Er:YAG and Er,Cr:YSGG seem to be unable to induce significant distinct morphological effects during cavity preparation.

In contrast, the use of high-speed drills for cavity preparation promotes enamel and dentin cavities flattened, with smooth internal walls and geometrically well-defined shapes, with closed dentinal tubules and presence of smear layer (Botta et al., 2009; Navarro et al., 2010). These characteristics, as well as the changes in chemical and crystalline structure in remaining tissue promoted by laser irradiation, must be taken into consideration in order to choose an appropriate adhesive system for composite restoration, since the adhesive systems interact in a different way with laser or bur treated tissues (Moretto et al., 2011).

Erbium lasers are also effective on removal of dental caries. *In vitro* studies revealed that Er:YAG and Er,Cr:YSGG can selectively remove dental caries due to the higher amount of water and organic content when compared to sound tissues (Eberhard et al., 2008; Tachibana et al., 2008); in this way, it is possible to obtain a conservative therapy, with no removal of sound tissue and lack of thermal damages. However, the adjustment of laser energy density in commercial equipments is sometimes difficult to promote the selective ablation of infected dentin and in order to preserve the affected dentin, and the clinical results still depend on the experience and knowledge of the professional, added to the use of manual instruments for correct diagnosis of remaining tissue. In fact, clinical trials report the well acceptance of patients (Dommisch et al., 2008; Krause et al., 2008), the maintenance of pulp vitality and marginal seal, the good quality of restorations and the absence of secondary caries even after two years (Yazici et al., 2010). Also, it is reported that these lasers can fulfill the requirements of Minimal Invasive Dentistry, due to the possibility of conservation of the sound tissue structure during caries removal and to the possibility of surface decontamination of affected dentin (Kornblit et al., 2008).

To determine an end point for caries removal, there are some equipments that associate Er:YAG laser irradiation to the diagnosis by laser fluorescence (Dommisch et al., 2008; Eberhard et al., 2008; Jepsen et al., 2008; Krause et al., 2008;). The essential principle of this application is that the fluorescence of sound tissue differs from the fluorescence of carious tissue due to the variation in chemical composition, such as the presence of proteins, bacteria and other contents. In this equipment, the fluorescence is induced by red laser that emits at the wavelength of 655 nm, and the Er:YAG laser is turned off when significant changes on fluorescence are detected during caries removal, established by a cut-off value that indicates that all decayed tissue was removed. Some *in vitro* (Eberhard et al., 2008; Jepsen et al., 2008) and *in vivo* (Dommisch et al., 2008; Krause et al., 2008) studies showed the feasibility of this equipment; however, there is no consensus about the correct values of cut-off in different clinical conditions. Also, it must be emphasized that there are limitations of this technique mainly in dentin (Eberhard et al., 2008; Krause et al., 2008), when false-positive can be reported due to the presence of pigments in affected or tertiary dentin, for instance, which should not be removed. In this way, the association of manual instruments and is still necessary to assure a safe and correct clinical removal of dental caries.

Clinical trials have demonstrated that Er:YAG and Er,Cr:YSGG lasers can be considered a safe and efficient treatment for caries removal, since it is reported pulpal response and histological effects similar to those obtained by the use of conventional bur. Also, due to the lack of noise, pressure, discomfort and sometimes the necessity of local anesthesia, it is reported a good compliance of patients, mainly the pediatric ones. However, it must be emphasized that the time necessary to remove caries by laser irradiation is almost two or three times longer than the bur treatment, depending on the repetition rate and energy density (Navarro et al., 2010; Yamada et al., 2001). The increase of energy density and repetition rate can lead to discomfort and pain to patients, besides increasing the surface temperatures. For this reason the strategies used for improving the laser ablation speed are limited (Navarro et al., 2010).

4. Influence of pulse width on tissue removal

Although the pulse duration of most commercial lasers (range of μs) is shorter than the thermal relaxation time of dental hard tissues, laser ablation promotes irregular cavities (depending on composition of target tissue), desiccation of the surface (due to the removal of underlying water) and the presence of few microcracks (related to the energy density), the amount of water coolant and the repetition rate must be adjusted during the clinical procedure.

The adjustment of repetition rate is important to assure that the inter-pulse period is longer than the thermal relaxation time of tissues; in this way, it is possible that the temperature of the irradiated tissues decrease between laser pulses (McDonald et al., 2001). Another strategy for cooling the tissue during laser irradiation is reducing the pulse duration (Seka et al., 1995). Depending on the pulse duration (<1 ps), the process of ablation is changed and the non-linear processes (or non-thermal ones) take place (Ana et al., 2006; Freitas et al., 2010; Kruger et al., 2008; McDonald et al., 2001; Niemz, 2004; Strassl et al., 2008).

According to Niemz (1995), lasers with pulse durations in the range of ms (10^{-3} s), μs (10^{-6} s) or ns (10^{-9} s) generate considerable heat during ablation of dental hard tissues, in a mechanism mediated by *thermal interaction*. On the other hand, lasers with pulse durations of ps (10^{-12} s) and fs (10^{-15} s) ablate the tissues by forming an ionizing plasma. These lasers, commonly called as USPL (ultra short pulse lasers), operates at very high repetition rate (larger than 15 kHz) and energy per pulse typically of hundreds of μJ (Wieger et al., 2006).

Although USPLs have extremely higher repetition rate (> KHz) and peak power (up to TW), previous studies relate that a single ultra short laser pulse removes significantly less volume of dental tissue when compared to conventional Er:YAG laser removal (Strassl et al., 2008). This fact occurs due to the differences in focal size and penetration depth of USPLs (which are severely lower when compared to Er:YAG lasers that operate at pulse width of μs); in this way, the pulse repetition rate had to be increased in USPLs to obtain a similar ablation volume than those obtained by Er:YAG (Wieger et al., 2006).

Some literature studies compared the morphological aspects, as well the depth of craters during ablation of dental hard tissues with lasers operating with distinct pulse widths. Niemz (1995) relates that the Nd:YLF laser (λ = 1053 nm) operating with pulse duration of 30 ps provide cavity preparation on sound and decayed enamel without severe thermal or mechanical damages, with negligible shock-wave effects. Also, in the same paper, they showed that the ablation of carious enamel was 10 times more efficient than the ablation of sound enamel. A study performed by McDonald et al. (2001) showed that the total deposited energy on tissue as well the laser pulse duration change the crater depth generated on dentin, and the Nd:YAG with pulse width of 35 ps is unable to promote carbonization of dentin in comparison with a Nd:YAG laser with pulse width of ms.

The heating of dental hard tissues can induce composition and crystallographic changes on these tissues which are dependent on temperature rises. In this way, both morphological aspects and chemical analysis are indicative of thermal effects of lasers on enamel and dentin. A study performed by Kamata et al. (2004) showed that the chemical properties of hydroxyapatite (HAp) are unchanged after ablation with lasers operating with pulse widths of 50 fs, 500 fs and 2 ps. These results suggest that USPLs do not significantly increase the temperature of HAp. On the other hand, the use of Nd:YAG operating with pulse duration of 6 ns and 200 ns on enamel promote melting and recrystallization of this tissue (Antunes et al., 2005), indicating temperature rises up to 1200° C. Also, with the pulse duration of 6 ns, Nd:YAG promoted changes on organic content of enamel and dentin (Antunes et al., 2006).

Thermal measurements were performed using a laser with pulse width of fs on enamel using thermocouples, and it was detected temperature rises about 2° C on enamel surfaces after a 8 ms train of 70 fs pulses (Pike et al., 2007). This fact indicates that the USPLs do not induce significant thermal rises on surfaces and on surrounding tissues and can be used with safety even without refrigeration.

5. The use of Ultra Short Pulse Lasers (USPLs) in dentistry

Even with the higher repetition rates and the application of air-water coolant during the cutting process, commercially high intensity infrared lasers still cannot cut dental hard tissues with the same speed or the same precision than those promoted by drills (White et al., 1994). In this way, studies were performed to verify the possibility of using ultra short pulse lasers (USPLs) for cutting dental hard tissues, considering the success of using the USPL for precise cutting in industry and in medicine (ophthalmology) (Niemz, 2004).

The USPLs were first developed to allow spectroscopic and electrical conductivity measurements (Strickland & Mourou, 1985) and, according to Strassl et al. (2008), studies concerning the use of USPLs for medical applications started more than 15 years ago. In fact, one of the first studies that report the use of lasers with pulse widths of ps and fs was performed by Stern et al. (1989), relating applications for corneal ablation. Since then, efforts were made to understand the effects of these lasers on biological tissues and to develop of practically applicable systems. Although the majority of the studies report the use of laboratorial equipments for biological purposes, nowadays it is possible to find commercially available equipments for ophthalmology and for laboratorial use; this fact indicates that, in a near future, commercial equipments can be available for dentistry applications too.

The USPLs are lasers with pulse duration ranging from 100 fs to 500 ps, with power densities above 10^{11} W/cm^2 in solids (Niemz, 2004). The main characteristics of these complex systems (Freitas et al., 2010) are the very low pulse duration and the high precision that can be acquired due to the extremely small focalization area, in which a peak power up to 1.5 TW (Freitas et al., 2010) can be obtained. Also, these lasers can operate at repetition rates higher than 15 kHz and energy per pulse of hundreds of μJ (Wieger et al., 2006). In this way, these lasers offer the advantage of promoting precise smooth ablation without a heat-affected zone, effects that cannot be controlled when using lasers with pulse duration of μs or ns. Some researchers report that the main advantage of using the USPLs in dentistry is to achieve a controlled material removal and, as a consequence, reducing the pain caused by the vibration and friction heat (Kruger et al., 1999). According to Neev et al. (1996), the main advantages of USPLs are: the decreased energy density to ablate the material; minimal mechanical and thermal damages due to the extremely short laser pulses; minimal dependence of the tissue composition for ablation; precision in the ablation depth; low noise level in comparison with high-speed bur; ability to texture surface and precise spatial control.

The USPLs are solid-state lasers, such as Nd:YLF, Ti:Al$_2$O$_3$, Cr:LiSAF (Alexandrite), Cr:BeAl$_2$O$_4$, Cr:LiSGaF, Cn:LiCAF, Cr:YAG, Ti:Al$_2$O$_3$/Nd:glass, Er:glass. These lasers interact with the tissues by a mechanism called *plasma-induced ablation* or *plasma mediated ablation*, in which the phenomenon of *optical breakdown* occurs. In a few words, the ablation is caused by plasma ionization, in which laser irradiation produces an extremely high electric field that forces the ionization of the molecules and atoms, promoting a breakdown and, then, the ablation or ejection of target tissue (Niemz, 2004). During the cutting, it is possible to observe the formation of a bright plasma spark, and a typical low noise, characteristic of plasma formation.

Considering the strictly short pulse durations and the low energy per pulse in USPLs systems, it is possible to infer that the ablation process is practically not dependent on the wavelength or the composition and absorption characteristics of the tissue (Perry et al., 1999). Also, the removal of ablated material is faster than the heat propagation on the tissue, i.e., the pulse length is lower than the heat conduction time of target tissue (Perry et al., 1999); in this way, there is no transmission of heat to pulp or surrounding tissues, for example, as well, no thermal damages to the irradiated tissues. Other advantage of using USPLs in dentistry is that these systems can remove any kind of restorative material, including amalgam (Freitas et al., 2010), which is not possible using other systems due to the reflection of light or overheating of the material.

Although they are characterized by extremely high peak powers, the USPLs uses lower energy densities when compared to laser with pulse width of μs. The reduction of the energy density is because the femtosecond laser energy densities necessary for micromachining are an order of magnitude lower than those in the nanosecond-laser case for equal wavelength and repetition rate (Kruger et al., 1999).

The ablation of dental hard tissues with USPLs were investigated by Niemz et al. (1995), using a system with pulse length of 30 ps. These authors reported enamel cavities with good precision and absence of thermal damages when compared with cavities performed by lasers operating with pulse length of μs and ns. Further researches confirmed that the application of USPLs with pulse length of few femtoseconds almost completely avoids thermal damages and the formation of microcracks on irradiated tissues and on surrounding ones (Kruger et al., 1999; Freitas et al., 2010). It must be pointed out that lasers that operate with pulse length of μs can generate the formation of microcracks on irradiated tissue depending on the energy density, and these thermal damages can be responsible for the development of secondary caries (Apel et al., 2005).

Other studies were performed to verify the feasibility of removing restorative materials with USPLs, since these lasers can ablate any kind of material. Also, the literature reports the selectivity on removing different materials due to the different nature of interaction of USPLs with dielectric or metal materials, for instance (Freitas et al., 2010). In this way, it is easier to adjust a laser fluence that can be bellow or above the ablation threshold of a specific material. Literature studies determined that the threshold fluence for ablating enamel with USPL is higher than the fluence for ablating dentin and, in the same way that using erbium lasers, it is easier and faster to ablate dentin than enamel, which suggests selectivity to the tissue removal (Lizarelli et al., 2008; Niemz et al., 2004; Strassl et al., 2008; Wieger et al., 2006;). In 2006, Wieger et al. used a picosecond Nd:YVO$_4$ laser for ablation of sound dentin, and it was observed the production of a microretentive pattern with opened tubules and the absence of microcracks or melting. These authors also compared the ablation rate (i.e. the ablation volume per laser pulse) of seven types of composite resins, and showed that the ablation rates of restorative materials are much higher than that measured on dentin, demonstrating that the removal of restorative materials is faster than dental hard tissue. Another study performed by Freitas et al. (2010) determined the ablation threshold fluence for removal of amalgam and composite resin restorations by a femtosecond chirped Ti:sapphire laser. In this work it was also demonstrated the selectivity of USPLs in the material removal process suggesting a selective preparation, preserving health tooth structure.

Concerning the removal of dental caries, literature studies reported that the threshold fluence for carious dentin is lower than that for sound dentin, also suggesting a selective removal of caries (Niemz, 2004). A recent study (Schelle et al., 2011) that used a Nd:YAG laser with 8 ps pulse duration confirm that the ablation threshold for carious dentin is lower than that for sound dentin and it was obtained good precision even when removing caries. These findings suggest that the USPLs are promising tools for selective removal of dental caries; however, the literature is scarce considering the applications of USPLs for selective removal of dental caries in order to establish suitable equipments and parameters. Also, there are no studies that relate the possibility of selective removal of infected dentin and preserving the affected dentin, for instance.

Although it is reported the possibility of precise removal of tissue with USPLs, it should be pointed out that the time required for a cavity preparation with USPLs is higher than the time required when using a laser with pulse duration of μs or a drill, even with the higher repetition rate of the available systems (Kruger et al., 1999). Although there is some commercially available equipment for ophthalmology, the application of USPLs in dentistry for cavity preparation and caries removal is not yet a routine technique, and the cost and complexity of systems still represent a problem to be solved.

6. Adhesion to caries affected dentine

Carious lesions have different characteristics depending on diverse factors such as host, diet, period of time and injury severity. Controversial results can be observed in the literature of adhesion to caries-affected dentine. While some studies claim that the bond strength obtained in caries affected dentine is similar to the attained in sound tissue (Mobarak et al., 2010; Zanchi et al., 2011; Zawaideh et al., 2011), other researchers detected lower bond strength when adhesives were applied on caries affected dentine (Kunawarote et al., 2011; Marquesan et al., 2009; Perdigão, 2010). Basically, these diverse results can be due to the use of natural carious human molars to compose the sample. Although some studies use artificial caries affected dentine (Zanchi et al., 2011) results are still controversial. Also, using natural carious substrate in experimental studies can induce results with high variability; consequently, they do not allow direct comparison between studies.

Bonding to standard artificially obtained caries affected laser irradiated dentine could not be detected in literature. The following figures present the differences observed in caries affected dentin irradiated by distinct types of lasers. Also, a comparison between these surfaces and the sound ones is essential, because adhesive systems were developed to interact with smear layer covered dentine.

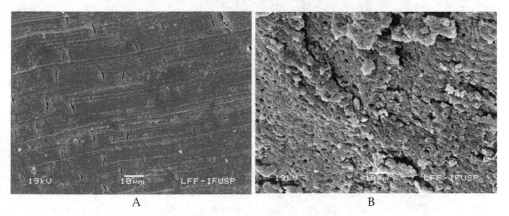

A   B

Fig. 3. Scanning electron micrographs of sound (A) and carious (B) human dentine. A-Typical smear layer image, with clear indication of tubules apertures position by the presence of microcracks, suggesting a thin smear layer; B - Presence of biofilm on dentine surface, areas with exposed open tubules, while other regions are considered free of debris. Original magnification: A = 1000 X; B = 500 X.

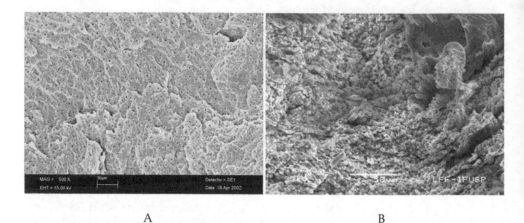

A   B

Fig. 4. Scanning electron micrographs of sound (A) and carious (B) human dentin after irradiation with Er:YAG laser (λ = 2940 nm, pulse width of 400 μs, beam diameter of 1 mm, repetition rate of 10 Hz). A - sound dentin. Typical Er:YAG laser ablation where we can see open dentinal tubules in a irregular dentinal surface ; B - when carious dentin is irradiated the surface is absolutely irregular, completely covered by debris and biofilm, indicating that carious tissue remains on the surface. Original magnification: 500 X.

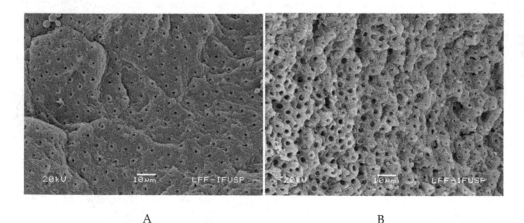

A   B

Fig. 5. Scanning electron micrographs of sound (A) and carious (B) human dentin after irradiation with a Er,Cr:YSGG laser (λ = 2078 nm, pulsed width of 140 μs, repetition rate of 20 Hz, beam diameter of 750 μm). A - As sound dentin is irradiated by Er,Cr:YSGG laser an irregular dentinal surface is created by the ablation process. Dentinal tubules are open and peritubular dentine can be easily detected around all dentinal tubules; B - Carious irradiated dentin still presents open dentinal tubules, but are larger in diameter and filled with debris from the carious tissue. Note that these features are completely distinct from the irradiation by Er:YAG laser. Original magnification: 1000 X.

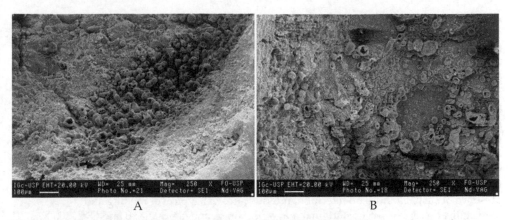

Fig. 6. Scanning electron micrographs of sound (A) and carious (B) human dentin after irradiation with a Nd:YAG laser (λ = 1064 nm, pulse width of 100 μs, repetition rate of 20 Hz, beam diameter of 300 μs). A - When sound dentin is irradiated by Nd:YAG laser melting and carbonization can be detected covering all the irradiated area, no dentinal tubules can be observed; B - Carious Nd:YAG irradiated dentin also presents melting and carbonization areas, very similar to the sound irradiated dentine. Original magnification: 250 X.

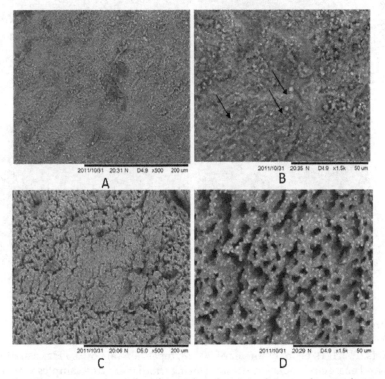

Fig. 7. Scanning electron micrographs of sound and carious human dentin after irradiation with a Nd:YAG (λ = 1064 nm), operating at pulse width of 5 ns, beam diameter of 900 μm,

repetition rate of 20 Hz, scanning speed of 2 mm/s, energy per pulse of 280 mJ and energy density of 0.44 J/cm². During irradiations, the samples were positioned and moved with a linear translation stage with 10 μm resolution, and it was performed 10 scans. In A, after irradiation on sound dentin, it is possible to evidence fully occlusion of dentinal tubules. In B, a higher magnification of image A, the presence of fine globules and glazed areas (arrows), typical of melting and recrystallization of tissue can be detected. It is not observed the presence of smear layer or any signal of carbonization and cracks. In C a representative image of carious dentin after irradiation is showed, and the presence of an irregular tissue, with some projections of dentinal tubules and absence of biofilm and smear layer is evidenced. It is not observed thermal damages such as cracks or carbonization of tissue. Some areas present dentinal tubules completely opened, while other areas present closed dentinal tubules. In D, a higher magnification of image C, dentinal tubules are completely opened and the presence of small globules on intertubular tissue (arrows), typical of melting and recrystalization are observed. Original magnification: A and C = 500 X; B and D = 1500 X.

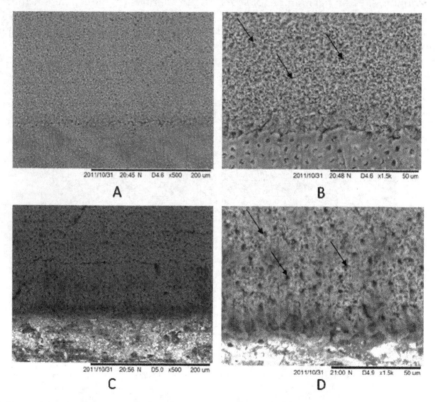

Fig. 8. Scanning electron micrographs of sound (A and B) and carious (C and D) human dentin after irradiation with a Ti:sapphire laser (Ti:Al₂O₃, λ = 830 nm), operating at pulse width of 40 fs (FWHM), beam diameter of 20 μm, repetition rate of 100 Hz, scanning speed of 5 mm/s and energy per pulse of 104 mJ. During irradiations, the samples were positioned and moved with a linear translation stage with 10 μm resolution, and it was performed 10 scans. In A, it is possible to evidence the ablation of sound dentin (upper), with a regular

edge with non irradiated dentin (bottom). It is observed a clear and uniform ablation, with absence of cracks, melting or carbonization. As well, it is not observed the presence of projections or conical craters, indicating that the laser interaction with sound dentin is not influenced by the composition or the presence of dentinal tubules. In B, it is showed a higher magnification of the same image, evidencing the ablation of sound dentin (upper), in contrast with non irradiated dentin (bottom). It is also noted the presence of opened dentinal tubules (arrows), and absence of smear layer. In C, it is observed a clear and uniform ablation of carious dentin, with the creation of a regular ablated surface and absence of cracks, melting or carbonization. In D, it is showed a higher magnification of image C, showing that the biofilm was removed and it was exposed the openings of dentinal tubules (arrows). It is also observed the higher depth and the precise edge of ablated area, indicating that it was removed a higher amount of carious tissue when compared to sound dentin irradiation. Original magnification: A and C = 500 X; B and D = 1500 X.

Based on the figures presented above, we can conclude that it is fundamental to investigate bond strength to irradiated caries-affected dentine, which is a clinically relevant tissue, as lasers are a contemporaneous tool in daily clinical practice. In this way, it is obvious that the performance of the adhesive systems is different when applied in irradiated dentin. To obtain a long lasting clinical result, specific adhesive systems should be developed to be used in irradiated dental surfaces, especially in caries-affected dentine.

Methods of inducing artificial caries lesions have been used to standardize the decayed substrate for laboratory testing. Cariology studies using artificial caries lesions have been performed to assess preventive effect of fluoride agents, test methods of caries removal and adhesion on caries affected dentine.

Some in vitro caries models have been reported. In the chemical method, the acidified gel technique and pH-cycling method are included; in contrast, microorganism strains with known cariogenicity are used in the microbiological method in a way whereby the acid from bacterial metabolism demineralizes the dental structure (Steiner-Oliveira et al., 2011). More elaborate systems involving chemostats, flowcells, artificial mouths, and constant-depth film fermenter have been developed in an attempt to better mimic the environment of the oral cavity. However, their high cost and complex apparatus requirements are often limiting factors (Gilmour et al., 1990).

Some authors believe that the bacterial model is the closest to the conditions found in vivo (Gilmour et al., 1990). The steps of an example of a microbiological method are described, as follows. Initially, the dental specimens need to be sterilized with gamma ray irradiation (25 KGy) since the teeth should be free of microorganisms. A microorganism strain with known cariogenicity, for example, Streptococcus mutans ATCC 25175 or UA159 must be incubated in Tryptic Soy Broth (TSB) media supplemented with 5% sucrose to obtain bacterial growth. After growth, the colonies will be transferred into tubes containing TSB (with 5% sucrose) to initiate microorganism preconditioning. The dental specimen should be immersed in a solution (TSB with 5% sucrose and a quantity of the inoculums broth) and will be maintained therein for at least 7 days, being transferred to a fresh solution every 24 h. During the incubation periods, tests should be performed to check for the presence of bacterial contaminants with the use of a solid culture medium (Tryptic Soy Agar – TSA)(Azevedo et al., 2011).

Caries-affected substrate obtained in vitro by the microbiological method significantly contributes to the field of adhesion, because it will allow laboratory tests to be performed on standard caries-affected dentine, which is a clinically relevant substrate. The microbiological method allows the production of artificial caries-affected dentine effectively induced for 7 days and demineralization depth is standardized and it is confirmed by optical coherence tomography (OCT) (Azevedo et al., 2011). Efforts have been made to produce artificial caries-affected dentine and bond strength studies must be conducted, especially in laser irradiated tissues, to associate the use of laser to remove caries and long lasting clinical treatments.

7. Conclusion

This chapter presented laser technology as an alternative to caries removal, attending the conservative principals of dentistry, assuring that minimally invasive procedures can be used to treat caries lesions.

8. Acknowledgement

The authors would like to thank to Dr. Wagner de Rossi, Dr. Marcus Paulo Raele, Prof Moises O. Santos, Leandro Matiolli Machado and Prof. Carolina Benetti for their kind assistance during irradiations; and also to Prof. Dr. Alessandra Pereira de Andrade for her assistance with figures management. Authors also wish to thank FAPESP (#2010/10126-3) for partially supporting the project of writing this book chapter.

9. References

Altshuler, G.B., Belikov, A.V. & Erofeev, A.V. (1994). Laser treatment of enamel and dentin by different er-lasers. Proceedings of SPIE, Vol. 2128, pp. 273-281, Los Angeles, CA, Jan 1994.

Ana, P.A., Bachmann, L. & Zezell, D.M. (2006) Lasers effects on enamel for caries prevention. *Laser Physics*, Vol.16, No.5, pp. 865-75.

Ana, P.A., Blay, A., Miyakawa, W. & Zezell, D.M. (2007) Thermal analysis of teeth irradiated with Er,Cr:YSGG at low fluences. *Laser Physics Letters*, Vol.4, No.11, pp.827-834.

Antunes, A., de Rossi, W. & Zezell, D.M. (2006) Spectroscopic alterations on enamel and dentin after nanosecond Nd:YAG laser irradiation. *Spectrochim Acta A Mol Biomol Spectroscopy*, Vol.64, No.5, pp.1142-6.

Antunes, A., Vianna, S.S., Gomes, A.S.L., de Rossi, W. & Zezell, D.M. (2005). Surface morphology, elemental distribution, and spectroscopic changes subsequent the application of nanosecond pulsed Nd:YAG laser on dental enamel surface. *Laser Physics Letters*, Vol.2, No.3, pp.141-147.

Apel. C., Meister, J., Gotz, H., Duschner, H. & Gutknecht, N. (2005). Structural changes in human dental enamel after subablative erbium laser irradiation and its potential use for caries prevention. *Caries Research*, Vol.39, pp. 65-70.

Azevedo, C.S., Trung, L.C.E., Simionato, M.R.L., Freitas, A.Z.F. & Matos, A.B. (2011). Evaluation of caries-affected dentin with optical coherence tomography. Brazilian Oral Research. Vol. 25, No.5, pp.407-13.

Bachmann, L., Craievich, A.F. & Zezell, D.M. (2004). Crystalline structure of dental enamel after Ho:YLF laser irradiation. Archives of Oral Biology, Vol.49, No.11, pp.923-9.

Bachmann, L., Rosa, K.,, Ana, P.A., Zezell, D.M., Craievich, A.F. & Kellermann, G. (2009). Crystalline structure of human enamel irradiatedwith Er,Cr:YSGG laser. *Laser Physics Letters*, Vol.6, No.2, pp.159-162.

Benedicenti, S., Cassanelli, C., Signore, A, Ravera, G. & Angiero, F. (2008) Decontamination of root canals with the gallium-aluminum-arsenide laser: an in vitro study. *Photomedicine and Laser Surgery*, Vol.26, No.4, pp.367-70.

Boari, H.G.D., Ana, P.A., Eduardo, C.P., Powell, G.L. & Zezell, D.M. (2009). Absorption and thermal study of dental enamel when irradiated with Nd:YAG laser with the aim of caries prevention. *Laser Physics*, Vol.19, No.7, pp.1463-1469.

Botta, S.B., Ana, P.A., de Sa Teixeira, F., da Silveira Salvadori, M.C. & Matos, A.B. (2011) Relationship between surface topography and energy density distribution of Er,Cr:YSGG beam on irradiated dentin: an atomic force microscopy study. *Photomedicine and Laser Surgery*, Vol.29, No.4, pp.261-9.

Botta, S.B., Ana, P.A., Zezell, D.M., Powers, J.M. & Matos, A.B. (2009) Adhesion after erbium, chromium:yttrium-scandium-gallium-garnet laser application at three different irradiation conditions. *Lasers in Medical Science*, Vol.24, No.1, pp.67-73.

Botta, S.B., Vieira, S.N., Cordon, R., Marques, M.M. & Matos, A.B. (2009) Can the method of primer application influence adhesion to Er:YAG-laser irradiated dentin? *Journal of Contemporary Dental Practice*. Vol.10, No.1, pp.49-57.

De Moor, R.J. & Delme, K.I. (2010). Laser-assisted cavity preparation and adhesion to erbium-lased tooth structure: part 2. present-day adhesion to erbium-lased tooth structure in permanent teeth. *Journal of Adhesive Dentistry*, Vol.12, No.2, pp.91-102.

Dommisch, H., Peus, K., Kneist, S., Krause, F., Braun, A., Hedderich, J., Jepsen, S. & Eberhard, J. (2008) Fluorescence-controlled Er:YAG laser for caries removal in permanent teeth: a randomized clinical trial. *European Journal of Oral Science*, Vol.116, No.2, pp.170-6.

Dundar, B. & Guzel, K.G. (2011) An analysis of the shear strength of the bond between enamel and porcelain laminate veneers with different etching systems: acid and Er,Cr:YSGG laser separately and combined. *Lasers in Medical Science*. Vol.26, No.6, pp.777-82.

Eberhard, J., Bode, K., Hedderich, J. & Jepsen, S. (2008) Cavity size difference after caries removal by a fluorescence-controlled Er:YAG laser and by conventional bur treatment. *Clinical Oral Investigations*. Vol.12, No.4, pp.311-8.

Eberhard, J., Eisenbeiss, A.K., Braun, A., Hedderich, J. & Jepsen, S. (2005) Evaluation of selective caries removal by a fluorescence feedback-controlled Er:YAG laser in vitro. *Caries Research*. Vol.39, No.6, pp.496-504.

Featherstone, J.D.B. (2000) The science and practice of caries prevention. *Journal of the American Dental Association.* 131(7): 887-899.

Freitas, A.Z., Freschi, L.R., Samad, R.E., Zezell, D.M., Gouw-Soares, S.C. & Vieira ND. (2010) Determination of ablation threshold for composite resins and amalgam irradiated with femtosecond laser pulses. *Laser Physics Letters.* Vol. 7, No.3, pp.236-241.

Fried, D. (2000) IR laser ablation of dental enamel. Lasers in dentistry VI. Proceedings of SPIE, Vol. 1, No.4, pp. 136-148, San Jose, CA, Jan 2000.

Fried, D., Ashouri, N., Breunig, T. & Shori, R. (2002) Mechanism of water augmentation during IR laser ablation of dental enamel. *Lasers in Surgery and Medicine.* Vol.31, No.3, pp.186-93.

Fried, D., Featherstone, J.D.B., Visuri, S.R., Seka, W. & Walsh, J.T. The caries inhibition potential of Er:YAG and Er:YSGG laser radiation. Lasers in dentistry II, Proceedings of SPIE, Vol. 2672, pp.73-78, San Jose, CA, Jan 1996.

Gilmour, A.S.M, Edmunds, D.G. & Dummer, P.M.H. (1990) The production of secondary caries-like lesions on cavity walls and the assessment of microleakage using an in vitro microbial caries system. *Journal of Oral Rehabilitation.* Vol.17, No.6, p.573-8.

Gwinnett, AJ. (1992) Structure and composition of enamel. *Operative Dentistry.* Vol. 5, pp. 10-17.

Hibst, R. & Keller, U. (1989) Experimental studies of the application of the Er:YAG laser on dental hard substances: I. Measurement of the ablation rate. *Lasers in Surgery and Medicine.* Vol.9, No.4, pp.338-44.

Jepsen, S., Açil, Y., Peschel, T., Kargas, K. & Eberhard, J. (2008) Biochemical and morphological analysis of dentin following selective caries removal with a fluorescence-controlled Er:YAG laser. *Lasers in Surgery and Medicine.* Vol.40, No.5, pp.350-7.

Kamata, M., Imahoko, T., Ozono, K. & Obara, M. (2004). Materials processing by use of a Ti : Sapphire laser with automatically-adjustable pulse duration. *Applied Physics A-Materials Science & Processing.* Vol. 79, No. 7, pp.1679-1685.

Koba, K., Kimura, Y., Matsumoto, K., Takeuchi, T., Ikarugi, T. & Shimizu, T. (1998) A histopathological study of the morphological changes at the apical seat and in the periapical region after irradiation with a pulsed Nd:YAG laser. *International Endodontic Journal.* Vol.31, No.6, pp.415-20.

Kornblit, R., Trapani, D., Bossù, M., Muller-Bolla, M., Rocca, J.P. & Polimeni, A. (2008) The use of Erbium:YAG laser for caries removal in paediatric patients following Minimally Invasive Dentistry concepts. *European Journal of Paediatric Dentistry.* Vol.9, No.2, pp.81-7.

Krause, F., Braun, A., Lotz, G., Kneist, S., Jepsen, S. & Eberhard, J. (2008). Evaluation of selective caries removal in deciduous teeth by a fluorescence feedback-controlled Er:YAG laser in vivo. Clinical *Oral Investigations.* Vol. 12, No.3, pp.209-15.

Kruger, J., Kautek, W. & Newesely, H. (1999). Femtosecond-pulse laser ablation of dental hydroxyapatite and single-crystalline fluoroapatite. *Applied physics A-material science procedure.* Vol.69, pp.S403-S407.

Kunawarote, S., Nakajima, M., Foxton, R.M. & Tagami, J. (2011) Effect of pretreatment with mildly acidic hypochlorous acid on adhesion to caries-affected dentin using a self-etch adhesive. *European Journal of Oral Science*. Vol. 119, pp.86–92.

Lang-Bicudo, L., Eduardo, F.P., Eduardo, C.P. & Zezell, D.M. (2008) LED phototherapy to prevent mucositis: a case report. *Photomedicine and Laser Surgery*. Vol.26, No.6, pp.609-13.

Lizarelli, R.F.Z., Costa, M.M., Carvalho-Filho, E., Nunes, F.D. & Bagnato, V.S. (2008). Selective ablation of dental enamel and dentin using femtosecond laser pulses. *Laser Physics Letters*, Vol. 5, No.1, pp.63-69.

Marquezan, M., Corrêa, F.N.P., Sanabe, M.E., Filho, L.E.R., Hebling, J. & Guedes Pinto A.C. (2009) Artificial methods of dentine caries induction: A hardness and morphological comparative study. Archives of Oral Biology. Vol.54, No.12, pp.1111-7.

McDonald, A., Claffey, N., Pearson, G., Blau, W. & Setchell, D. (2001). The effect of Nd:YAG pulse duration on dentine crater depth. *Journal of Dentistry*. Vol.29, No.1, pp.43-53.

Mobarak, E.H., El-Korashy, D.I. & Pashley, D.H. (2010). Effect of Chlorhexidine concentrations on micro-shear bond strength of self-etch adhesive to normal and caries-affected dentin. *American Journal of Dentistry*. Vol.23, No.4, pp.217-222.

Moldes, V.L., Capp, C.I., Navarro, R.S., Matos, A.B., Youssef, M.N. & Cassoni, A. (2009) In vitro microleakage of composite restorations prepared by Er:YAG/Er,Cr:YSGG lasers and conventional drills associated with two adhesive systems. *Journal of Adhesive Dentistry*, Vol. 11, No.3, pp.221-229.

Moretto, S.G., Azambuja Jr., N., Arana-Chavez, V.E., Reis, A.F., Giannini, M., Eduardo C.P. & De Freitas, P.M. (2011). Effects of ultramorphological changes on adhesion to lased dentin-Scanning electron microscopy and transmission electron microscopy analysis. *Microscopy Research and Technique*. Vol.74, No.8, pp.720-6.

Nammour, S., Rocca, J.P., Pireaux, J.J., Powell, G.L., Morciaux, Y. & Demortier, G. (2005) Increase of enamel fluoride retention by low fluence argon laser beam: a 6-month follow-up study in vivo. *Lasers in Surgery and Medicine*. Vol.36, No.3, pp.220-4.

Nammour, S., Zeinoun, T., Bogaerts, I., Lamy, M., Geerts, S.O., Bou Saba, S., Lamard, L., Peremans, A. & Limme, M. (2010). Evaluation of dental pulp temperature rise during photo-activated decontamination (PAD) of caries: an in vitro study. *Lasers in Medical Science*. Vol.25, No.5, pp.651-4.

Navarro, R.S., Gouw-Soares, S., Cassoni, A., Haypek, P., Zezell, D.M. & Eduardo, C.P. (2010). The influence of erbium:yttrium-aluminum-garnet laser ablation with variable pulse width on morphology and microleakage of composite restorations. *Lasers in Medical Science*. Vol.25, No.6, pp.881-9.

Neev, J., Da Silva, L.B., Feit, M.D., Perry, M.D., Rubenchik, A.M. & Stuart, B.C. (1996) Ultrashort pulse lasers for hard tissue ablation. *Eee Journal of Selected Topics in Quantum Electronics*. Vol.2., No.4, pp. 790-800.

Neves, A.A., Coutinho, E., De Munck, J. & Van Meerbeek B. (2010). Caries-removal effectiveness and minimal-invasiveness potential of caries-excavation techniques: a micro-CT investigation. *Journal of Dentistry*. Vol.39, No.2, pp.154-62.

Niemz M.H. (1995). Cavity preparation with the Nd:YLF picosecond laser. *Journal of Dental Research*. Vol.74, No.5, pp.1194-9.

Niemz, M.H. (2004). Laser-tissue interactions – fundamentals and applications. Springer-Verlang, ISBN 3-540-40553-4, Leipzig, Germany.

Obeidi, A., McCracken, M.S., Liu, P.R., Litaker, M.S., Beck, P. & Rahemtulla, F. (2009) Enhancement of bonding to enamel and dentin prepared by Er,Cr:YSGG laser. *Lasers Surgery and Medicine*. Vol.41, No.6, p.454-62.

Olivi, G., Angiero, F., Benedicenti, S., Iaria, G., Signore, A. & Kaitsas, V. (2010) Use of the erbium, chromium:yttrium-scandium-gallium-garnet laser on human enamel tissues. Influence of the air-water spray on the laser-tissue interaction: scanning electron microscope evaluations. *Lasers in Medical Science*. Vol.25, No.6, pp.793-7.

Perdigão, J. (2010). Dentin bonding—Variables related to the clinical situation and the substrate treatment. *Dental Materials*. Vol. 26, No.2, pp.e24-e37.

Perry, M.D., Stuart, B.C., Banks, P.S., Feit, M.D., Yanovsky, V. & Rubenchik, A. M. (1999) Ultrashort-pulse laser machining of dielectric materials. *Journal of Applied Physics*. Vol.85, No.9, pp.6803-10.

Pike, P., Parigger, C., Splinter, R. & Lockhart, P. (2007). Temperature distribution in dental tissue after interaction with femtosecond laser pulses. *Applied Optics*. Vol.46, No.34, pp.8374-8378.

Rechmann, P., Fried, D., Le, C.Q., Nelson, G., Rapozo-Hilo, M., Rechmann, B.M. & Featherstone, J.D. (2011). Caries inhibition in vital teeth using 9.6-μm CO_2-laser irradiation. *Journal of Biomedical Optics*. Vol.16, No.7, pp.071405.

Schelle, F., Engelbach, C., Brede, O., Braun, A., Frentzen, M. (2011). Ablation of caries using an ultra short pulsed laser system. *Journal of Dental Research*. Vol. 90, Spec Issue B: abstract 722.

Seka, W., Featherstone, J.D.B., Fried, D., Visuri, S.R. & Walsh JT. (1996) Laser ablation of dental hard tissue: From explosive ablation to plasma-mediated ablation. Lasers in Dentistry, Proceedings of SPIE, Vol. 2672, pp. 144-158, Los Angeles, CA, Jan 1996.

Seka,W., Fried, D., Featherstone, JDB. (1995). Light deposition in dental hard tissue and simulated thermal response. *Journal of Dental Research*. Vol.74, pp.1086-92.

Serbin, J., Bauer, T., Fallnich, C., Kasenbacher, A. & Arnold, W.H. (2002). Femtosecond lasers as novel tool in dental surgery. *Applied Surface Science*. Vol.197, pp. 737-740.

Sperandio, F.F., Meneguzzo, D.T., Ferreira, L.S., Ana, P.A., Azevedo, L.H. & Sousa, S.C. (2011) Different air-water spray regulations affect the healing of Er,Cr:YSGG laser incisions. *Lasers in Medical Science*. Vol.26, No.2, pp.257-65.

Steiner-Oliveira, C., Rodrigues, L.K.A., Zanin, I.C.J., de Carvalho, C.L., Kamiya, R.U., Hara, A.T. et al. (2011). An in vitro microbial model associated with sucrose to produce dentin caries lesions. *Cent European Journal Biology*. Vol. 6, No.3, pp.414:21.

Stern, R.H. & Sognnaes, R.F. (1964). Laser beam effect on dental hard tissue. *Journal of Dental Research.* Vol. 43, No.5, pp. 873.

Stern, D., Puliafito, C.A., Dobi, E.T., Reidy, W.T. (1989). Corneal ablation by nanosecond, picosecond and femtosecond lasers at 532 nm and 625 nm. *Archives of Ophthalmology.* Vol.107, pp.587- 592.

Stock, M., Hibst, R. & Keller, U. (1997). Comparison of Er:YAG and Er:YSGG laser ablation of dental hard tissues. Proceedings of SPIE. Vol. 3192, pp. 88-95, Los Angeles, CA, Jan 1997.

Strassl, M., Wieger, V., Brodoceanu, D., Beer, F., Moritz, A. & Wintner, E. (2008). Ultra-Short Pulse Laser Ablation of Biological Hard Tissue and Biocompatibles. *Journal of Laser Micro Nanoengineering.* Vol.3, No.1, pp.30-40.

Strickland, P. & Mourou, G. (1985) Compression of amplified chirped optical pulses. *Optics Community.* Vol. 56, pp. 219.

Tachibana, A., Marques, M.M., Soler, J.M. & Matos, A.B. (2008). Erbium, chromium:yttrium scandium gallium garnet laser for caries removal: influence on bonding of a self-etching adhesive system. *Lasers in Medical Science.* Vol.23, No.4, pp.435-41.

White, J.M., Goodis, H.E., Hennings, D., Ho, W. & Hipona, C.T. (1994). Dentin ablation rate using Nd:YAG and Er:YAG lasers. *Journal of Dental Research.* Vol. 73, abs 1733, pp.318.

White, J.M., Goodis, H.E., Setcos, J.C., Eakle, S., Hulscher, B.E. & Rose, C.L. (1993). Effects of pulsed Nd:YAG laser energy on human teeth: a three-year follow-up study. *Journal of the American Dental Association.* Vol.124, No.7, pp.45-51.

Wieger, V., Strassl, M. & Wintner, E. (2006). Pico- and microsecond laser ablation of dental restorative materials. *Laser and Particle Beams.* Vol. 24, pp.41-45.

Yamada, Y., Hossain, M., Nakamura, Y., Suzuki, N. & Matsumoto, K. (2001). Comparison between the removal effect of mechanical, Nd:YAG, and Er:YAG laser systems in carious dentin. *Journal of Clinical Laser Medicine Surgery.* Vol.19, No.5, pp.239-43.

Yazici, A.R., Baseren, M. &, Gorucu, J. (2010). Clinical comparison of bur- and laser-prepared minimally invasive occlusal resin composite restorations: two-year follow-up. *Operative Dentistry.* Vol.35, No.5, pp.500-7.

Yilmaz, H.G., Kurtulmus-Yilmaz, S., Cengiz, E., Bayindir, H. & Aykac, Y. (2011).Clinical evaluation of Er,Cr:YSGG and GaAlAs laser therapy for treating dentine hypersensitivity: A randomized controlled clinical trial. *Journal of Dentistry.* Vol.39, No.3, pp.249-54.

Zanchi, C.H., Lund, R.G., Perrone, L.R., Ribeiro, G.A., Del Pino, F.A.B., Pinto, M.B. & Demarco FF. (2011). Microtensile bond strength of two-step etch-and-rinse adhesive systems on sound and artificial caries-affected dentin. *American Journal of Dentistry.* Vol. 23, No.3, pp.152-6.

Zawaideh, F., Palamara, J.E.A., Messer, L.B. (2011). Bonding of resin composite to caries-affected dentin after Carisolv® treatment. *Pediatric Dentistry.* Vol. 33, No.3, pp.213-220.

Zezell, D.M., Boari, H.G., Ana, P.A., Eduardo, C.P. & Powell, GL. (2009) Nd:YAG laser in caries prevention: a clinical trial. *Lasers Surgery and Medicine.* Vol.41, No.1, pp.31-5.

Zijp, J.R. & Bosch, J.J. (1993). Theoretical model for the scattering of light by dentin and comparison with measurements. *Applied Optics*. Vol.32, No.4, pp.411-5.

Part 3

Dental Caries in Children

9

Caries Incidence in School Children Included in a Caries Preventive Program: A Longitudinal Study

Laura Emma Rodríguez-Vilchis, Rosalía Contreras-Bulnes,
Felipe González-Solano, Judith Arjona-Serrano,
María del Rocío Soto-Mendieta and Blanca Silvia González-López
Centro de Investigación y Estudios Avanzados en Odontología,
Facultad de Odontología de la Universidad Autónoma del Estado de México
México

1. Introduction

Several epidemiological studies (Okawa, et al., 1992; Marthaler & O'Mullane, 1996; Beltrán-Aguilar, et al. 1999; Vrbič, 1996; Brown, et al., 2000; Carvalho, et al., 2001; Estupiñan-Day, et al., 2001; Bönecker, et al., 2003) on dental caries experience in children and adolescents have been carried out around the world for the last three decades. Most of the reports agree that caries has been reduced, and these data have been confirmed by the Global Data Bank of the World Health Organization; however, the distribution and severity of dental caries varies in different parts of the world and within the same region or country.

Caries decline has been observed in children and adolescents from industrialized countries while those living in some less developed countries show a tending to increase. The reported caries reduction is the result of a number of public health measures, coupled with changing living conditions, lifestyles and improved self-care practices. (Petersen, et al., 2005)

It has been shown that schools provide an important setting for promoting health. (Kwan, et al., 2005) In Mexico, a school-based caries preventive program was established in the 1970's in the State of Mexico as a pioneer program. This program is focused on oral health education and mouth rinse (0.2% NaF) twice a month; however, there are no previous reports that assess the impact of this local program on dental caries prevention. It is assumed that caries will be reduced.

The aim of this study was to evaluate annually the impact of a school-based caries preventive program on the dental status and caries incidence, in Mexican schoolchildren within a three year period.

2. Dental caries

There is now extensive knowledge about the etiology, prevention, diagnostic and treatment of dental caries. Regarding the etiology, the role of bacteria in the production of acid by fermenting carbohydrates causes the decrease in pH, with the subsequent loss of tooth minerals. The preventive measures include: diet and plaque control (mechanical and chemical methods), use of fluorides (systemic and topical), pit and fissure sealants (Harris & García-Godoy, 1999; Featherstone, 2000; Axelsson, 2000, 2004; Gussy, et al., 2006). Furthermore, strategies to control the disease through risk assessment have been developed, which have also been extensively investigated (Vanobbergen, et al., 2001; Pearce, et al., 2002; Bratthall & Hänsel Petersson, 2005; Featherstone, et al., 2007; Ramos-Gomez, et al., 2010; Gao, et al., 2010). On the other hand, the advance of technology has also developed tools for the proper diagnosis of the lesion incipient such as DIAGNOdent and QLF (Stookey, 2004; Berg, 2007; Trænæus, et al., 2007) as well as the need to detect in epidemiological studies noncavitated lesions (Ismail, et al., 2007). In the treatment of lesion there is a large amount of literature, resources and works focused on prevention of the formation of cavities. Despite all the existing measures for caries control there are no populations free of dental caries in the world.

3. Trends in dental caries

Caries epidemiology continues to be an important issue in both oral health surveillance and research into refined methods for caries diagnosis (Marthaler, 2004). The changing on caries disease patterns throughout the world are closely linked to number of public health measures, including effective use of fluorides, together with changing living conditions, lifestyles and improved self- care practices (Petersen, et al., 2005).

In Europe and specifically in Western Europe the decline in caries prevalence has been very substantial. It has not received much attention until recently but is now often taken for granted. However, caries prevalence is still very different when looking at various parts of Europe, and may undergo unexpected changes due to various factors. Increasing immigration has been identified as a new factor, leading to increases of the overall dental caries prevalence in Switzerland (20% non-Swiss residents), the Netherlands and Germany (Marthaler, 2004). Furthermore, there has been a decline in caries prevalence between 1993 and 2003 in all age groups apart from 3-year-old Sweden children (Jacobsson, et al., 2011).

As levels of oral disease decreased in the 1980s and 1990s, the oral health of children and adults in the UK has been improving steadily since the 1970s. The average number of decayed missing and filled permanent teeth (DMFT; a measure of the severity of caries attack in the permanent dentition) at 12 years fell rapidly in the 1980s and has since shown a further steady decline. This has been matched by an increase in the proportion of children who have no evidence of decay. Thus by 2009, only 33% of 12-year-old children had a mean DMFT>0 (a measure of caries prevalence) and the average decay experience was 0.74 DMFT. Nonetheless, those children with treated or untreated dental caries had, on average, 2.21 DMFT and the care index, which is the proportion of that decay which is filled, was only 47%. In addition there was a marked geographic gradient with the north of England showing higher levels of decay than the south of England. For 5-year-olds there has been an overall decline in the average level of dental disease and an increase in the proportion of children who are decay-free, but the change is less pronounced. Over 20 years, the average number of decayed, missing and filled primary teeth has fallen from 1.80 in 1983 to 1.55 in 2004 (Drugan & Downer, 2011).

On the other hand in the United States of America the caries continues to decline in the permanent dentition for many children but is increasing among poor non-Hispanic whites aged 6–8 years (8–22%) and poor Mexican-Americans aged 9–11 years (38–55%). Although dental caries in older children continues to decline or remain unchanged, increasing tooth decay among some young children is a concern. Moreover, it is also troublesome that paediatric caries appears to be disproportionately affecting young boys compared with girls considering that here has not been a difference in prevalence of caries between boys and girls observed in national surveys prior to NHANES 1999-2004. Although the increasing prevalence of dental caries appears to be occurring in some of our traditionally 'low-risk' groups such as the nonpoor, primary caries is also increasing in a small number of 'high-risk' groups as well. Our findings suggest that future caries research should be expanded towards better understanding of not only the factors that promote paediatric dental caries among traditionally high-risk children, but also among those once considered low-risk for tooth decay (Dye, et al., 2010).

The prevalence of dental caries in primary teeth of children aged 2–4 years increased from 18% in 1988-1994 to 24% in 1999-2004. Racial disparities persisted in that age group, with caries significantly more prevalent among non-Hispanic black and Mexican American children than among non-Hispanic white children. Caries prevalence in primary teeth of non-Hispanic white children aged 6–8 years remained unchanged, but increased among non-Hispanic black and Mexican American children. State-specific prevalence of caries among third-graders ranged from 40.6% to 72.2%. Caries in permanent teeth declined among children and adolescents, while the prevalence of dental sealants increased significantly. State oral health programs' funding and staffing remained modest, although the proportion of states with sealant programs increased 75% in 2000 to 85% in 2007 and the proportion with fluoride varnish programs increased from 13% to 53% (Tomar & Reeves, 2009).

For most Americans, oral health status has improved since 1988–1994. Dental caries continues to decrease in the permanent dentition for youths, adolescents, and most adults. Among seniors, the prevalence of root caries decreased, but there was no change in the prevalence of coronal caries. However, the prevalence of dental caries in the primary dentition for youths aged 2–5 years increased from 1988–1994 to 1999–2004. The prevalence of dental sealants among youths and adolescents increased. Tooth retention and periodontal health improved for both adults and seniors, and edentulism among seniors continued to decline. Dental utilization (experiencing a dental visit within the past 12 months) remained unchanged between 1988–1994 and 1999–2004 for youths, adolescents, and seniors; however, dental utilization declined for most adults (Dye, et al., 2007).

According to the World Health Organization the dental caries is still a major public health problem in most industrialized countries, affecting 60–90% of schoolchildren and the vast majority of adults. It is also a most prevalent oral disease in several Asian and Latin American countries while it appears to be less common and less severe in most African countries. Currently, the disease level is high in the Americas but relatively low in Africa. In light of changing living conditions; however, it is expected that the incidence of dental caries will increase in the near future in many developing countries in Africa, particularly as a result of growing consumption of sugars and inadequate exposure to fluorides (Petersen, 2003).

Whelton estimated that changes in the progression of caries have been problematic due to the shortage of longitudinal data in the literature for children, adolescents, and young and older adults. The cohort effect, combined with sampling effects and diagnostic differences, confounds the investigation of the true changes in caries progression with time. The elucidation of the age-related pattern and rate of caries development in successive age cohorts will be important in informing future clinical trial design. In summary, the changes in caries patterns which have an impact on the design of caries clinical trials are:

- the lower caries incidence in children,
- the relatively greater effect of fluorides in preventing caries on approximal surfaces;
- the slower rate of progression of caries,
- the increased risk of primary caries in adults, and
- the increased use of fissure sealants.

These changes indicate that caries continues to be a challenge throughout life. The conduct of clinical trials of caries-preventive agents must now incorporate more sensitive diagnostic methods capable of valid and reliable measurement of caries initiation and progression in its early stages. The application of sophisticated statistical analysis which takes account of the pattern of caries attack will also help to overcome the difficulties posed by these changes in caries patterns. The application of such techniques to dental datasets which have large numbers of tooth-surface variables and multiple observations has been made possible by the increasing capacity of and accessibility to high-speed computers (Whelton, 2004).

4. Fluorides

Fluoride as a caries-preventive agent was discovered as the side effect of fluorosis in teeth in areas with elevated levels of fluoride in the drinking water (Ten Cate, 2004). Research on the oral health effects of fluoride started around 100 years ago. For the first 50 years or so it focused on the link between water borne fluoride – both natural and artificial – and dental caries and fluorosis (Petersen, et al., 2004). It was difficult to determine small (sub-ppm) concentrations of fluoride in drinking water. Nevertheless, the early studies on fluoridation of the drinking water were convincing and initiatives were taken to add various types of fluorides to other oral hygiene products (Ten Cate, 2004). In the second half of the 20thcentury, fluoride research was focused on the development and evaluation of fluoride toothpastes and rinses and, to a lesser extent, alternatives to water fluoridation such as salt and milk fluoridation.

Fluoride mouthrinses were commonly used in school-based programs with 0.2% NaF solution weekly or fortnightly during the 1960's-1980's, but have now, to great extent, been withdrawn since most children are using fluoride toothpaste. The effect of the rinsing programs was in the range of 20-40% caries reduction (Koch & Poulsen, 2006).

The first test of a fluoride mouthrinse was conducted in the 1940s. An acidified NaF mouthrinse used three times a week, for 1 year by dental students failed to achieve a significant caries reduction, possibly because of very low fluoride concentrations. Fluoride mouthrinse received little attention until the early 1960s, when the effect was extensively evaluated in well-controlled clinical studies as well as in field trials on schoolchildren in Scandinavia, particularly in Sweden. Most of these studies and programs were based on weekly supervised rising with a neutral 0.2% NaF solution.

Drinking water is not fluoridated in Sweden, and during the early 1960s effective fluoride toothpaste had not yet become available. In addition, the standard of oral hygiene was very low. Few schoolchildren cleaned their teeth every day. Therefore, caries prevalence among children was very high, and most children developed several new caries lesions every year. Under these conditions, the introduction of a simple preventive measure, supervised rinsing with 0.2% NaF solutions once a week, resulted in very significant caries reductions (25% to 40%) (Axelsson, 2004).

Several efforts have been made to summarize these extensive data sets through systematic reviews, such as those conducted on water fluoridation by the UK University of York Centre for Reviews and Dissemination; on fluoride ingestion and bone fractures; and on fluoride toothpastes and rinses through the Cochrane Collaboration Oral Health Group. These systematic reviews concluded that:

1. Water fluoridation reduces the prevalence of dental caries (% with dmft /DMFT > 0) by 15% and in absolute terms by 2.2 dmft/DMFT.
2. Fluoride toothpastes and mouth rinses reduce the DMFS 3-year increment by 24–26%.
3. There is no credible evidence that water fluoridation is associated with any adverse health effects.
4. At certain concentrations of fluoride, water fluoridation is associated with an increased risk of unaesthetic dental fluorosis although further analysis suggested that the risk might be substantially greater in naturally fluoridated areas and less in artificially fluoridated areas.
5. There was a paucity of research into any possible adverse effects of fluoride toothpastes and rinses.

Although these findings are important, it must be acknowledged that a lack of fluoride does not cause dental caries (Petersen, et al., 2004).

Not all fluoride agents and treatments are equal. Different fluoride compounds, different vehicles, and vastly different concentrations have been used with different frequencies and durations of application. These variables can influence the clinical outcome with respect to caries prevention and management. The efficacy of topical fluoride in caries prevention depends on a) the concentration of fluoride used, b) the frequency and duration of application, and, to a certain extent, c) the specific fluoride compound used. The more concentrated the fluoride and the greater the frequency of application, the greater the caries reduction (Newbrum, 2001).

In recent years, an increasing number of reports have been published in which the observed caries- preventive effect of fluoride has been lower than could have been expected on the basis of the earlier literature. This is true for both systemic and topical methods such as water fluoridation, fluoridated school milk, fluoride mouthrinses and professional applications of topical fluoride including fluoride varnish applications. The current low levels of caries occurrence and the wide spread use of fluoridated toothpastes as well as other fluoride products and methods have been suggested as reasons for the reduced relative effect of water fluoridation. In the same way, the fact that people are today commonly exposed to fluoride from multiple sources is likely to dilute the effect of fluoride from any single source. The moderate usefulness of added fluoride exposure at the population level today may also be due to the fact that individually applicable fluoride regimes are most likely to reach people who least need them. The individuals whose dental health-related lifestyles are most unfavorable and who are not visiting a dentist regularly are likely to be least exposed to fluoride, and it is not easy to provide them with any individual protection against caries. The advantage of community water fluoridation is that it reaches even the least advantaged segments of the population. If the risk for caries is high, however, water fluoridation alone cannot provide full protection against the onset of cavities (Hausen, 2004).

The WHO report is quite clear that the post-eruptive effect of sugar consumption is one of the main etiological factors for dental caries and notes in particular the damaging effects of:

1. Refined or processed foods in general.
2. The consumption of sugary soft drinks.
3. Children going to bed with a bottle of a sweetened drink or drinking at will from a bottle during the day.

A WHO/FAO analysis of the evidence on the role of diet in chronic disease recommends that free (added) sugars should remain below 10% of energy intake and the consumption of foods/drinks containing free sugars should be limited to a maximum of four times per day. For countries with high consumption levels it is recommended that national health authorities and decision-makers formulate country-specific and community-specific goals for reduction of consumption of free sugars. However, WHO also notes that many countries currently undergoing nutrition transition do not have adequate fluoride exposure. It is the responsibility of national health authorities to ensure implementation of feasible fluoride programs for their country.

First, it is clear that all countries and communities should advocate a diet low in sugars in accordance with the WHO/FAO recommendations. This has been emphasized most recently in May 2004 at the World Health Assembly by the confirmation of the WHO Global Strategy on Diet, Physical Activity and Health. Secondly, countries with excessive levels of fluoride ingestion, particularly where there is a risk of severe dental fluorosis or of skeletal fluorosis, should maintain a maximum fluoride level of 1.5 mg/l as recommended by WHO Water Quality Guidelines, although this objective is admittedly not always technically easy to achieve. Thirdly, where sugar consumption is high or increasing, the caries-preventive effects of fluorides need to be enhanced.

WHO recommends that every effort must be made to develop affordable fluoride toothpastes for use in developing countries. As a public health measure, it would be in the interest of countries to exempt these toothpastes from the duties and taxation imposed on cosmetics (Petersen, et al., 2004).

Twetman reported strong evidence for a caries-preventive effect of daily use of fluoride toothpaste compared with placebo in the young permanent dentition (PF, 24.9%), that toothpastes containing 1500 ppm of fluoride had a superior preventive effect (additional PF, 9.7%) compared with standard dentifrices of 1000 ppm of fluoride. Also, strong evidence for higher caries reductions with supervised toothbrushing compared with unsupervised brushing was founded. There was incomplete evidence regarding the effect of fluoride toothpaste in the primary dentition. This systematic review reinforces the importance of daily toothbrushing with fluoridated toothpastes for preventing dental caries, although long-term studies in age groups other than children and adolescents are still lacking (Twetman, et al., 2003).

Water fluoridation, where technically feasible and culturally acceptable, has substantial advantages particularly for subgroups at high risk of caries. Alternatively, fluoridated salt, which retains consumer choice, can also be recommended. WHO is currently in the process of developing guidelines for milk fluoridation programs, based on experiences from community trials carried out in both developed and developing countries (Petersen, et al., 2004).

The proposal of salt as a vehicle for fluoride in caries prevention is attributed to Wespi (1948, 1950). In the mid-1950s, domestic salt supplemented by potassium fluoride, up to 90 mg/kg, became available in various cantons of Switzerland.

The first 5-years results following consumption of fluoride-rich domestic salt were published by Marthaler and Schenardi (1962). The documented caries reduction of 32% fewer DMFSs in the permanent teeth of 7-to 9-year-old children was not statistically significant. Only with the subsequent caries data that became available from studies in Colombia (250 mg F/kg as NaF), and Hungary (250 mg F/kg as NaF) was it shown that fluoride-induced caries reductions could reach 50%.

A prerequisite was the availability of domestic salt with a high fluoride concentration. The state of knowledge on the subject, up to the mid-1970s, was summarized by Marthaler (1978). The conclusions were that fluoride ingested via salt prevents dental caries in man, the cariostatic effect being similar to water fluoridation: The fluoride content of salt is adjusted so that urinary fluoride excretion levels are similar to those in areas with optimal water fluoride content (Axelsson, 2004).

Based on the successful results of caries prevention obtained by salt fluoridation program in Switzerland, Hungary, Colombia and other countries, fluoride has been added to the table salt in Mexico from the late 1980s. The Mexican Sanitary Norm indicated that a concentration of 250 mg F/kg of salt should be added. Irigoyen (Irigoyen & Sanchez Hinojosa, 2000) reported that the caries prevalence and the treatment needs experienced in the State of Mexico population have decreased over the last decade. However, dental health is far from optimal, and the state has not achieved the low caries index observed in many developed countries. It is necessary to continue the work with caries prevention programs and to improve access to dental care services. Since there is a National Salt Fluoridation Program already established, no additional systemic sources of fluoride should be implemented; nevertheless, to continue the promotion of the use of fluoridated dentifrices, fluoride rinses and gels, fissure sealants and health education activities could be benefit to the population's oral health status.

Recent literature has revealed instances where a considerable reduction of the level of preventive efforts has not been followed by an increase in caries frequency and vice versa. This must have been due to the fact that the studied preventive methods, that had proved to be effective elsewhere, were not effective and efficient in those particular settings. Since conditions strongly determine the usefulness of caries prevention including different fluoride regimes, more research is still needed to monitor the effectiveness of caries-preventive programs and their components in variable conditions of today and tomorrow (Hausen, 2004).

5. Dental programs for caries prevention

Oral Health is fundamental to general health and well-being. A healthy mouth enables and individual to speak, eat and socialize without experiencing active disease, discomfort or embarrassments. Children who suffer from poor oral health are 12 times more likely to have restricted-activity days than those who do not. More than 50 million school hours are lost annually because of oral health problems which affect children´s performance at school and success in later life (Kawan, et al., 2005).

Basically, erupting teeth are healthy. The first carious lesion and the first restoration in a tooth means the start of series of treatments that during the tooth's lifetime will end up in more and more complicated restorations or treatments if the caries process is not controlled. Today there is enough scientific knowledge about factors that might interfere in this process in order to develop preventive strategies. Operative treatment per se will never control caries. (Koch & Poulsen, 2006).

Minimal intervention is a key phrase in today´s dental practice. Minimal intervention dentistry (MID) focuses on the least invasive treatment options possible in order to minimize tissue loss and patient discomfort. Concentrating mainly on prevention and early intervention of caries, MID´s first basic principle is the remineralization of early carious lesions, advocating a biological or therapeutic approach rather than traditional surgical approach for early surface lesions. One of the key elements of a biological approach is the usage and application of remineralizing agents to tooth structure (enamel and dentin lesions). These agents are part of a new era of dentistry aimed at controlling the demineralization/remineralization cycle, depending upon the microenvironment around the tooth (Rao & Malhotra, 2011).

School provide man effective platform for promoting oral health because they reach over 1 billion children worldwide. The health and well-being of school staff, families and community members can also be enhanced by programs based in schools. Oral health messages can be reinforced throughout the school years, which are the most influential stages of children's lives, and during which lifelong beliefs, attitudes and skill are developed (Kwan, et al., 2005).

After caries decline of about 80% in children in Western Europe and other industrialized countries, there should be a critical debate about the best way for future caries prevention (Splieth, et al., 2004).

In Europe and Asia, positive results have come from implementing supervised toothbrushing programs in kindergartens and providing free fluoridated toothpaste to high risk children from underprivileged and multicultural groups. Furthermore, a comprehensive staged dental health program and professional fluoride varnish applications proved the possibility of a reduction in early childhood caries in vulnerable groups (Wennhall, et al., 2008).

Multiple fluoride use played an important role in caries reductions achieved in the 1980s and 1990s, but it also resulted in a polarization of lesion distribution in young people: the majority consists of low caries or even lesion-free individuals, while a minority is a so-called high caries risk group which seems not to be open to preventive programs. Last decade studies indicate that frequent fluoride applications (>6 times/year) in conjunction with effective plaque removal can be a successful approach for effective future caries prevention in high caries risk groups. Health promotion programs that are merely educational and do not provide fluoride do not seem to be effective. Alternatively, preventive measures could be performed at home or in a private practice, but only minimal compliance is reached in high risk groups compared with out-reaching group programs. Thus, group programs are instrumental in providing effective and efficient caries-preventive measures in children. The more expensive time of a dental practice team should be limited to procedures where costly equipment is needed (professional tooth cleaning, sealants, etc.). For efficient caries prevention, measures formerly targeted specifically at either populations, groups, or individuals should be remodeled and aimed to interact in order to achieve optimal oral health in children at a reasonable cost (Splieth, et al., 2004).

School dental screening is a popular public health intervention in many countries throughout the world. In the United Kingdom, school dental screening is a statutory function of local National Health Service (NHS) bodies and has been a feature of children's dental services for the past hundred years (Education Act, 1918).

The process involves a visual dental examination of children in the school setting to identify the presence of dental disease and conditions; parents of children who are screened positive are informed and encouraged to take their child to primary care services for further investigation. The WHO has recently endorsed dental screening of children in the school setting, stating that, "Screening of teeth and mouth enables early detection, and timely interventions towards oral diseases and conditions, leading to substantial cost savings. It plays an important role in the planning and provision of school oral health services as well as health services." Due to the long history of school dental screening in the UK, the aims of this cluster-randomized controlled trial conducted in the UK failed to show that the intervention used in a national school dental screening program significantly reduces active dental caries levels or increases dental attendance rates at the public health level. Milsom, et al. reported that school dental screening delivered according to 3 different models in the northwest of England children aged 6-9 years derived little benefit in terms of attending the dentist, and receiving treatment for their carious permanent teeth. The current method of school dental screening is no longer tenable, alternative ways to ensure that vulnerable children receive adequate dental care need to be explored (Milsom, et al., 2006).

Oral health education program in Belgian primary schoolchildren has been effective in improving reported dietary habits and the proper use of topical fluorides and resulted in a higher care index.

The implemented yearly based extra oral health promotional program did not result in a significant reduction of caries prevalence. The effectiveness on plaque level and gingival health was inconclusive. However, the favorable reported behavioral changes and the increased restoration level together with the educational responsibility of the profession justify the efforts and costs of this program (Vanobbergen, et al., 2004).

In the same way, supervised daily toothbrushing using fluoridate toothpaste in schools and intensive oral hygiene instructions sessions program was successful in controlling dental caries in children, as reported by Al-Jundi, et al. in a school-based caries preventive program in children from Jordan over a period of 4 years (Al-Jundi, et al., 2006).

The evaluation of caries incidence after 7.5 years of follow-up, in an infant population under a dental health preventive program in Mostoles (Madrid), which consisted of preventive measures included health education, a weekly mouth rinse using sodium fluoride (NaFl) at 0·2% concentration, fissure sealants to first permanent molars and topical application of fluoride gel, showed that the preventive program had been effective and had a clear protective effect on permanent teeth (Tapias, et al., 2001).

The six months evaluation of a comprehensive preventive care from dental hygienists implemented in children at six Massachusetts elementary schools, grades 1 through 3, with pupil populations at high risk of developing caries indicates that this care model relatively quickly can overcome multiple barriers to care and improve children's oral health. If widely implemented, comprehensive caries prevention programs could accomplish national health goals and reduce the need for new care providers and clinics.

To increase access to care, improve oral health and reduce disparities in oral health care for children, treatments must be safe, effective, efficient, personalized, timely and equitable. This program can be implemented locally and can reduce the incidence of dental caries in school-aged children (Niederman, et al., 2008).

Sealants application programs have been suggested as an effective measurement for caries prevention. Khurshid reported that preventive oral health care as measured by the presence of dental sealants can significantly reduce the occurrence of dental caries in Hispanic children in underserved areas such as the US–Mexico border in Texas. The study confirms the strong effect of low house hold income and lack of health insurance in increasing the likelihood of dental caries in children. The old adage that prevention is better than cure applies to dental health as much as to any other public health issue (Khurshid, 2010).

6. Dental programs in Mexico

In Mexico, a school-based caries preventive program was established in the 1970's in the State of Mexico; it was a pioneer program, and later in 1988 the program of salt fluoridation was implemented for the first time as a pilot program in the state. The program was carried out with technical support from the Pan American Health Organization (PAHO) and financial from W.K. Kellogg. Then, the salt fluoridation program is positioned as a nation-wide policy in 1992. Because in the country there are five states and other municipalities with concentrations of fluoride in drinking water above the optimum amount, steps were taken to prevent consumption in these regions.

The preventive educational program developed in preschool and primary school nationwide currently includes various activities, constituted in the "basic scheme of oral health" prevention that consists of 14 applications of sodium fluoride 0.2%, 4 detections of plaque, 4 brushing technique instructions, 4 flossing instructions (from 8 years old) and 4 educational talks. All the activities are developed in every school year; in addition, there is a curative care program that is not always free.

Great efforts have been made for the abatement of oral diseases of highest incidence and prevalence and major achievements have been accomplished, but it is necessary to strengthen the activities implemented with the purpose to achieve caries-free communities program so the action 2001-2006 oral health includes in its coverage of 4 to 15 years of age (Secretaria de Salud, 2011).

In Mexico State, the coverage of preventive educational program is around 75%, yet there are limited healing care facilities for school children; only a few dental schools have these services available, and many times children are channeled to public institutions' clinics. The Autonomous University of Mexico State is involved in the implementation of the program as part of the training curriculum for students with some adjustments in regard to the educational component, and all other activities are performed according to the provisions of the educational program-including preventive fluoride 14 applications per year. This chapter includes the results of the incidence of caries within a 3 years follow-up of certain schools under the care of the University.

7. Study design

The present study is a 3-year longitudinal analysis of a school-based caries prevention program. The study protocol was reviewed and approved by the Research and Ethics Committee of Autonomous University of the State of Mexico (UAEM from its initials in Spanish). The inclusion criteria were children without orthodontic treatment and all children whose parents signed an informed consent form prior to the examinations. The sample was selected by a convenience non-probability sampling method, and included 145 schoolchildren (66 boys and 79 girls), 6-7 years of age, who attended from the first to the third school year in four public elementary schools at Toluca city, where the School of Dentistry of the Autonomous University of the State of Mexico is responsible for the implementation of the program. The program included 20 minute sessions of oral health education for children and teachers (five per school year), and parents (one per school year). The curriculum included information about caries etiology and prevention (oral hygiene, diet counseling, fluorides, pit and fissures sealants), 0.2% NaF mouth rinse (fourteen per school year), toothbrushing technique instructions (four per school year), flossing instructions in children up to 8 years old, and disclosing solution application (four per school year).

To motivate the children, oral health educational material was designed and adapted to their chronological age, using a puppet theater among other resources. The oral examination was performed on site (public elementary schools) in daylight conditions by two examiners, who used a dental mirror and a WHO/CPITN-type E probe (World Health Organization, 1997). No radiographs were taken. To ensure satisfactory inter-examiner reproducibility, the examiners were calibrated twice a week during the six months previous to the start of sampling (Kappa 0.95) by examining the same group of people and comparing their findings.

The oral health of children was evaluated by using deft/s and DMFT/S index. A tooth or surface was considered carious (D) if there was visible evidence of a cavity, including untreated dental caries and filled teeth with recurrent caries. The M component included missing teeth and / or decayed teeth with indication for extraction due to caries, or teeth missing as a result of caries. The F component was filled teeth; the sum of the three figures forms the DMFT/S-value. For primary dentition, deft/s index was used, where e indicates extracted teeth. Cumulative incidence was expressed as the proportion of new children with caries over the 3 years period. For caries incidence data were collected on DMFT and deft recording forms. Information to the parents about the oral health status of the children was provided by means of an advice/referral letter.

7.1 Statistical analysis

All data were analyzed using the SPSS 13.0 statistical package for Windows (SPSS Inc., Chicago, IL, USA). The measurements were analyzed using Kolmogorov-Smirnov test at a (p ≤ 0.05) level of significance to assess distribution of data. The measurements were analyzed using Wilcoxon test was used with a level of significance of p ≤ 0.05.

8. Results

The mean age of the 145 children at the baseline was 6.5 years old, while during final examination was 9.5 years old. After 3 years follow up mean dmf/s and DMFT/S (Table I). DMFT scores showed increased 0.1 a 0.9 with differences statistically significantly. The percentage of caries-free children is showed in Table 2. At the be beginning of the study 93% of the children was caries-free for permanent teeth, decreasing to 57% while only 17% was healthy in both dentitions at the end of the study. Cumulative incidence was 0.39.

Year	dmft Mean (SD)	dmfs Mean (SD)	DMFT Mean (SD)	DMFS Mean (SD)
2007	4.2 (3.8)[A]	10.2 (12.1)[AB]	0.1 (0.4)[A]	0.1 (0.5)[A]
2008	4.2 (3.2)[A]	10.3 (10.4)[A]	0.5 (1.0)[B]	0.6 (1.5)[B]
2009	3.8 (2.9)[B]	9.3 (9.20)[B]	0.7 (1.2)[C]	0.9 (1.7)[C]
2010	2.8 (2.4)[C]	6.3 (6.60)[C]	0.9 (1.3)[D]	1.4 (2.2)[D]

* Groups with different letters are significantly different (p ≤ 0.05).

Table 1. Caries experience of the study population in a three-year long follow up

Year	dmft≠0 no.	dmft≠0 %	dmft=0 no.	dmft=0 %	DMFT≠0 no.	DMFT≠0 %	DMFT=0 no.	DMFT=0 %	dmft=0 DMFT=0 no.	dmft=0 DMFT=0 %
2007	111	77	34	23	10	7	135	93	34	23
2008	116	80	29	20	36	25	109	75	27	19
2009	118	81	27	19	51	35	94	65	24	17
2010	110	76	35	24	63	63	82	57	25	17

Table 2. Percentage of children with caries and caries-free for dentition

Period	Caries-free permanent teeth	New decay permanent teeth	Cumulative Incidence
2007-2008	765	51	0.07
2008-2009	1403	37	0.03
2009-2010	1698	31	0.02

Table 3. Caries incidence changes from first to third year for study group

9. Conclusion

According to 1999-2004 survey in the United States, the mean dfs for children 2-8 years was 3.7, although for 6-11 years of age was 4.30 and 1.84 for dft. The same study reported 51.17% caries prevalence in primary dentition for 6-11 years old children. However, caries experience for permanent teeth was 21% while DFS index was 0.65. Additionally, a prevalence of 10.16%, 0.19 DFT and 0.29 DFS were reported in children from 6 to 8 years old (Dye, et al., 2010; National Institute of Dental and Craniofacial Research, 2011).

In 2004, 5 years-old children in the United Kingdom showed a 1.55 dmft, later in 2009, 33% from 12-years-old children had a mean DMFT>0 and the decay experience average was 0.74, showing that the proportion of children without decay has risen to 61% (Drugan & Downer, 2011).

Reports from Värmland, Sweden indicate that 76% of 6 years-old children are caries free in primary dentition, while 7,8,9 and 10 years old children were 98%, 96%, 94% and 92% caries free for permanent dentition, respectively. (Axelson, 2004). In Europe, some reports have indicated a 79-93% dmfs or DMFS, or equal to zero (Marthaler, et al., 2004)

In 2001, caries prevalence in Chinese children aged 5-6 years was 78 -86%, and dmft was 4.8 - 7.0. A lower prevalence of caries was reported (41-42%) in 12 years old children, and a 0.9% DMFT, according to WHO criteria (Wong, et al., 2001).

The results of this study, showed a high caries prevalence and also higher dmft, dmfs, DMFT and DMFS index compared with well developed countries such as United States, United Kingdom, Sweden and other countries in Europe, but similar to those in China.

It seems that the efforts to diminish dental caries through the evaluated preventive and educational program have do not had the expected impact though these children are under salt fluoridation program. It is necessary to reconsider the implementation of additional measures according to caries risk group as has been reported previously, as well as to evaluate the cost and the effectiveness of mouthwashes.

10. Acknowledgment

This study was financially supported by the Universidad Autónoma del Estado de Mexico. The authors would like to thank the staff of the three primary schools for their kind collaboration during the data collection.

11. References

Al-Jundi, S.H., Hammad, M. & Alwaeli, H. (2006). The efficacy of a school-based caries preventive program: a 4-year study. *International Journal of Dental Hygiene*, 4, 1, 30-4.

Axelsson, P. *Diagnosis and risk prediction of dental caries.* (2000). Quintessence, ISBN 0-86715-362-8, Germany.

Axelsson, P. *Preventive materials , methods and programs.* (2004). Quintessence, ISBN 0- 86715-364-4, Slovakia.

Beltrán-Aguilar, E.D., Estupiñán-Day, S. & Báez R. (1999). Analysis of prevalence and trends of dental caries in the Americas between the 1970s and 1990s. *International Dental Journal*, 49, 322-329.

Berg, J.H. (2007). Dental caries detection and caries management by risk assessment. *Journal Esthetic Restorative Dentistry*. 19, 1, 49-55.

Bönecker, M., & Cleaton-Jones, P. (2003). Trends in dental caries in Latin American and Caribbean 5-6 and 11-13-year-old children: a systematic review. *Community Dentistry and Oral Epidemiology*, 31, 152-7.

Bratthall, D. & Hänsel Petersson, G. (2005). Cariogram – a multifactorial risk assessment model for a multifactorial disease. *Community Dentistry and Oral Epidemiology*, 33, 4, 256–64.

Brown, L.J., Wall, T.P., & Lazar, V. (2000). Trends in total caries experience: permanent and primary teeth. *Journal of the American Dental Association*, 131, 223-231.

Carvalho, J.C., Van Nieuwenhuysen, J.P., & D'Hoore, W. (2001). The decline in dental caries among Belgian children between 1983 and 1998. *Community Dentistry and Oral Epidemiology*, 29, 55-61.

Drugan, C.S. & Downer, M.C. (2011). Dental health in the United Kingdom and influencing variables. *Bundesgesundheitsblatt Gesundheitsforschung Gesundheitsschutz*, 54, 9, 1027-34.

Dye, B.A., Tan, S., Smith, V., Lewis, B.G., Baker L.k., Thornton-Evan, G., Eke P.I., Beltran-Aguilar, E., Horowitz, A.M. & Li, C-H. (2007). Trends in oral health status: United States, 1988–1994 and 1999–2004. *Vital Health Statistics*, 11, 248, 1-92.

Dye, B.A., Arevalo, O. & Vargas, C.M. (2010). Trends in paediatric dental caries by poverty status in the United States, 1988–1994 and 1999–2004. *International Journal of Paediatric Dentistry*, 20, 132-143.

Estupiñan-Day, S.R., Baez, R., Horowitz, H., Warpeha, R., Sutherland, B. & Thamer M. (2001). Salt fluoration and dental caries in Jamaica. *Community Dentistry and Oral Epidemiology*, 29, 247-52.

Featherstone, J.D. (2000). The science and practice of caries prevention. *Journal of the American Dental Association*, 131, 7, 887-99.

Featherstone, J.D., Domejean-Orliaguet, S., Jenson, L., Wolff, M. & Young, D.A. (2007). Caries risk assessment in practice for age 6 through adult. *Journal of the California Dental Association*, 35, 10, 703-713.

Gao, X.L., Hsu, C.Y., Xu, Y., Hwarng, H.B., Loh, T. & Koh, D. (2010). Building caries risk assessment models for children. *Journal of Dental Research*, 89, 6, 637-43.

Gussy, M.G., Waters, E.G., Walsh, O. & Kilpatrick, N.M. (2006). Early childhood caries: current evidence for aetiology and prevention. *Journal of Paediatrics Child Health*, 42, 1-2, 37-43.

Harris, N.O. & García-Godoy F. *Primary preventive dentistry*. (1999). 5 th. Appleton & Lange, ISBN 0-8385-8129-3, USA, 41-47, 279-285.

Hausen, H. (2004). How to improve the effectiveness of caries-preventive programs based on fluoride. *Caries Research*, 38, 3, 263-7.

Irigoyen, M.E. & Sánchez-Hinojosa, G. (2000). Changes in dental caries prevalence in 12-year-old students in the State of Mexico after 9 years of salt fluoridation. *Caries Research*, 34, 4, 303-7.

Ismail, A.I., Sohn, W., Tellez, M., Amaya, A., Sen, A., Hasson, H. & Pitts, N.B. (2007). The International Caries Detection and Assessment System (ICDAS): an integrated system for measuring dental caries, *Community Dentistry and Oral Epidemiology*, 35, 170–178

Jacobsson, B., Koch, G., Magnusson, T. & Hugoson, A. (2011). Oral health in young individuals with foreign and Swedish backgrounds-a ten-year perspective. *European Archives of Paediatric Dentistry*, 12, 3, 151-8.

Khurshid, A. (2010). Effectiveness of preventive oral health care in Hispanic children living near US–Mexico border. *International Journal of Public Health*, 55, 291–298.

Koch, G. & Poulsen, S. (2006). *Pediatric dentistry-a clinical approach*. Blackwell, ISBN 10-87-16-12271-2, Denmark ,119, 134.

Kwan, S.Y.L., Petersen, P.E., Pine, C.M. & Borutta, A. (2005). Health-promoting schools: an opportunity for oral health promotion. *Bulletin of the World Health Organization*, 83, 9, 677-65.

Marthaler, T.M. & O'Mullane, D.M. (1996). The prevalence of dental caries in Europe 1990-1995. Symposium Report. *Caries Research*, 30, 237-255.

Marthaler, T.M. Changes in dental caries 1953–2003. (2004). Caries Research, 38, 173-181.

Milsom, K., Blinkhorn, A., Worthington, H., Threlfall,A., Buchanan, K., Kearney-Mitchell P. & Tickle, M. (2006). Effectiveness of school dental screening: a cluster-randomized control trial. *Journal of Dental Research*, 85, 10, 924-928.

National Institute of Dental and Craniofacial Research (NIDCR). (2011). Dental Caries (Tooth Decay) in Children (Age 2 to 11) Data Source: The National Health and Nutrition Examination Survey (NHANES) (collected between 1999 and 2004) data regarding dental caries in children. Available from: http://www.nidcr.nih.gov/DataStatistics/FindDataByTopic/DentalCaries/DentalCariesChildren2to11 Link

Newbrum, E. (2001). Topical fluorides in caries prevention and management: a North American perspective. Journal of Dental Education, 2001, 65, 10, 1078-83.

Niederman, R., Gould, E., Soncini, J., Tavares, M. Osborn, V. & Goodson, M. (2008). A model for extending the reach of the program traditional dental practice: the forsythkids *Journal of the American Dental Association*, 139, 1040-1050.

Okawa, Y., Takahashi, Y., Sazuka, J., Matsukubo, T. & Takaesu, Y. (1992). Decline in caries prevalence in 6-14-year-old schoolchildren during 1975-85 in Shizouka, Japan. *Community Dentistry and Oral Epidemiology*, 20, 246-9.

Pearce, E.I.F., Dong, Y-M., Yue, L., Gao, X-J., Purdie, G.L. & Wang J-D. (2002). Plaque minerals in the prediction of caries activity. Community Dentistry and Oral Epidemiology, 30, 61–9.

Petersen, PE. (2003). The World Oral Health Report 2003: continuous improvement of oral health in the 21st century-the approach of the Who Global Oral Health Programme. *Community Dent Oral Epidemiology*, 31, 3-23.

Petersen, P.E., & Lennon, MA. (2004). Effective use of fluorides for the prevention of dental caries in the 21st century: the WHO approach. *Community Dentistry and Oral Epidemiology*, 32, 319–21.

Petersen, P.E., Bourgeois, D., Ogawa, H., Estupinan-Day, S. & Ndiaye C. (2005). The global burder of oral diseases and risks to oral health. *Bulletin of the World Health Organization*, 83, 9, 661-9.

Ramos-Gomez, F., Crystal, Y.O., Ng, M.W., Tinanoff, N., & Featherstone, J.D. (2010). Caries risk assessment, prevention, and management in pediatric dental care. *General Dentistry*, 58, 6, 505-17.

Rao, A. & Malhotra, N. (2011). The role of remineralizing agents in dentistry: a review. *Compendium of Continuing Education in Dentistry*, 32, 6, 26-33.

Secretaria de Salud y Subsecretaria de Prevención y Protección a la Salud. (2001). *Programa de Acción: Salud Bucal*. ISBN 968-811 999-7, México, 7-45.

Splieth, C.H., Nourallah, A.W. &, König, K.G.(2004). Caries prevention programs for groups: out of fashion or up to date? *Clinical Oral Investigations*, 8, 1, 6-10.

Stookey, G.K. (2004). Optical methods-quantitative light fluorescence. *Journal of Dental Research*, 83 Spec No C:C 84-8.

Tapias, M.A., De Miguel, G, Jiménez-Garcia R, González A, Dominguez V. (2001). Incidence of caries in an infant population in Mostoles, Madrid. Evaluation of a preventive program after 7.5 years of follow-up. *International Journal of Paediatric Dentistry*, 11, 6, 440-6.

Ten Cate, J.M. (2004). Fluorides in caries prevention and control: empiricism or science. *Caries Research*, 38, 3, 254-7.

Tomar, S.L. & Reeves, A. F. (2009). Changes in the oral health of US children and adolescents and dental public health infrastructure since the release of the healthy people 2010 objectives. *Academic Pediatrics*, 9, 388-95.

Tranaeus, S, Shi., X-Q. & Angmar-Månsson B. (2005).Caries risk assessment: methods available to clinicians for caries detection. *Community Dentistry and Oral Epidemiology*, 33, 265–73.

Twetman, S., Axelsson, S., Dahlgren, H., Holm, A.K., Källestål, C., Lagerlöf , F., Lingström, P., Mejàre, I., Nordenram, G., Norlund, A., Petersson, L.G. &, Söder B. (2003). Caries-preventive effect of fluoride toothpaste:a systematic review. *Acta Odontologica Scandinavica*, 2003, 61, 347–355.

Vanobbergen, J., Martens, L., Lesaffre, E., Bogaerts, K. & Declerck D. (2001). The value of a baseline caries risk assessment model in the primary dentition for the prediction of caries incidence in the permanent dentition. Caries Research, 35, 6, 442-50.

Vanobbergen, J., Declerck, D., Mwalili, S. & Martens L. (2004).The effectiveness of a 6-year oral health education programme for primary schoolchildren. *Community Dentistry and Oral Epidemiology*, 32, 173–82.

Vrbič V. (1996). Oral health in Slovenia, 1987-1993. *Community Dentistry and Oral Epidemiology*, 24, 364-5.

Wennhall, I., Matsson, L., Schröder, U. & Twetman, S. (2008). Outcome of an oral health outreach programme for preschool children in a low socioeconomic multicultural area. *International Journal of Paediatric Dentistry*, 18, 2, 84-90.

Whelton, H. (2004). Overview of the impact of changing global patterns of dental caries experience on caries clinical trials. *Journal of Dental Research*, 83 (Spec Iss C), C29-C34.

Wong, M.C., Lo, E.C., Schwarz, E. & Zhang, H.G. (2001). Oral health status and oral health behaviors in Chinese Children. Journal of Dental Research, 80, 5, 1459-65.

World Health Organization. (1997). Oral Health Surveys: Basic Methods. 4th ed. Ed. Geneve.

10

The Effects of Plant Extracts on Dental Plaque and Caries

Hamidreza Poureslami

Associate Professor, Department of Paediatric Dentistry, Dental School, Kerman, University of Medical Sciences, Iran

1. Introduction

Daily use of an efficient anti-plaque compound, especially a formulated form in toothpaste, can be very beneficial in plaque control. Some groups of antimicrobial compounds have been studied thus far. The most important of these compounds are herbal extracts, metallic salts and phenol compounds. Each of these three groups has demonstrated positive results in clinical and laboratory studies. Herbal extracts have received special attention because of being non-chemical and non-synthetic, and they have been long used in traditional medicine (Elvin 1980, Marsh & Bradshaw 1993).

In this section will be discussed about most important of plant extracts that have shown good effects on dental plaque and caries.

2. Salvadora Persica

The Salvadora Persica tree drives its Persian name, Darakht-e-Miswak or tooth brush tree. South of Iran, next to Persian Gulf, is the main growing area of this plant. This plant belongs to the Salvadoraceae family, a crowded evergreen shrub that has a soft inclined to a white wood. Since the brushes made of its wood strengthen the gums, it has been called "Miswak tree" (Meswak tree) in traditional medicine (Poureslami 2007).

Chemical compounds such as sodium chloride, calcium oxalate, silica, fluoride, sulfated compounds, vitamin C and tannic acid have been found in this plant. Moreover, this plant contains saponin, flavonoid, an alkaloid named Salvadorin, Trim ethylamine, an herbal steroid named beta-sit sterol and benzyl isothiocyanate. It is claimed that the vitamin C and sit sterol content of this plant have great roles in strengthening the gum capillaries and preventing gum inflammation. calcium salts and fluoride are quite effective in preventing dental caries. Moreover, the silica and calcium salts in the plant act as grinder and detergent. Trim ethylamine is known to be effective in reducing surface adhesion and also in decreasing plaque accumulation. Tannins, tannic acid, Sulfated compounds and benzyl isothiocyanate, are reported to have antimicrobial effects and help the healing of gum inflammation. Leaves, fruits and seeds of this plant have been used in traditional medicine as appetizer, mild laxative, diuretic and anti-fungal medication and people in some Asian and African countries have used it for many years (Akhtar & Ajmal 1981 , Al Sadhan &

Almas 1999 , Almas et al 2005 , Ezmirly et al 1981 , Darmani et al 2006 , Darout et al 2002 , Al-Otaibi et al 2003).

During recent years, many researchers throughout the world have studied Miswak as a helpful plant in oral hygiene. Clinical trials have shown that regular use of chewing stick of Salvadora Persica reduces plaque. It has been reported that incidence of caries among users of chewing sticks is low despite the intake of a carbohydrate rich diet and a lack of modern dental prophylactic measures. The Arabian researchers concluded from a comprehensive survey of several thousands of Saudi school children that the low incidence of gingival inflammation was attributable to the practice of using Miswak for teeth cleaning (Gazi et al 1992).

In vitro studies indicate that, of a variety of common oral bacteria, members of the genus streptococcus (including the mutans streptococci) are especially sensitive to the antimicrobial activities of S. Persica (Al-lafi & Ababneh 1995).

In a study the efficacy of Miswak in the prevention of dental caries has been investigated and compared with the efficacy of ordinary toothbrush and toothpaste. The data collected at the end of the study showed that the risk of dental caries for each tooth in the control group was 9.35 times more than the case group (Aldini & Ardakani 2007).

It has been told rinsing with Miswak extract stimulated parotid gland secretion and raised the plaque PH, suggesting a potential role in caries prevention (Sofrata et al 2007).

It has been observed that miswak was as effective as a toothbrush for reducing plaque on buccal surfaces of teeth both experimentally and clinically (Mohammed et al 2006).

Another study compared the oral health efficacy of persica mouthwash with that of a placebo. The results showed that use of persica mouthwash improves gingival health and lower carriage rate of cariogenic bacteria when compared with the pretreatment values (Khalessi et al 2004).

Scientific evaluation of use of miswak revealed that it is at least as effective as toothbrushing for reducing plaque and gingivitis and that the antimicrobial effect of S. persica is beneficial for prevention/treatment of periodontal diseases (Al- Otaibi 2004).

A clinical study was conducted using patients` saliva and measuring the effect of miswak (chewing stick), miswak extract, toothbrush, and normal saline on mutans and lactobacilli. The results showed that there was a marked reduction in Strep. Mutans among all groups. When the groups were compared, the reduction in Strep. Mutans was significantly greater using miswak in comparison to toothbrushing and there was no significant differences for lactobacilli reduction. The investigators concluded that miswak has an immediate antimicrobial effect. Strep. Mutans were more susceptible to miswak antimicrobial activity than lactobacilli (Almas & Al-Zeid 2004).

It seems persica mouthwash doesn`t have any side effects. Results of a study has shown the mouthwash significantly lowers the gingival index, plaque index, and bleeding index in case group without any reported side effects (Kaur et al 2004).

The results of the three serial studies showed that miswak extract, alone or in combination with toothpaste, can affect the growth of plaque bacteria. The investigators concluded that miswak extract can be used in mouth rinses and toothpastes for control dental plaque and caries (Poureslami 2007).

The results of a study showed that miswak extract could be a promised natural material as an additive to glass ionomer cements (El-Tatari et al 2011).

Almas and co-workers compared the antibacterial effects of Miswak extract with eight commercial mouth rinses. They evaluated the antimicrobial effects on Pyogenes Faecalis, Mutans Streptococci, Candida Albicans plus Aureus and Epidermidis staphylococci by determining the inhibition zones. In their study, none of the solutions was considered a gold standard; they compared the antimicrobial effect of Miswak with that of each mouth rinse and the antimicrobial effects of the eight mouth rinses with each other. According to their results, mouth rinses containing chlorhexidine had the greatest antibacterial effects, while mouth rinses containing cetylpyridinium had moderate effect; Miswak extract had a low effect (Almas et al 2005).

3. Bloodroot plant (Sanguinarine)

Chemically, sanguinarine is a benzophenanthridine alkaloid derived from the alcoholic extraction of powdered rhizomes of the bloodroot plant, Sanguinaria Canadensis, that grow in central and south America and Canada. Sanguinarine contains the chemically reactive iminium ion which is probably responsible for its activity. It appears to be retained in plaque for several hours after use, and is poorly absorbed from the gastrointestinal tract. Several clinical studies have been carried out into its effects. A sanguinarine mouth rinse and toothpaste regime given for 6 months during orthodontic treatment reduced plaque by 57% and gingival inflammation by 60% compared with figures of 27% and 21% for the placebo control group. Reviews on antimicrobial mouth rinses including sanguinarine conclude that short-term studies have shown variable but significant plaque inhibitory effects but the effect on gingivitis appears to be equivocal. In respect of its possible modes of action, it has also been shown that sanguinarine at a concentration of 16 microgram per milliliter completely inhibited 98% of microbial isolates from human dental plaque and that sanguinarine and zinc act synergistically in suppressing the growth of various oral strains of streptococci (Eley1999).

4. Sage & Myrrh

A wide range of toothpastes are commercially available and recently interest in naturally based products ,such as Qualimiswak and Prodontax, has increased. Parodontax (Madaus. Cologne. Germany)is composed of sodium bicarbonate and various herbal extracts including Camomile, Echinacea, Sage, Myrrh, Rhatany, and Peppermint oil. The individual components are reputed to have a variety of medicinal properties. Chamomile is claimed to have anti-inflammatory characteristics and Echinacea to have activating effect on leukocytes. Sage is reputed to be an antiseptic while both Myrrh and Rhatany are astringents that have been recommended for incorporation in to dentifrices and mouthwashes. The antibacterial effect of these herbal extracts on anaerobes has been reported (Yankell 1988).

Mullally and colleagues reported that Parodontax toothpaste was as effective as the conventionally formulated dentifrice in the control of plaque (Mullally et al 1995).

5. Licorice root

Licorice is the name applied to the roots and stolons of Glycyrrhiza species. Licorice roots extract contains Glycyrrhizol A, a compound that has strong antimicrobial activity against cariogenic bacteria,. Two pilot human studies indicate that a brief application of Licorice roots extract lollipop led to a marked reduction of cariogenic bacteria in oral cavity among most human subjects tested (Hu et al 2011).

6. Quercus infectoria gall

Quercus infectoria (Fabaceae) is a small tree, the galls arise on young branches of this tree as a result of attack by the gall-wasp, Adleria gallae-tinctoria. The plant is known as Mayaphal and Majufal in Hindi. Quercus infectoria gall extract has the potential to generate herbal metabolites. the crude extracts demonstrating anti-dental caries activity could result in the discovery of new chemical classes of antibiotics. These chemical classes of antibiotics could serve as selective agents for the maintenance of human health and provide bio-chemical tools for the study of infectious diseases (Vermani & Navneet 2009).

7. Nidus Vespae

Nidus Vespae is widely distributed in China and is typically harvested in the autumn & winter seasons and dried in the open air, after removal of dead wasps, for use in traditional Chinese medicine, where it has been used in the treatment of a variety of diseases, including cardiovascular, digestive and urinary disorders. The well-known pharmacopoeia of traditional Chinese medicine also lists the use of Nidus vespae For toothaches, through tooth brushing. A study showed significant inhabitation of glucosyltransferases activity and biofilm formation by Nidus Vespa extract. The researchers concluded it to be a promising natural product for the prevention of dental caries. Nidus Vespa have been extensively used in traditional Chinese medicine, given their multiple pharmacological activities, including antimicrobial, anti-inflammatory, anti-virus and anesthetic properties (Xiao et al 2007).

8. Cratoxylum formosum gum

The gum of Cratoxylum formosum, commonly known as mempat, is a natural agent that has been used extensively for caries prevention by hill tribe people residing in Thailand. A research showed Cratoxylum formosum gum has high antimicrobial activity against S. mutans and may become a promising herbal varnish against caries (Suddhasthira et al 2006).

9. Acacia Arabica

This evergreen tree is of medium height around 25 to 30 feet. It looks like a bush and is commonly foun in dry forest areas. This ayurvedic herb is great astringent and is equally useful as dentifrice, anti-hemorrhagic agent, and anti-diarrheal.A clinical trial was designed to evaluate the short-term clinical effects of Gumtone ,a commercially available gel containing Acacia Arabica in the reduction of plaque and gingival inflammation. Gumtone gel showed significant clinical improvement in gingival and plaque index scores as compared to a placebo gel. Gumtone gel was not associated with any discoloration of teeth or unpleasant taste (Pradeep et al 2010).

10. Chicory

Ancient ayurevedic literature contains several references on the medicinal uses of Cichorium intibus Linn (Chicory). Its usage has been for topical application in the treatment of acne, ophthalmia and inflammation of throat. The root is supposed to have aromatic cooling and healing properties. It is believed to purify and enrich blood, reduce inflammation of soft tissues and prevents pain in the joints. Some pharmacological actions of aqueous and alcoholic extracts of roots of chicory were reported. It was found that the extracts of chicory possess therapeutic properties in animal experimental models. In an *in vitro* study per formed by Patel on the anti-plaque effects of chicory extract, after adding herbal extract to the combination of four different commercial toothpastes, the anti-plaque effects of the mentioned toothpastes in comparison with the same toothpastes without herbal extract were evaluated using bacterial sensitivity tests and discs. Results of this study demonstrated a greater anti-plaque effect in all toothpastes containing herbal extract in comparison to the same toothpastes without extract. In another study, Patel compared the antiplaque activity of chicory extract with the antiplaque activity of penicillin, tetracycline, chloramphenicol, and streptomycin using microbial sensitivity tests and discs. In his study, bacteria in plaque samples showed high sensitivity to chloramphenicol and streptomycin, and their sensitivity to chicory extract was between the sensitivity to chloramphenicol and streptomycin (Patel & Venkatakrishna-Bhatt 1983).

11. Prunella vulgaris & Macleya cordata

In recent years has studied the biological activity of an extract of Prunella vulgaris L. (Labiatae), and it found marked cytoprotective, antioxidant/radical scavenging, antiviral and anti-inflammatory effects both in vitro and in vivo. This plant, known as the "self-heal", was popular in traditional European medicine during the 17th century as a remedy for alleviating sore throat, reducing fever, and accelerating wound healing. A major constituent of P. vulgaris is rosmarinic acid, a phenolic antioxidant whose content can be as high as 6 %. Phytochemical studies indicate that P. vulgaris further contains oleanolic, betulinic, ursolic, $2\alpha,3\alpha$-dihydroxyurs-12-en-28-oic and $2\alpha,3\alpha$-ursolic acids, triterpenoids, flavonoids, tannins and anionic polysaccharide prunelline. Isoquinoline alkaloids from Macleya cordata R. Br. (Papaveraceae) are another group of biologically active components studied recently. The main alkaloids of this plant, quaternary benzo[c]phenanthridines (QBA) sanguinarine and chelerythrine, are among the most active of antimicrobials natural substances. These alkaloids display a plethora of species- and tissue-specific actions but the molecular basis of their pharmacological activities remains obscure. They exhibit antimicrobial, anti-inflammatory, antimitotic, adrenolytic, sympatholytic, cytostatic and local anesthetic effects. A double blind, placebo-controlled clinical trial was performed to investigate the effectiveness of a herbal-based dentifrice, containing Prunella vulgaris and Macleya cordata, in the control gingivitis. The result showed the dentifrice was effective in reducing plaque and symptoms of gingivitis (Adamkova et al 2004).

12. Chitosan plus herbal extracts

Chitosan, an abundant natural polymer, is obtained by alkaline N-deacetylation of chitin. Chitosan being a binding agent, bio-adhesive, bio-compatible, bio-degradable, and non-toxic polymer also possessing medicinal activities, such as antifungal, antibacterial, antiprotozoal, anticancer, antiplaque, ant tartar, hemostatic, wound healing, and potentiates anti-inflammatory response, inhibits the growth of cariogenic bacteria, immunopotentiation, antihypertensive, serum cholesterol lowering, increases salivary secretion (anti-xerostomia), and helps in the formation of bone substitute materials. The adherence of oral bacteria on the tooth surface leads to plaque formation. It is believed that the adhesion between the bacteria and the tooth surface is due to electrostatic and hydrophobic interactions. These interactions are disrupted by chitosan derivatives because of competition by the positively charged amine group. The antibacterial activity of chitosan could be due to the electrostatic interactions between the amine groups of chitosan and the anionic sites on bacterial cell wall because of the presence of carboxylic acid residues and phospholipids. Use of most of the currently used gelling agents, such as tragacanth, Irish moss, and sodium alginate mucilage, in the toothpaste was limited only to their gelling capacity and also require antimicrobial preservatives due to their carbohydrate nature, whereas chitosan being a good gelling agent, does not require any preservatives as chitosan possess antimicrobial activities. Chitosan nanoparticles have found as drug carriers. In a study was evaluated anti-plaque activity a chitosan-based poly herbal toothpaste. The toothpaste significantly reduced the plaque index by 70.47% and bacterial count by 85.29%(34). (Mohire & Yadav 2010).

13. Conclusion

In conclusion, the herbal extracts can be effect on the growth of dental plaque bacteria and dental caries. Therefore, the herbal extracts can be used in mouth rinses and toothpastes and can be beneficial in controlling dental caries.

14. References

Adamkova H, Vicar J, Palasova J, Ulrichova J, Simanek V. (2004) Macleya cordata and Prunella vulgaris in oral hygiene products- their efficacy in the control of gingivitis. *Biomed Pap Med Fac Univ Palacky Olomouc Czech Repub*,148:103-5.

Akhtar MS, Ajmal M. (1981) Significance of chewingsticks (miswaks) in oral hygiene from a pharmacological view-point. *J Pak Med Assoc* , 31(4):89-95.

Aldini EZ, Ardakani F. (2007) Efficacy of miswak (Salvadora persica) in prevention of dental caries, *J Shahid Sadoughi Univ Med Sci Hlth Serv* ,14:24-31.

Al-lafi T, Ababneh H. (1995) The effect of the extract of the Miswak (chewing sticks) used in Jordan and the Middle East on oral bacteria. *Int Dent J* , 45:218-22.

Almas K, Al-Zeid Z. (2004) The immediate antimicrobial effect of a toothbrush and Miswak on cariogenic bacteria: A clinical study. *J Contemp Dent Pract* , 155:105-14.

Almas K, Skaug N, Ahmad I. (2005) An in vitro antimicrobial comparison of miswak extract with commercially available non-alcohol mouth rinses. *Int J Dent Hyg* , 3(1):18-24.

Al Otaibi M. (2004) The Miswak (chewing stick) and oral health. Studies on oral hygiene practices of urban Saudi Arabians. *Swed Dent J Suppl* , 167:2-75.

Al-Otaibi M, Al-Harthy M, Soder B, Gustafsson A, Mansson B. (2003) Comparative effect of chewing sticks and toothbrushing on plaque removal and gingival health. *Oral Health Prev Dent* , 1(4):301-7.

Al Sadhan RI, Almas K. (1999) Miswak (chewing stick): A cultural and scientific heritage. *Saudi Dent J* , 11(2):80-88.

Darmani H, Nusayr T, Al-Hiyasat AS. (2006) Effects of extracts of miswak and derum on proliferation of Balb/C 3T3 fibroblasts and viability of cariogenic bacteria. *Int J Dent Hyg* , 4(2):62-66.

Darout IA, Christy AA, Skuag N, Egeberg PK. (2002) Identification and qualification of some potentially antimicrobial anionic components in miswak extract. *Ind J Pharmacol* , 32(1):11-4.

Eley BM. (1999) Antibacterial agents in the control of supragingival plaque- a review. *British Dent J* , 186:286-96.

El- Tatari A, de Soet JJ, de Gee AJ, Abou Shelib M, van Amerongen WE. (2011) Influence of salvadora persica extract on physical and antimicrobial properties of glass ionomer cement. *Eur Arch Paediatr Dent.* , 12:22-25.

Elvin-Lewis M. (1980) Plants used for teeth cleaning throughout the world. *J Prevent Dent* , 6(1):61-70.

Ezmirly ST, Chen JC, Wilson SR. (1981) Isolation of glucotropaeolin from Salvadora persica L. *J Chem Soc Pak* , 3(1):9.

Gazi MI, Davies TJ, Al-Bagieh N, Cox SW. (1992) The immediate-and medium-term effects of Meswak on the composition of mixed saliva. *J Clin Periodontol* , 19:113-17.

Hu CH, et al. (2011) Development and evaluation of a safe and effective sugarfree herbal lollipop that kills cavity-causing bacteria. *Int J Oral Sci* , 3:13-20.

Kaur S, Abdul Jalil R, Akmar SI. (2004) The immediate Term effect of chewing commercially available Meswak (Salvadora persica) on levels of Calcium, Chloride, Phosphate and Thiocyanate in whole saliva. *Ann Dent* , 11:51-9.

Khalessi AM, Pack AR, Thomson WM, Tompkins GR. (2004) An in vivo study of the plaque control efficacy of Persica a commercially available herbal mouthwash containing extracts of Salvadora persica. *Int Dent J* , 54:279-83.

Marsh PD, Bradshaw DJ. (1993) Microbiological effects of new agents in dentifrices for plaque control. *Int Dent J* , 43(4 Suppl 1):399-406.

Mohammed B, Jan B, Sarah B, Meshari F, Otaibi AL. (2006) The effectiveness of chewing stick Miswak on plaque removal. *Saudi Dent J* , 18:125-33.

Mohire NC, Yadav AV. (2010) Chitosan-based polyherbal toothpaste: as novel oral hygiene product. *Indian J Dent Res* , 21: 380-84.

Mullally BH, James JA, Coulter WA, Liden GJ. (1995) The efficacy of a herbal-based toothpaste on the control of plaque and gingivitis. *J Clin Periodontol* , 22:686-89.

Patel VK. Venkatakrishna-Bhatt H. (1983) Cichorium intibus: A novel herbal preparation as a gum massage, dentifrice, anti-inflammatory and anti-plaque agent. *Therapie* , 38:405-14.

Poureslami HR, Makarem A, Mojab F. (2007) Paraclinical effects of Miswak extract on dental plaque. *Dent Res J* , 4:106-10.

Pradeep AR, Happy D, Garg G. (2010) Short-term clinical effects of commercially available gel containing Acacia Arabica: a randomized controlled clinical trial. *Aust Dent J* , 55:65-69.

Sofrata A, Lingström P, Baljoon M, Gustafsson A. (2007) The effect of miswak extract on plaque PH: An in vivo study. *Caries Res* , 41:451-54.

Suddhasthira T, Thaweboon S, Dendoung N, Thaweboon B, Dechkunakorn S. (2006) Antimicrobial activity of Cratoxylum formosum on streptococcus mutans. *Southeast Asian J Trop Med Public Health,* 37:1156-59.

Vermani A, Navneet P. (2009) Screening of Quercus infectoria gall extracts as antibacterial agents against dental pathogens. *Indian J Dent Res,* 20:337-39.

Xiao J, et al. (2007) Effects of Nidus vespae extract and chemical fractions on glucosyltransferases, adherence and biofilm formation of streptococcus mutans. *Arch Oral Biol ,* 52:869-75.

Yankell SL. (1988) The role of natural products in modern oral hygiene. *J of Clin Dent ,* 1.(suppl.A):1-44.

11

Effect of Dental Caries on Children Growth

Tayebeh Malek Mohammadi[1] and Elizabeth Jane Kay[2]
[1]Kerman University of Medical Sciences,
[2]Peninsula Dental School,
[1]Iran
[2]UK

1. Introduction

Abnormal growth/ weight gain in young children is a substantial public health problem which causes much concern among parents and health professionals.

Recent reports suggest that in many established market economies changes in dietary practices have resulted in a change in children and adolescents' body mass index. Among the reported dietary changes are alterations in the pattern of intake of carbohydrates. It would seem entirely consistent with current knowledge to assume that such changes may also impact upon dental caries in the child population.

Dental caries is a disease which attacks the dental hard tissues by demineralising the enamel. If oral conditions are favourable then this demineralisation can progress from the outer enamel layer of the tooth into the softer underlying dentine, resulting in decay. Dental decay is more common in individuals who have frequent intakes of dietary sugars (fermentable carbohydrates). Frequency of intake of carbohydrate is more predictive of the decay process than the absolute amount. Dental caries is also an extremely widespread childhood disease. It is particularly prevalent among deprived populations (Wright, 2000).

Dental caries is the most common reason for children undergoing general anaesthesia and thereby is therefore a major cause of exposure of small children to the medical risks associated with general anaesthesia (Whittle, 2000).

A number of nutritional factors, which may be factors in growth and development such as Vitamins A and D, water hardness and protein, have been hypothesised as potentially linked to dental caries (Mellanby & Pattison, 1928; East, 1941; Aptone-Merced & Navia, 1980). However, there is little evidence to substantiate that the systemic effects of poor nutrition increase the risk of dental decay, and it is generally accepted that while diet can have a profound local effect on erupted teeth, it has much less effect while the teeth are forming(Rugg-Gunn, 2000).

It has been demonstrated that low birth weight children more frequently have hypo plastic defects in the enamel of their teeth than normal weight babies, but that dental caries is also less frequent (Fearne et al, 1990).

An association between physical problems affecting the mouth, and childhood growth, has been hypothesized and it has been suggested that dentists may be ideally placed to recognize children at risk of poor growth and development (Boyd, 1998).

The concept that dental disease and child's body weight may be related was raised as early as 1982, when a retrospective case-note study examined the body weights of children attending for general anaesthetic tooth extractions, were compared to children attending for routine dental care (Miller et al 1982) and subsequent studies have suggested that treatment of caries may lead to improvement in weight gain (Acs et al, 1998, 1999; Malek Mohammadi et al, 2009) at least in children whose growth is below average.

This chapter presents evidence which strongly suggests that children's growth is affected by the state of their dental health. These relatively simple observations are very important, as they provides yet another reason for policy makers and Governments to invest time, resources and expertise in improving both children's diets, and their dental health. It is essential to remember that dental caries is one of only very few common childhood diseases which cause large numbers of the child population to undergo general anaesthesia. Children who are allowed to develop dental decay therefore suffer, not only in terms of potential effects on their growth and development, but also directly, as the treatment, if it is carried out using general anaesthesia poses a serious health risk to the children involved.

2. Principles of normal growth

Growth is a critical indicator of child health and its importance is recognized by the World Health Organization, which identifies growth assessment as the best single measure for defining the nutritional status and health of children, as well as being an indicator of quality of life in whole populations (Hall, 1996).

Normal growth is a sign of good health, and ill children often grow slowly. Growth in children is not simply an increase in height and weight, but is a complex process involving increases in both the size and number of cells. It is influenced by genetic factors, but a number of other factors are also relevant, including nutrition, and these may act to prevent the individual achieving his or her genetic potential. Measurement of growth indicators, such as weight, height and head circumference can give valuable information about a child's nutritional well-being and growth pattern.

3. Growth monitoring

Health professionals accept that routine growth monitoring in children is a standard component of community child health services (Department of Health and Social Security,UK, (HMSO), 1974). In both developing and developed countries, health workers monitor growth in order to detect problems, and where possible, intervene if there is evidence of malnutrition and growth problem. Health workers and mothers spend considerable time on this activity, because early detection of growth failure depends on effective monitoring (Reid, 1984). Monitoring requires accurate, regular measurements, accurate transcription of data to a growth chart and appropriate action if poor growth is identified. It is also important to ensure that measurements are performed consistently, using appropriate equipment and also using trained staff (Garner et al 2000). Inconsistencies can occur at a number of stages, including in the setting up and calibration of equipment, the measuring techniques used, and the recording of data.

Growth monitoring may be done through height and weight measurements but a variety of other indices such as supine length, standing height, height velocity, weight velocity, weight for height, height for weight, Body Mass Index(BMI) and many more other measurements are also considered relevant.

In order to interpret biological variables such as height and weight, it is important to compare them with normal data for children of the same age and, where appropriate, sex. Accurate measurement and the use of standard growth charts are important tools for monitoring a child's growth.

4. Growth problems

Assessment of growth and nutrition is important, both in the diagnosis of primary nutritional and growth disorders and also in the diagnosis of chronic disorders. Because of some background disturbances, sometimes a child may be abnormally short or tall and light or heavy from infancy onwards, whereas in others initial normal growth is followed by growth failure or acceleration.

5. Nutrition and growth

Food consumption has a tremendous influence on human lives and is essential to life itself. Eating appropriate amounts of a wide variety of foods helps to maintain optimal health. Prolonged periods of poor food choices may cause impaired health. People need approximately 50 nutrients for growth and maintenance of health. These nutrients are present in a wide variety of different types of foods. Carbohydrates, lipids and proteins are energy nutrients which give the human body the energy it needs for moving and doing work, as well as for such vital activity as breathing and pumping blood. Minerals, a category made up of more than 20 nutrients perform a variety of functions, although they are not sources of energy. Vitamins are regulatory substances needed in even smaller amounts than minerals. At present, 13 vitamins are recognized as essential nutrients. Every person, (whether a child or mature adult), needs good nutrition in order to maintain good health and this can be supplied by a well-balanced healthy diet taken in regular meals and in appropriate surroundings (Wright, 2000).

The evidence in the World Health Organization (WHO) Global Database on Child Growth (De Onis et al, 2000) and Malnutrition gives a description of the magnitude and geographical distribution of childhood under- and over-nutrition worldwide. Analyses based on the database's information confirm that child under-nutrition remains a major public health problem in many countries, and can hamper children's physical growth and mental development. Indeed, it may even be a major threat to their survival. Despite an overall decrease in poor growth in developing countries, in some, poor growth is increasing in prevalence and in many others the incidence of growth faltering remains disturbingly high(De Onis et al, 2000, 1993). An important observation which has been made, is that the pattern of growth faltering in developing countries, not only within a region but also globally, are remarkably similar even though different instruments and measuring methods were used in the surveys. This suggests that interventions during the earliest periods of life are likely to have the greatest impact in promoting good nutrition and preventing poor growth and development in children.

6. Healthy eating habits in preschool children

Good preschool eating patterns are important because they influence both energy and nutrient intake, and dental health. An optimum eating pattern would be regular meals and nutritious, low fat, low sugar snacks. Young children have small appetites but large nutrient needs relative to their body size, therefore regular refueling is required. An eating pattern based on distinct meals is generally beneficial and also promotes dental health. Dental caries is prevalent in preschool children and it is directly related to the amount and frequency of consumption of non-milk extrinsic sugars in the diet (Holt, 1991). Family meal patterns are inevitably affected by family routines, parents working hours and the child's appetite at different times of day. Regular meals allow opportunities for socializing and for parents to set a good example with respect to food choices and eating behavior (Graham, 1972).

A suitable snack should provide nutrients other than calories and should be low in non-milk extrinsic sugar and not interfere with the child's appetite for meals (Sims & Morris, 1974). Snacks high in non-milk extrinsic sugars greatly increase the risk of dental caries and an excessive intake of high fat, high sugar snacks will lead to an energy intake in excess of need (Splett & Strory, 1991). Many snacks will reduce the appetite for meals, often to the detriment of total nutrient intake (Beaton & Chery, 1988). The best snacks are bread and cereals, or fruit and vegetables. They need to be readily available, affordable and appealing to a child (Ministry of Agriculture, Food and Farming, (MAFF), 1997).

7. Feeding problems in pre-school children

Feeding problems are remarkably common in pre-school children. The incidence of feeding problems has been estimated to vary from 16% to 75 %(Eppright et al, 1969; Minde & Minde, 1986). This is a time of growing individuality for children, a time when a child's personality and temperament is demonstrated. Most cases of food refusal and feeding problems are minor and have no effect on growth or the child's weight gain but occasionally the problems can be very severe. Feeding problems may relate to the choosing of foods, or to eating behaviors. Both of these may be accompanied with food refusal or food fads which have psychological and other underlying causes (Harrise & Booth, 1992).

Medical conditions must always be considered and excluded as a reason for a child failing to eat. In the absence of underlying disease, psychological problems should be considered. Many young children pass through a phase of being faddy about food and refusing to eat certain foods. Food faddiness tends to reflect the extremes of young children's food likes and dislikes and often has a psychological cause. Food like and dislikes are influenced by taste, familiarity, parents attitudes to food, and food appeal. In this respect, refusal to eat meat and vegetables and also refusal to drink milk have been reported in young children. Poor appetite, limited food appeal, emotional upset and manipulative behavior are said to be the most common reasons for food refusal in young children(Harrise & Booth, 1992).

Excessive intake of snacks, milk and drinks, particularly squash, may be a reason for poor appetite in young children (Houlihane & Rolls 1995). Snacks close to mealtimes may also suppress appetite (Sims & Morris, 1974). Irregular frequent meals are a common feeding pattern in young children. This behavior may influence both the appetite and dental health of children. In a study in 1991 Holt showed that between-meal snacking was prevalent in 4 year-old children (Holt, 1991). Small children may be over-whelmed by a large plate of food. Small portions, of colorful, attractively presented food are more tempting (Harrise & Booth, 1992).

Toddler behavior is strongly influenced by past experience. Any negative experience with food might result in future food refusal. Transient food refusal may occur after birth of a sibling or other event, in an attempt to redirect attention to themselves (Harrise & Booth, 1992). Refusal to chew due to failure to introduce texture and lumps before 6-7 months of age can result in children rejecting lumpy food later (K & R Minde, 1986).

8. Assessment of diet, nutrition and feeding problems

One of the most important indicators of suitable and adequate nutrition is normal growth. Therefore, prolonged food refusal, even due to non-organic causes can result in impaired growth. Regular weight and height measurement is therefore necessary. Taking a detailed diet history is also an important part of growth assessment (HMSO, 1992). Diet questions should include a food diary describing all food and drink consumed, with details of meal pattern, location of eating time and supervision received(HMSO, 1992). There are different types of diaries available. Food frequency tables are one type which includes information about frequency of consumption as well as the type of foods usually eaten. Details of nutrient intake can be made by analysis of the type and amount of reported foods, but reporting problems can make such analysis unreliable.

9. Early Childhood Caries (ECC)

Dental caries is a complex, multi-factorial disease and is a significant health and social problem which affects people of all ages and is responsible for a vast amount of pain, misery and economic loss. It is a major problem in young children. Caries of the primary teeth "Early Childhood Caries" or ECC is one of the most prevalent health problems in infants and toddlers (Mayanagi et al, 1995). It can be considered an epidemic in lower-income families and in under developed parts of the world (Ismail & Sohn 1999). ECC is one of the major causes of hospitalization in young children, who often need to receive general anaesthesia for extraction or tooth restoration (Sheller et al, 1996).

10. Public health aspects of dental caries

Despite improvements in the oral health of children in recent decades, early childhood caries (ECC) remains a serious threat to child welfare. ECC is manifested by severe decay of primary teeth. This can be a debilitating condition that can not only affect the children but also their families and the communities in which they live. Toothache leads to school absence, which is a ready indicator of children's health. In the USA, where caries is lower than elsewhere, visits or dental problems accounted for 117 000 hours of school lost per 100 000 children (Gift et al, 1992). Because most school dental services work mainly during school hours, loss of schooling among the poor, who have higher caries rates, is high. Other manifestations of ECC include pain, infection, abscesses, chewing difficulty, malnutrition, gastrointestinal disorders, and low self-esteem (Ripa, 1988). ECC might also lead to malocclusion and poor speech articulation, and is associated with caries in the permanent dentition (Kaste et al, 1992).

The problems associated with this disease often generate fear and aversion to treatment, and severely affected patients may require extensive restorative treatment, stainless steel crowns or tooth extraction, which may involve sedation or general anesthesia(Ripa, 1988; Weinstein et al, 1992).

Treatment of ECC is expensive and if general anaesthesia is used, the cost can increase along with the medical risk to which the children involved are exposed. ECC is the most prevalent infectious disease among children, 5 times more common than asthma and 7 times more prevalent than hay fever (Rockville, 2000).

In the absence of widely accepted standards for diagnosing ECC, various diagnostic criteria have been used(Derkson, 1982; Ripa, 1988; Kelly & Bruerd, 1987; Winter, 1966). The lack of standard diagnostic criteria affects reported prevalence rates and makes it difficult to compare data from different studies (Kaste et al, 1992). Nevertheless, ECC is clearly a common problem in the United States and other countries particularly among economically disadvantaged children (Milnes, 1996; Kelly & Bruerd, 1987; Winter, 1966; Broderick et al, 1989) . Five to 10 percent of young children and twenty percent of children from families with low income have ECC and the rate is higher among the families from ethnic and racial minorities.

Most studies of ECC have focused on clarifying disease etiology by investigating demographic variables and by characterizing risk behaviours (Barnes et al, 1992; Dilley et al, 1980; Goepferd, 1986; Babeely et al, 1989). Some investigators have conducted several studies that are directly relevant to the proposed project, including evaluation of risk factors for ECC in underserved ethnic groups, the use of different criteria to diagnose ECC, the cost of treating ECC, laboratory analysis of salivary risk factors for cariogenesis, and development of caries risk assessment models. However, most studies failed to investigate the role of childhood caries in the quality of life and well-being in this vulnerable group and the effects of it later in the affected individuals' lives.

Therefore ECC is undoubtedly an important issue from public health point of view as it is so widespread, is preventable, and can impact on general well being and perhaps overall health. The accepted model for the development of caries consists of three categories of risk factors: micro-organisms, substrate/oral environment, and host/teeth. Recent scientific evidence strongly suggests that the first step in the development of ECC is primary infection by Mutans Streptococci.

The most important predisposing factors for ECC are listed as diet, nutrition and feeding behaviour. Certain inappropriate feeding practices have also been associated with ECC. The bottle contents, the frequency and duration of feeding, and how long the child is bottle-dependent, are especially important. Bottle-feeding with liquids such as Jello water and soda-pop is particularly harmful because these drinks contain sucrose, a highly cariogenic substrate. Prolonged use of a bottle containing high-fructose liquid at naptime or bedtime is strongly associated with ECC (Reisines & Douglass, 1998).

There are many studies concerning the role of type, frequency and content of consumed foods; however a reliable and valid instrument has not been developed to reliably measure dict in relation to caries development in individuals. However there is no doubt that the frequent consumption of sugary food plays a role in the development of ECC.

Other studies have shown that lack of oral hygiene and certain family characteristics also increase the risk of ECC: parents of children with ECC had less education and more caries, were more obese, were more likely to be overindulgent and less likely to say "no" to their children, and cleaned their children's teeth less frequently than parents of children without ECC (Acs et al, 1992; Winter, 1966).

Although the type of sugar consumed is an important factor in the development of caries, the frequency of sugar consumption is of greater significance. Several studies support this hypothesis (Amiutis, 2004; Zita & McDonald, 1959). Since the publication of the Vipeholm study, (Gustafsson et al, 1954) it has been accepted that the frequency of ingestion of sugar-containing foods is directly proportional to caries experience. In addition a study by Konig showed a positive correlation between the frequency with which animals ate cariogenic foods and dental caries severity (Konig et al, 1968) and Holt found that the pre-children with caries have between meal snacks approximately four times each day(Holt, 1991) .

There are many studies which suggest that children with ECC have a high frequency of sugar consumption, not only in fluids given in the nursing bottle, but also of sweetened solid foods. Results of clinical studies suggest that this dietary characteristic is likely to be one of the most significant caries risk factors in ECC (Konig et al, 1968; Sheiham, 1991). Increased frequency of eating sucrose increases the acidity of plaque and enhances the establishment and dominance of aciduric Mutans Streptococci.

The increased total time sugar is in the mouth increases the potential for enamel demineralization, and there is inadequate time for demineralization by the buffering action of saliva (Loesche, 1986). There is also evidence that the amount of sugar consumed is an important factor in caries development, although it is very likely that the frequency of eating sugar rises as the amount of sugar consumed rises. A high positive correlation between amount and frequency of eating sugary foods can therefore be assumed (Burt, 1986).

11. Feeding pattern in children with ECC

The relationship between sugar consumption and dental caries is one of cause and effect. The evidence to support such a relationship is generally considered overwhelming (Burt, 1986). Epidemiological studies have shown that caries prevalence was highest among children who ingested a diet high in sugar (Sheiham, 1991). Surveys have also shown that high consumption of cariogenic drinks and foods at bed time by pre-school children is an important factor in risk of caries (Palmer, 1971). Holt's study in 1991 on a group of preschool children showed that children consume sweets, biscuits and sweet drinks regularly and that mean dmft increases significantly with a higher rate of sugar consumption (Holt, 1991).

12. Diet, nutrition and dental health

It has been well-documented in animals that early malnutrition affects tooth development and eruption (Mellanby, 1928) and can result in increased dental caries later in life. But in humans, a causal relationship between nutritional status and dental health has not been directly demonstrated (Alvarez & Navia 1989). However two separate cross-sectional studies in Peruvian children have shown that malnutrition is associated with delayed tooth development and increased caries experience (Alvarez et al, 1988, 1990). However it has been shown beyond reasonable doubt that there is a distinct relationship between diet and dental caries (Gustafsson et al, 1954). These effects are accepted, but there are two important aspects to the relationship; food choice and nutrient intake, both may affect and be affected by, poor dental health.

The role of nutrition in the maintenance of health is well known. Nutritional deficiencies in the growing child, whether due to deprivation, over-indulgence, or mal-absorption syndrome may have significant impact on somatic growth (Root et al, 1971). The potential impacts of eating disorders on overall health have also been established (Gross et al, 1986). The constellation of poor dietary habits which result in early childhood caries is currently most recognized for its impact on the dentition, rather than on overall health. However recently, some reports have claimed that severe dental decay could be a contributing factor for poor growth in children (Miller et al, 1982; Acs, 1992; Ayhan et al, 1996; Malek Mohammadi et al, 2009).

One of the most important indicators of health is normal growth and normal growth is an indicator of nutrition. The health of the dentition would appear to have some effects on nutrition. Therefore, there may be a relationship between the health of the dentition and growth. Miller's study (as mentioned above), showed that 1105 children with severe dental caries who needed extractions of deciduous teeth under general anaesthesia (GA) were significantly lighter than 527 control children (Miller et al, 1982). One part of the study was a retrospective comparison of clinical records. The children were weighed as a routine and their height measured as well. A control group was selected from children who were attending for routine dental care (DC). The children in the GA group were lighter than those in the DC group and in the GA group 31.3% were below the 23rd percentile compared with only 17.1% in the DC groups. The second part of the study compared the diet history of the two groups. The frequency of eating was higher in GA group. The DC group ate animal protein more frequently than the GA group and the GA group had a higher fat intake. There was a significant difference between the groups, in their intake of refined solid carbohydrate between meals.

Another retrospective case control study was conducted in a paediatric population by Acs in 1992 and a review of anaesthesia records of children with nursing caries was undertaken (Acs, 1992). The weights of 115 children with no special medical history were compared to subjects matched for age, gender, race and socioeconomic status. The study group had at least one pulpally involved tooth and the comparison subjects had no gross carious lesions. The weight of children with caries was significantly lower than the control group and 8.7% of children with caries weighed less than 80% their ideal weight, compared with only 1.7% of the comparison group. The mean age of the low weight children with caries was significantly greater than for children at or above their ideal weights. This was interpreted as indicating that progression of caries may affect growth adversely.

In a similar study in Ankara similar results were obtained (Ayhan et al, 1996). In this study, the mean weight of 126 children, aged 3 to 5 years old with caries was compared with the mean weight of children with no caries but similar age and sex. The mean weight of case children was between 25th and 50th percentiles while the mean weight of control group was between 50th and 75th percentiles. Seven percent of children with caries weighed less than 80% of their ideal weight compared 0.7% of the control group children. Evaluation of height showed that it was similar to weight but head circumference was not statistically different in the two groups.

In a recent published study, data analysis from National Oral Health Survey in Philippines (Benzian et al, 2011) showed that prevalence of low BMI was significantly higher in children with odontogenic infections as compared with children without odontogenic infections.

The regression coefficient between BMI and caries was highly significant (p < 0.001). Children with odontogenic infections (PUFA + pufa > 0) [PUFA/pufa is an index used to assess the presence of oral conditions and infections resulting from untreated caries in the primary (pufa) and permanent (PUFA) dentition] as compared to those without odontogenic infections had an increased risk of a below normal BMI.

13. Effect of improved dentition on nutrition and growth in children

The reported association between chronic malnutrition, growth, and dental caries suggests that dental decay might contribute to poor weight gain in children (Alvarez et al, 1990). Four cases of children with early childhood caries and subsequent dental rehabilitation were published by Acs in 1998 (Acs et al, 1998). Regardless of the presumptive aetiology of the poor weight gain, all of these children demonstrated an immediate increase in weight, propelling them to higher weight percentile categories with increased adjusted 6-month increments of growth after their carious teeth had been repaired. At the end of the observation, none of these children continued to satisfy the criteria for the designation of faltering growth. These observations were consistent with the phenomenon of catch-up growth that has been observed in faltering growth children (Prader et al, 1963).

The effect of dental health improvement on growth was evaluated through another study by Acs in 1999 (Acs et al, 1999). The percentile weight categories of children with non-contributory medical histories and early childhood caries were compared to caries free patients, before and after comprehensive dental treatment under general anaesthesia. Percentile weight categories of the test subject were significantly less than that of the comparison group and 13.7% of ECC patients weighed less than 80% of their ideal weight. Following complete dental rehabilitation, children with ECC exhibited significantly increased growth velocities through the course of the follow-up period. At the end of the follow-up period there were no longer any statistically significant differences in the percentile weight categories of the test and comparison groups.

In a longitudinal clinical trial study in Manchester treatment of severe caries resulted in weight gain in 5-6 year-old children. (Malek Mohammadi et al, 2009) One thousand two hundred children aged 2-12 year-old had carious teeth extracted under general anesthesia during the study period. Of these, 218 five and six year old children participated in the study. Most of the children recruited to the study had a high caries rate, as expected. The mean (SD) dmft was 7.18 (3.27). Fifty-eight per cent of children had dmft >6. Ninety-six (44%) children had signs of dental abscesses or oral fistula when they were examined. The children as a group were of average height, weight and BMI. The proportion of the study population who weighed below the standards tenth percentile at baseline was 6.9% (15), whilst 8.3% (18) were below the standard's 10th percentile for height. Frequency distribution of the study population's weight, height and BMI at baseline and follow up indicated a decrease in the proportion of children in the lower percentiles for BMI, six months after extraction of carious teeth. On average the children showed a clear gain in weight at follow up and a slight gain in height. The 15 children with low weight (<10th percentile) at baseline also had significant increases in SD scores for weight and BMI (p<0.001) at follow up.

These studies suggest that children's ability to gain weight may be negatively affected by the presence of carious teeth in their mouths and that weight is gained more quickly than normal in the six months after tooth extractions.

In another longitudinal birth cohort, children who had caries at 61 months had slower increases in weight and height between birth and 61 months than those without decay at 61 months (Kay et al, 2010). It is possible that the chronicity of ECC may have a similar influence like other chronic diseases on a child, making them unable to sustain normal growth, and therefore, impacting on general health and well being.

Whilst nutrition is very important in growth and development, recently it has been suggested that children who do not have any medical problems, but who are deficient in growth, may have higher levels of caries. Growth deficiency and ECC may therefore be related in some way. Oral health affects people physically and psychologically and influences how they grow, enjoy life, look, speak, chew, taste food and socialize, as well as their feelings of social well-being (Locker, 1997).

If dietary intake alters as a result of caries this could result in an alteration of established growth patterns which are then re-established once the carious teeth are removed. The potential for increased glucocorticoid production in response to pain, decreased growth hormone secretion in response to disturbed sleep pattern, and overall increased metabolic rate during the course of infection are all possible explanations of the observed association between growth and caries. An alternative explanation for the observation would be that pain and infection alter eating habits e.g. if carious teeth become pulpitic, the eating of refined carbohydrates will cause pain and children may avoid such foods resulting in reduced calorific intake. Whichever explanation is accepted for the observed association, the hypothesis that dental disease and growth are related through the common factor of diet are supported by the studies presented and also seem plausible, both biologically, and behaviorally.

Severe caries detracts from children's quality of life: they experience pain, discomfort, disfigurement, acute and chronic infections, and eating and sleep disruption as well as higher risk of hospitalization, high treatment costs and loss of school days with the consequently diminished ability to learn. Caries may also affect nutrition, growth and weight gain. Children of three years of age with nursing caries weighed about 1 kg less than control children probably because toothache and infection alter eating and sleeping habits, dietary intake and metabolic processes. Disturbed sleep affects glucosteroid production (Acs, 1992).

Dental problems which cause chewing to be painful may affect the intake of dietary fibre and some nutrient-rich foods; consequently, serum levels of beta carotene, folate and vitamin C have been observed to be significantly lower in those with poorer oral status (Sheiham & Steele, 2001).

It is likely that younger children, with early caries, prior to the onset of pain and infection have poor feeding habits, particularly high carbohydrate intake. However as the children age and caries progresses, the onset of pain and infection may alter eating habits eg. If carious teeth become pulpitic, the eating of refined carbohydrates will cause pain and the child would therefore be more likely to avoid such foods. Altered dietary intake secondary to pain could therefore result in an alteration of established growth patterns.

Because oral and other chronic diseases have determinants in common, more emphasis should be on the common risk factor approach. The hypothesis that ECC and growth may be related through the common factors of diet and nutrition seems plausible. While there are many studies which have investigated the role of diet in children's growth and in dental caries, diet as a common casual factor for poor growth and dental caries has not previously been fully investigated.

Dental caries, which is associated with what children eat, poses a real, and potentially life threatening danger to the children affected by it, because it frequently results in general anaesthesia quite apart from any other effects it may have on child wellbeing. Diseases which do not cause small children to undergo general anaesthesia and all the risks and problems it entails, but which affect individuals' health many years later cause disquiet amongst nutritionists and paediatricians. It is unfortunate that a disease such as dental caries, which causes extreme pain and leads to outpatient general anaesthesia, does not seem to engender the same levels of worry and concern. It would seem that the impact of the caries on children's general health and well-being has largely been ignored.

14. Summary and conclusion

Good nutrition is essential for good physical health. Nutrition also plays a key role in the development and maintenance of a healthy mouth, especially the teeth and gums. The food we eat affects our teeth both before and after their eruption into the mouth. The relation of dental caries and periodontal diseases to the type and frequency of diet and to intake nutritional elements is well-known. At the same time, the health or lack of health of our teeth and gums can affect what we eat. Missing teeth are a factor in food choices and may affect individuals' ability to consume the necessary nutritional elements. Nutritional deficiencies in growing children, whether due to deprivation or mal-absorption syndromes may have significant impact on their natural development and somatic growth. The potential impact of eating disorders, chronic diseases and infection on overall health via physiologic and hormonal mechanisms has also been well established.

-   Early childhood caries is a chronic disease with a form of rampant decay of the primary dentition distinguished by the specificity of tooth surfaces involved and the rapid progression of carious lesions on those surfaces. It is usually associated with the onset of acute or chronic pain and infection. It appears that the chronicity of childhood caries might have the same influence on a child's ability to sustain normal growth patterns as any other chronic disease or infection, and therefore caries may impact upon general health and well being. Numerous studies have reported the prevalence of the disease as to affect up to 70% of the childhood population, especially in socio-economically deprived population.

- Inadequacy of the host's immune-defences may play a role in the acquisition of carious lesions. However, feeding habits are more important, especially in early childhood, and the role of feeding habits and behaviors in producing dental decay in childhood has been established by numerous studies.
- It has been reported that childhood caries inhibits adequate nutrition, thereby adversely affecting the growth of the body, specifically weight. Children with childhood caries have been noted to be significantly more likely to weigh less than 80% of their age-adjusted ideal weight, thereby satisfying one of the criteria for failure to thrive.
- The phenomenon of catch-up growth has been reported to occur in children whose growth had been slowed by illness or malnutrition and a case report has suggested that children with low weight and carious teeth demonstrated significant weight gain following dental rehabilitation.
- However, although many studies of the role of a healthy mouth in dietary intake pattern and nutritional intake have been reported, but there are very few epidemiological or intervention studies concerning the association between the growth of children and their oral health or the role of diet and nutrition in this association.
- The most important issue to be gleaned from the literature is that health professionals, especially paediatricians, do not routinely consider the effect of oral health in growth due to lack of dental knowledge or awareness of the importance of a healthy dentition in overall health. It seems that dental health professionals could play an important role in highlighting this issue and like other primary health carers, could perhaps be helpful in diagnosing and managing these two important health problems through dietary advice and encouragement of appropriate feeding behavior. Therefore, by preventing one it may be possible to prevent, or at least reduce, the risk of the other.

15. References

Acs G, Lodolini G, Kaminsky S, Cisneros GJ. (1992). Effect of nursing caries on body weight in a pediatric population. *Pediatrc Dent*, 14: 302-305.

Acs G, Loddine G, Shulman R, Cussid S. (1998). The effect of dental rehabilitation on the body weight of children with failure to thrive: case report. *Compend Contin Educ Dent*, 19: 164-8.

Acs G, Shulman R, Ng M, Chussid S. (1999). The effect of dental rehabilitation on the body weight of children with early child hood caries. *Pediatr Dent*, 21: 109-13.

Alvarez JO, Lewis CA, Saman C, Caceda J, Montalvo J, Figueroa ML, Izquierdo J, Caravedo L, Navia JM. (1988). Chronic malnutrition, dental caries and tooth exfoliation in Peruvian children aged 3-9 years. *Am J Clin Nutr*, 48: 368-372.

Alvarez JO, Navia JM. (1989).Nutritional status, tooth eruption, and dental caries: A review. *Am J Clin Nut*, 49: 417-426.

Alvarez JO, Eguren JC, Caceda J, Navia JM.. (1990). The effect of nutritional status on the age distribution of dental caries in the primary teeth. *J Dent Res*, 69: 1564-1566.

Amiutis WR. (2004). Bioactive properties of milk protein with particular focus on anticariogenicity. *J Nutr,* 134: 895-955.

Aptone-Merced L, Navia JM. (1980). Pre-eruptive protein malnutrition and acid solubility of rat molar enamel surfaces. *Arch Oral Bio*, 25: 701-705.

Ayhan H, Suskan E, Yildirim S. Ayhan H, Suskan E, Yildirim S. (1996).The effect of rampant caries on height, body weight and head circumference. *J Clin Pediat Dent*, 20: 209-212.

Babeely K, et al. (1989). Severity of nursing-bottle syndrome and feeding patterns in Kuwait. *Community Dent Oral Epidemiol*, 17: 237-9.

Barnes GP, Parker WA, Lyon TC Jr, Drum MA, Coleman GC. (1992). Ethnicity, location, age, and fluoridation factors in baby bottle tooth decay and caries prevalence of Head Start children. *Public Health Rep*, 107: 167-73.

Beaton GH, Chery A. (1988). Protein requirements of infants: a re-examination of concepts and approaches. *Am J Clin Nutr*, 48: 1403-12.

Benzian H, Monse B, Heinrich-Weltzien R, Hobdell M, Mulder J, van Palenstein Helderman W.(2011). Untreated severe dental decay: a neglected Determinant of low Body Mass Index in 12-year old Filipino children. *BMC Public Health*, 13. 07. 2011, Available from: http://www.biomedcentral.com/1471-2458/11/558.

Boyd LD, Palmer C, Dwyer JT. (1998). Managing oral health related nutrition issues of high risk infants and children. *J Clin Pediatr Dent*, 23: 31-6.

Broderick E, Mabry J, Robertson D, Thompson J. (1989). Baby bottle tooth decay in Native American children in Head Start centres. *Public Health Rep*, 104: 50-4.

Burt BA, Ismail Al. (1986). Diet, Nutrition and Food carieogenecity. *J Dent Res*, 65: 1475-1484.

De Onis M, Monteiro C, Akré J, Clugston G. (1993). The worldwide magnitude of protein energy malnutrition: an overview from the WHO Global Database on Child Growth. *Bull World Health Organ*, 71: 703-12.

De Onis M, Frongillo EA Jr, Blössner M. (2000). Is malnutrition declining? An analysis of changes in levels of child malnutrition since 1980. *Bull World Health Organ*, 78: 1222-33.

Department of Health and Social Security. (1996). present day practice in infant feeding. HMSO, London; N0 26.

Department of Health. The Health of the Nation. (1992). A Strategy for Health in England HMSO, London.

Derkson GD, Point P. (1982). Nursing bottle syndrome; prevalence and aetiology in a non-fluoridated city. *J Can Dent Assoc*, 48:389-93.

Dilley GJ, Dilley DH, Machen JB. (1980). Prolonged nursing habit: a profile of patients and their families. *ASDC J Dent Child*, 47: 102-8.

East BR. (1941).Association of dental caries in school children with hardness of communal water supplies. *J Dent Res*, 20: 323-326.

Eppright ES, Fox HM, Fryer BS, Lamkin CH, Vivian VM. (1969). Eating behaviour of preschool children. *J Nutr Educ Behav*; 1:16-19.

Fearne JM, Bryan EM, Elliman AM, Brook AH, Williams DM.(1990). Enamel defects in the primary dentition of children born weighing less than 2000 g. *Br Dent J*, 168: 433-7.

Garner P, Panpaich R, Logan S. (2000). Is routine growth monitoring effective? A systemic review of trial. *Arch Dis child*, 82: 197-201.

Gift HC, Reisine ST, Larach DC. (1992). The social impact of dental problems and visits. *Am J of Public Health*, 82: 1663-8.

Goepferd SJ. (1986). Infant oral health: a rationale. *ASDC J Dent Child*, 53: 257-60.

Graham GG. (1972). Environmental factors affecting the growth of children. *Am J Clin Nutr,* 25: 1184-8.

Gross KBW, Brough KM, Randolph PM. (1986). Eating disorders; anorexia and bulimia nervosa. *J Den child,* 53: 370-81.

Gustafsson BE, Quensel CE, Lanke LS, Lundqvist C, Grahne H, Bonow BE, Krasse B. (1954). The Vipeholm dental caries study; the effect of different levels of carbohydrate intake on caries activity in 436 individuals observed for five years. *Acta Odontol Scand,* 11: 232-64.

Hall DMB. (1996). *Growth Monitoring In: Health for all children.* Oxford University Press, Oxford.

Harrise G, Booth IW. (1992). The nature and management, eating problems in pre-school children. *Monographs in clin pediat,* 5: 61-84.

Holt RD. (1991). Foods and Drinks at four daily time intervals in a group of young children. *Br Dent J,* 170: 137-43.

Houlihane JOB, Rolls CJ. (1995) Morbidity from excessive intake of high energy fluids: the 'squash drinking syndrome' *Arch Dis Child,* 72: 141-43.

Ismail AI, Sohn W. (1999). A systematic review of clinical diagnostic criteria of early childhood caries. *J Pub Health Dent,* 59: 171-91.

Johansson I, Lummkari M, Ericson T. (1989). Effective of moderate vitamin A deficiency saliva secretion rate and salivary glycoproteins in adult rat. *Scand J Dent Res,* 97: 263-267.

Kaste LM, Marianos D, Chang R, Phipps KR. (1992). The assessment of nursing caries and its relationship to high caries in the permanent dentition. *J Public Health Dent,* 52: 64-8.

Katz L, Ripa LW, Petersen M.(1992). Nursing caries in Head Start children, St. Thomas U.S. Virgin Islands: assessed by examiners with different dental backgrounds. *J Clin Pediatr Dent,* 16: 124-8.

Kay, E. J., Northstone, K., Ness, A., Duncan, K. and Crean, S. J. (2010), Is there a relationship between Birth weight and subsequent growth on the development of Dental Caries at 5 years of age? A cohort study. *Communit Dent Oral Epidemiol,* 38: 408–414.

Kelly M, Bruerd B. (1987) The prevalence of baby bottle tooth decay among two native American populations. *J Public Health Dent,* 47: 94-7.

Konig KG, Schmid P and Schmid R. (1968).An apparatus for frequency- controlled feeding of small rodents and its use in dental caries experience. *Arch Oral Biol,* 13: 13-26.

Locker D. (1997). Concepts of oral health, disease and the quality of life. In: Slade GD, editor. *Measuring oral health and quality of life.* Chapel Hill: University of North Carolina, Dental Ecology, 8: 11-23.

Loesche WJ. (1986).Role of MS in human dental decay. *Microbial Rev,* 50: 353-80.

Louie R, Brunelle JA, Maggiore ED, Beck RW. (1990). Caries prevalence in Head Start children, 1986-87. *J Public Health Dent,* 50: 299-305.

Malek Mohammadi T, Wright CM, Kay EJ. (2009). Childhood growth and dental caries. *Communit Dent Health,* 26(1):38-42.

Mayanagi H, Saito T, Kamiyama K. (1995).Cross-sectional comparison of caries time trends in nursery school children in Sendia, Japan. *Communit Dent Oral Epidemio,* 23: 344-9.

Mellanby M, Pattison CL. (1928). The action of vitamin D in preventing the spread and promoting the arrest of caries in children. *Br Med J*, II: 1079-1082.

Mellanby M. (1928). The influence of diet on the structure of teeth. *Physiol Rev*, 8: 545-577.

Miller J, Vaughan-William E, Furlong R, Harrison L. (1982). Dental caries and children's weight. *J Epidemiol Community Health*, 36: 49-52.

Milnes AR. (1996). Description and epidemiology of nursing caries. *J Pub Health Dent*, 56: 38-50.

Minde k, Minde R.(1986) *Infant psychiatry; an introductory text*, London.

Ministry of Agriculture, Food and Farming. (1997). Healthy diets for young children, MAFF/DOH/Health Education Authority; London.

Palmer JD. (1971). Dietary habit at bed time in relation to dental caries in children. *Br Dent J*, 130: 288.

Prader A, Tanner JM, Von Haarnack G. (1963). Catch up growth following illness or starvation; an example of developmental canalization in man. *J Pediatr*, 62: 646-658.

Reid J. (1984).The role of maternal and child health clinic in Education and prevention: a case study from Papua New Guinea. *Soc Sci Med*, 19: 221-230.

Reisines A, Douglass JM. (1998). Psychosocial and behavioural issues in early childhood caries. *Community Dent Oral Epidemiol*, 26: 32-44.

Ripa LW. (1988) Nursing caries: a comprehensive review. *Pediatr Dent*, 10: 268-82.

Rockville, MD. (2000). Oral Health in America: A Report of the Surgeon General.:. US Department of Health and Human Services, *National Institute of Dental and Craniofacial Research, National Institutes of Health*.

Root AW, Bongiovanni AM, Eberlein WR. (1971). Diagnosis and management of growth retardation with special reference to the problem of hypopituitarism. J *Pediatr*, 78: 737-53.

Rugg-Gunn AJ. (2000). *Nutrition and Dental Health*. Oxford Medical Publication, Oxford.

Sheiham A. (1991). Why free sugar consumption should be below 15kg per person per year in industrialised countries, the dental evidence. *Br Dent J*, 171: 63-5.

Sheiham A, Steele J. (2001). Does the condition of the mouth and teeth affect the ability to eat certain foods, nutrient and dietary intake and nutritional status amongst older people? *Public Health Nutrition*, 4: 797-803.

Sheller B, Williams BJ, Lombardi SM.(1996).Diagnosis and treatment of dental caries related emergencies in a children's hospital. *J Clin Pediatr Dent*, 20: 313-16.

Sims LS, Morris PM. (1974)Nutritional status of preschoolers. An ecologic prospective. *Am Diet Assoc*, 64: 492-9.

Splett PL, Strory MC. (1991). Child nutrition: Objective for decade. *J Am Diet Assoc*, 91; 665-8.

Weinstein P, Domoto P, Wohlers K, Koday M. (1992). Mexican-American parents with children at risk for baby bottle tooth decay: pilot study at a migrant farm workers clinic. *J Dent Child*, 59: 376-83.

Whittle JG. (2000). The provision of primary care dental general anaesthesia and sedation in the North West region of England, 1996-1999. *Br Dent J*, 189: 500-2.

Winter GB. (1966). Symposium on aspects of the dental development of the child. 3. Local pathological conditions influencing the development of the upper labial segment. *Dent Pract Dent Rec*, 17:153-9.

Wright CM. (2000). Identification and management of failure to thrive: a community
perspective. *Arch Dis child*, 82: 5-9.

Zita AC, McDonald RE, Andrews AL. (1959). Dietary habits and the dental caries experience
in 200 children. *J Dent Res*, 38: 860-5.

Part 4

Others

12

Secondary Caries

Guang-yun Lai[1] and Ming-yu Li[2]

[1]Department of Restorative Dentistry and Periodontology,
Ludwig-Maximilians-University, Munich,
[2]Shanghai Key Laboratory of Stomatology, Shanghai Research Institute of Stomatology,
Ninth People's Hospital, Medical College, Shanghai Jiao Tong University, Shanghai,
[1]Germany
[2]P.R. China

1. Introduction

Secondary caries, the lesion at the margin of a restoration, has been widely considered as the most important and common reason for restoration replacement, regardless of the restorative material type [Collins et al., 1998; Dahl and Eriksen, 1978; Deligeorgi et al., 2001; Friedl et al., 1995; Mjör, 2005; Mjör and Toffenetti, 2000;]. As it develops after the initial caries has been removed and replaced by a restoration, 'secondary caries', which is often referred to as 'recurrent caries' by practitioners in North America, is used more commonly in Europe[Mjör, 2005]. The Fédération Dentaire Internationale defined secondary caries as a 'positively diagnosed carious lesion, which occurs at the margins of an existing restoration' [Fédération Dentaire Internationale, 1962]. Then two kinds of lesion may exist adjacent to the restorations: secondary caries and residual caries (remaining caries). The latter one is residual demineralized tissue left, due to the failure of eliminating all infected dentine or/and enamel during the cavity preparation. Therefore it is very difficult for clinicians to make an accurate diagnosis of secondary caries and provide a clear terminology. Nowadays it is generally acknowledged that secondary caries or recurrent caries is a primary carious lesion of tooth at the margin of an existing restoration, which occurs after the restoration has been used for some time [Mjör and Toffenetti, 2000].

Due to its importance to the longevity of the restorations and human oral health, over the past few decades, multiple of studies have been conducted both in vivo and in vitro to understand and prevent secondary caries, including the etiology and histopathology of secondary caries, the detective and diagnostic methods of secondary caries, the relationship between microleakage and secondary caries, as well as the cariostatic effects of various restorative materials. The purpose of this chapter is to present a systematic and brief review of secondary caries in order to draw people's attention to this common but also complicated dental disease.

2. Diagnosis of secondary caries

2.1 Histology of secondary caries

In the 1970s, Hals et al. did a comprehensive investigation of the secondary caries lesions around various restorative materials both in vitro and in vivo, and natural secondary caries on the extracted restored human teeth [Hals, 1975a, 1975b; Hals et al., 1974; Hals and Nernaes, 1971; Hals and Norderval, 1973; Hals and Simonsen1972]. According to their studies, whatever the restorative material type is, the secondary carious lesion displayed histologically the same basic pattern (Fig. 1): 1) an outer lesion, which is caused by the a new primary attack on the outer surface of the tooth; 2) a wall lesion, might be the consequence of the diffusion of bacteria, fluids or hydrogen ions between the restorations and the cavity wall. It is also supposed in their study that the fluoride released from the silicate material would be taken by both the cavity wall and the tooth surface around the restoration, which might reduce glycolysis and induce the remineralization [Hals, 1975a]. Thus, the individual caries patterns between the teeth with silicate materials and amalgam are different more or less. However, this described pattern of secondary caries including the outer lesion and wall lesion has been confirmed in later experiments [Diercke et al., 2009; Thomas et al., 2007; Totiam et al., 2007].

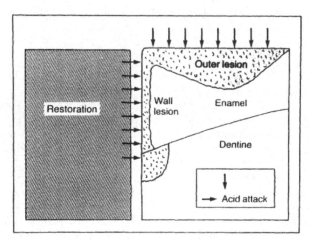

Fig. 1. A diagrammatic representation of secondary caries

The secondary caries lesion may occur in two parts: an outer lesion, formed on the surface of the tooth as a result of primary attack and a wall lesion formed as a result of diffusion of bacteria, fluids or hydrogen ions between the restorations and the cavity wall (From Kidd, 1990).

2.2 Frequency and location of diagnosed secondary caries

Since the early days of restorative dentistry, the phenomenon of secondary caries has been known and considered as the basis for the extension-for-prevention concept, the well-known principles of cavity preparation established by G.V. Black in the last century [Black, 1908]. The clinical diagnosed secondary caries has been shown to be principal cause for the replacement of all types of restorations both in permanent and primary teeth, 50%-60% of restorations are replaced as a result of the diagnosis of secondary caries [Mjör and Toffenetti, 2000]. As the development of restorative materials, some literatures regarding secondary caries indicated that the prevalence of secondary caries is associated with the restorative material type, although it may occur with all restorative materials [Burke et al.,

1999b; Forss and Widström E, 2004; Mjör, 1997; Mjör and Jokstadt, 1993]. Some published researches showed that compared to amalgam restorations, resin-based composite restorations represented a higher percentage of replacement because of the diagnosed secondary caries [Mjör and Jokstadt, 1993; Bernardo et al., 2007]. On the contrary, others reported that the amalgam was replaced because of the secondary caries more often than composite resin [Wilson et al., 1997; Burke et al., 1999a]. Compared with those studies, which acclaimed that a large proportion of restorations replaced as a result of diagnosis of secondary caries in general dental practice, one controlled clinical trials showed secondary caries represented in less than 1 percent of the restoration failures [Letzel et al., 1989], inversely, another controlled clinical trials by Bernardo et al. reported that secondary caries accounted for 66.7 percent and 87.6 percent of the failures that occurred in amalgam and composite restorations, respectively [Bernardo et al., 2007]. These controversies might be explained that the statistic results could be influenced by many factors, including the age of the population, the status of patients' oral health and dental care, examiner calibration and the duration of the experiment, etc.

Secondary caries, like other dental caries, is initially caused by the activities of microorganisms in dental plaque, so it is possible for any site on the restored teeth where is prone to the bacterial stagnation to develop secondary caries. General practitioners indicated that secondary caries was detected predominately on the gingival margins of Class II and Class I restorations, while seldom on the Class I restorations and the occlusal part of Class II restorations [Mjör, 1998; Mjör and Qvist, 1997]. A number of factors contribute to the more frequent occurrence of secondary caries on the gingival surface. First of all, the gingival aspect of any restorations is more difficult for patient to keep plaque free than any other parts, especially if it is located interproximally, while the occlusal surface is not a generally a plaque stagnation area and toothbrushing can easily reach this area to clean the plaque [Kidd, 2001; Mjör, 2005]. Secondly, during the restorative operation, the gingival surface is prone to contamination by gingival fluid and saliva, which causes the impossible visual inspection of the gingival floor and the deficiencies of insertion of restorative materials. And these deficiencies may lead to secondary caries more easily [Mjör, 2005]. Meanwhile, the less effective bonding of resin composite and the polymerization shrinkage at the gingival cavosurface may also influence the integrity of restoration at the gingival section and result in the development of secondary caries [Mjör, 2005].

2.3 The specific diagnostic problem and the diagnostic methods

As it was described above, while secondary caries accounts for more than half of replacing restorations regardless of the different materials in the general practice, around 50 percent, this high prevalence is not found in one controlled clinical trial in which only 2 among 2660 Class I or II restorations were replaced due to secondary caries [Letzel et al., 1989]. On the contrary, in another randomized controlled clinical trial 66.7% and 87.6% of the failures that occurred in amalgam and composite restorations because of the diagnosed secondary caries, respectively [Bernardo et al., 2007]. Are they correct or wrong? Why are there are huge differences between these studies? Are the practitioners involved in these studies poorly trained or ignorant about the criteria of secondary caries diagnosis? Indeed, until now it is very difficult to explain the above questions reasonably, however, except the variation between those studies themselves, it should be acknowledged that there are some specific diagnostic problems for secondary caries and it is very crucial to understand secondary caries correctly in order to make an accurate diagnosis.

In 1990 Kidd pointed out that there are several main specific diagnostic problems for secondary caries, including the difficulty of detecting the wall lesion; the relevance of a defective margin(e.g. ditched margin) to the longevity of a restoration and the difficulty of distinguishing secondary from residual caries [Kidd, 1990]. It is suggested that only frankly caries lesion at the margin of the restoration constitutes a dependable diagnosis of secondary caries [Kidd and Bieghton, 1996], whereas it is impossible to detect or see the wall lesion until it is so advanced that the overlying tissue collapses to reveal a large hole or the tooth tissue over it becomes grossly discoloured [Kidd, 1990]. Consequently, dentists often cannot detect or diagnose a secondary caries when a wall lesion is in progress under a sound surface.

Traditionally, the presence of clinically detectable defects in restoration margins has been associated with an increased risk of secondary caries occurring beneath such restorations [Hewlett et al., 1993]. Besides, marginal defects present between a restoration and the cavity wall, such as those occur in occlusal pits and fissures, may act as gathering points for bacterial plaque [Pimenta et al., 1995]. Surveys in which dental practitioners determine reasons for replacing restoration indicate that clinical evidence of defective margins is a commonly used criterion for replacing restorations [Boyd and Richardson, 1985; Qvist et al., 1986]. On the other hand, other studies showed the low relevance of defective margin to restoration replacement and secondary caries which supported the conclusion that the defective margin only can not be the reason to replace a restoration. Söderholm et al. suggested that the use of defected margin as the criterion for restoration replacement would have resulted in the unnecessary treatment of 34% of the teeth examined [Söderholm, 1989]. Kidd and O'Hara reported that caries incidence on the cavity wall adjacent to the margins was the same for both in the intact and defective restoration [Kidd and O'Hara, 1990]. Although, Hewelett et al. found the likelihood of radiographic secondary caries was much higher for defective restorations than for intact restorations through the investigation of radiographic secondary caries prevalence in 6285 teeth clinically defective restorations, it was still suggested that defective restoration status should be combined with radiographic examination [Hewlett et al., 1993]. Therefore, the presence of ditched margins where are plaque stagnation areas which might enhance the prevalence of secondary caries development, however, is not a sufficient factor to determine a possible process of secondary caries formation [Pimenta et al., 1995]. Furthermore, the progression of caries is determined by the dynamic balance between pathological factors that lead to demineralization and protective factors that lead to remineralization. If either the pathological factors are not sufficient or protective factor are present, caries will not develop regardless of tooth morphology [Featherstone, 2004].

According to the definition, secondary caries is a new primary caries and should be differentiated from residual caries. In the past, on the basis of the extension-for-prevention concept, the cavity preparation principles established by G.V. Black, students were taught to prepare the cavity as clean as possible. Nowadays, as the development of conservative dentistry and minimal intervention dentistry and remineralization, it is recommended that dentists should distinguish the affected tissue which could be healed by remineralization and infected tissue, only infected should be removed to preserve more dental tissue and increase the longevity of the teeth [Fusayama, 1988; Kidd, 2010; Massler, 1967;]. However, it is impossible to predict whether these residual lesions will progress. Thus, it is thought-provoking that the modern dentistry might increase the difficulty of distinguishing the secondary and residual caries. Or it might not be so important to differentiate the secondary and residual caries.

To diagnose the carious lesion, either primary or secondary, the dentists need good lighting, clean teeth, sharp eyes and even good bitewing radiography [kidd, 1984]. Secondary caries develops more frequently at the cervical and interproximal margins [Mjör, 1985; Mjör, 2005], more attention must be paid to find better methods or techniques to detect the secondary caries, despite of those difficulties to make an accurate diagnosis of secondary caries. The conventional visual and tactile methods using a sharp explorer have been advocated in the diagnosis of primary and secondary caries [kidd, 1990]. However, in recent years it has been shown that the sharp explorer seems to be an unwise instrument to detect secondary caries. On one hand, a sharp explorer could cause cavitation of an outer lesion, damage the margin of a restoration, or even become impacted in a marginal discrepancy which might then be misinterpreted as a carious lesion [Bergman and Lindén, 1969; Ekstrand et al, 1987]. On the other hand, wall lesions of secondary caries can not easily be detected until they have reached an advanced stage [Kidd, 1990], it is very difficult for explorer to contact the lesion and detect it at the early stage. And it is important to keep in mind that a sharp explorer will stick in any crevice, regardless of whether there is carious lesion [Mjör, 2005]. Additionally, discoloration around dental restorations may be due to the variety of factors such as the physical presence of amalgam, corrosion products, or secondary caries. It could be concluded that colors or stains next to restorations are not always predictive of secondary caries and not useful for the detection of secondary caries [kidd et al., 1995, Rudoolphy, 1995], whereas, it is very difficult to distinguish whether the discoloration originated from the restoration or was to due the demineralization [Ando et al., 2004]. Until now, besides the most common and traditional method of visual examination with a tactile instrument, there are some several other methods available to measure the mineral loss, such as microradiograph [Arends et al., 1987] and CLSM (confocal laser scanning microscopy), which measures the fluorescence area to determine the secondary caries [Fontana et al., 1996]. It is reported that QLF (light-induced fluorescence) might be a suitable technique for detection of early secondary carious lesions less than 400μm meanwhile LF (infrared laser fluorescence) might be a suitable technique for the detection of secondary caries, especially for lesions over 400μm or dentinal lesions [Ando et al., 2004].

3. Etiology of secondary caries

3.1 Microbiology of secondary caries

Dental caries is determined by the dynamic balance between pathological factors that lead to demineralization and protective factors that lead to remineralization [Featherstone, 2004]. As a major pathological factor, oral bacteria, especially acidogenic bacteria, can dissolve the tooth mineral. Those acidogenic bacteria are also aciduric and can live preferentially under acid conditions [Loesche, 1986].

Hitherto, it is unclear about the microbiology of secondary caries yet. Although secondary caries is described alike primary caries in histopathology, whether the etiology of secondary caries is the same as that of primary caries is a matter in dispute. Kidd et al. found no significant differences between the microflora in samples from cavity walls involving primary and secondary caries next to the amalgam [Kidd et al., 1993]. However, Thomas et al. investigated bacterial composition in relation to primary and secondary caries via an in situ model, and found a phenomenon of higher proportion of caries-associated bacteria on composite surfaces. Then they indicated that the microbiology on the surface of the primary caries differs from that on the surface of lesion around composite, and secondary caries around composite may differ from the primary lesions process [Thomas et al., 2008]. In addition, some studies focused on the ecology under the restorations. Mejàre et al. found the bacterial colonization beneath composite similar to that observed in dental plaque mainly including Streptococci and Actinomyces spp. [Mejàre et al., 1979]. Nevertheless, according to the experiment conducted by Splieth et al., it was the other way around [Splieth et al., 2003]. They compared the microbial spectrum under composite and amalgam fillings with special attention to the anaerobic flora. The results showed that bacterial composition under amalgam was similar to the flora of carious dentin and carious plaque, with anaerobic and facultative anaerobic gram-positive rods dominating. On the contrary, huge amounts of Bacteroides and Prevotella spp. were detected under many composite fillings, similar to the microflora of infected root canals with potentially pulpopathogenic microbes. Thus, the study suggested that the types of restorative materials seemed to have an effect on the composition of the microflora on the surface of secondary caries, and that beneath the restorations, and then the differences might exist between the microbial flora of secondary caries and primary caries. In this study, it was indicated that inadequate composite fillings might stimulate the growth of cariogenic as well as obligate anaerobic and potentially pulpopathogenic bacteria. This could be explained as follows: 1) The microspace between the restoration and the cavity floor favors the obligate anaerobic, and then leads to the detection of those bacteria; 2) It is not surprising to discover many obligate anaerobic normally colonize in human oral, even in oral of people without obvious endodontic diseases. 3) It doesn't mean that people without clinical symptoms of toothaches or pulpitis don't have chronic or arrested tooth diseases, so it is possible to detect those anaerobic bacteria. However, existence does not mean participation, so it is necessary to certify the participation of those obligate anaerobic in the progress of secondary caries in further studies.

According to the viewpoint of Marsh that any species with the ability producing acids and tolerating the cariogenic environment can contribute to the dental caries process [Marsh, 2006]. *Streptococci mutans (S. mutans), Lactobacilli* and *Actinomyces naeslundii* have been used by various models in vitro studying secondary caries for a long time. *S. mutants* and lactobacilli can produce a series of acid and stay in a low pH environment for a long time, leading to demineralization of teeth and caries lesion. It has been shown that the three bacteria were widely present and might play an important role in the development of secondary caries around amalgam [González-Cabezas, 1999]. However, in a recent in situ study, *S. mutants* were not detected in each sample, but *Lactobacilli*. Meanwhile, *A. Odontolyticus* and *Candida spp.* were also found in most samples [Thomas et al., 2008]. In addition, in recent years, Beighton put forward a point of view — *S. mutants* might be good makers of secondary caries but not necessarily the etiological agents [Beighton, 2005]. The experiment by Thomas et al. described before, in which *S. mutants* was not found in every sample, but *Lactobacilli* and *A. Odontolyticus*, seemed to support Beighton's view. And scientists conjectured that there might be unknown caries-associated bacteria, which can not grow on blood agar [Thomas et al., 2008]. In the past decade, the detection of *A. Odontolyticus* and *Candida spp.* has caused the serious concern to researchers. It has been found that *Candida albicans* can dissolve hydroxyapatite in a liquid culture at a 20-fold higher rate than *S. mutants*, despite the much lower growth rate [Nikawa et al., 2003]. Klinke et al. assumed that *Candida albicans* might make a significant contribution to caries pathogenesis in caries-active children, and it could be taken into account *Candida albicans* as an appraisal of caries pathogenicity [Klinke et al, 2009]. Besides, it should be noted that some people may have serious caries activities without S. mutants dominating in dental plaque. Therefore, further research need to be carried out to determine the microbiology of secondary caries, such as the role of *S. mutants*, *A. Odontolyticus* and *Candida spp.* in the development of secondary caries and the relationship between restorations and microorganism of secondary caries.

3.2 The relevance of microleakage to secondary caries

Microleakage refers to the clinically undetectable leakage between the cavity wall and the filling [Kidd, 1976]. Irie et al. found that a gap of 6-10μm formed immediately even after applying an acid etch and a bonding agent [Irie et al., 2002]. Iwami et al. have confirmed that any restorative material can completely eliminate the microleakage between restoration and the cavity wall [Iwami et al., 2005], supported by other researches [Irie and Suzuki, 1999; Huang et al., 2002; Piwowarczyk et al, 2005]. A study in vitro showed that there was no significant difference in the degree of microleakage between conventional caries removal and chemo-mechanical removal [Mousavinenasab and Jafary, 2004]. Those above all show us that microleakage is inevitable.

The microspace between the restoration wall and tooth can allow salivary pellicle accumulation and bacterial invasion [González-Cabezas et al., 1999; González-Cabezas et al., 2002; Splieth et al., 2003]. In a sense, it provides a favorable environment for the oral bacteria, especially cariogenic bacteria, such as S. mutants and Lacotobacilli, to demineralize the tooth structure along the cavity wall, as long as conditions are adequate and suitable. The histopathological appearance of the wall lesion in the secondary caries is also explained by hydrogen ions due to the diffusion of bacteria into the space between restoration and cavity wall and its acdiogenic activities afterwards [Hals and Nernaes, 1971]. So microleakage has been considered as a potential predictor for secondary caries and has caused serious concern to many researchers. In some article, the wall lesion was described as the consequence of microleakge [Diercke et al., 2009].

Up to now, there has been no conclusive statement about the relationship between microleakage and secondary caries. Several studies in vitro have shown a positive relationship between the two things. Jørgensen and Wakumoto in a 1968 research found that there was an increasing likelihood of secondary caries with the increasing size of the microspace [Jørgensen and Wakumoto, 1968], which is in agreement with that reported by some other researches [Goldbeg et al., 1981; Dérand et al., 1991]. In a recent in vitro study on relationship of gap size and secondary caries, the findings suggested that the gap size between tooth and restoration affected the development of secondary caries along the cavity wall [Totiam et al., 2007], for which the rationale was that bigger gaps would provide necessary space for bacterial colonization and enough nutrients for cariogenic microorganisms leading to the creation of larger wall lesions. On the other hand, within smaller spaces, minerals dissolved from the tooth structure due to the acid attacks would supersaturate the space immediately and create the remineralization of tooth tissue and smaller wall lesions.

In contrast, other studies have not stated any association between gap presence and secondary caries [Kidd and O'Hara, 1990; Pimenta et al., 1995]. Some suggested that there was no caries lesion along the cavity wall, unless large voids or gaps of $\geq 250\mu m$ [Ozer and Thylstrup, 1995] or even $\geq 400\mu m$ [Kidd et al., 1995]. Jørgensen and Wakumoto found poor correlation between the two only when gaps was $\geq 50\mu m$ [Jørgensen and Wakumoto, 1968]. Thomas et al. found no clear caries along the cavity wall next to composite, but to acrylic resin through an in situ study [Thomas et al., 2007]. Besides, observed cracks in teeth might be the best clinical evidence for microleakage does not lead to dental caries. These cracks and the adjacent areas can be stained over time, however, there is no caries development. The stained component is considered to be the proteinaceous material in the crack or crevice, and similar in composition to that of the biofilm which normally covers all teeth and restorations [Mjör, 2005].

Recently, a few studies have been conducted concerning the relationship between gap size and secondary caries in the presence or absence of fluoride. Cenci et al. in 2008 suggested that microleakage did not seem to influence secondary caries while the presence of fluoride in the plaque like biofilm (PLB) provided either by glass ionomer cement (GIC) or fluoride dentifrice (FD) [Cenci et al., 2008]. In 2009, Cenci et al. demonstrated that carious lesion depth increased with gap size for composite resin (CR) and suggested that the gap width affected secondary caries formation at the cavity wall, but only in the absence of fluoride released from fluoride-containing materials, such as GIC [Cenci et al., 2009]. Thus, these findings give implications for clinical caries treatment choices and further studies in vivo or clinical experiments are needed to investigate the relationship between the gap size, fluoride presence and secondary caries.

In sum, up to the present, there is no specific conclusion on the relationship between microleakage and secondary caries, specially the wall lesion of the cavity. The possible reasons are as follows: 1) Oral cavity is such an extremely complex that it is impossible to simulate completely, so the research results may be not all-inclusive. 2) Secondary caries is caused by various factors, so it might be difficult for researchers to consider fully when designing their experiments. Thus, in consequence, different experiments bring out different results, and sometimes those results are even conflicting. 3) For individual differences, people have varying degrees of susceptibility to caries. Therefore, different clinical studies may lead to different results and conclusions. 4) Some clinical studies may lack reasonable designs, which lead to incomprehensive results. However, there is a consensus that microleakage is indeed associated with secondary caries due to the existence of bacteria. It seems that microleakage is just a necessary but not a sufficient condition for the formation of a wall lesion [Kidd et al., 1995; Thomas et al., 2007], although in 2009, Diercke et al. carried out a pure in vitro experiment, in which the development of the outer lesion in the secondary caries was inhibited to study the relation between the gap size and the wall lesion independently, and confirmed the occurrence of wall lesions without the presence of outer lesion and indicated the extent of wall lesion increased with increasing gap width ranging from 50 to 250µm [Diercke et al., 2009]. Therefore, more in-depth studies are needed to get a thorough understanding about the relationship between microleakage and secondary caries.

4. Prevention and treatment of secondary caries

4.1 Prevention of secondary caries

As secondary caries is one of the major reasons for restoration replacement, a large number of clinical dentists and scientists have placed great emphasis on preventing or slowing down the procession of secondary caries lesion from many aspects, so as to increase clinical restoration durability. Secondary caries, the same as other types of dental caries, is determined by the dynamic balance between pathological factors that lead to demineralization and protective factors that lead to remineralization. It is also considered that bacteria are an important etiologic factor leading to demineralization for secondary caries. Generally, the rationales of all the modification of restorative material or prevention of secondary caries normally include two fundamental points: one is the decrease of demineralization and/or increase of remineralization of the hard tooth tissues; the other is to interfere the metabolism of caries-related bacteria and/or to decrease the amount of bacteria/inhibit bacteria growth in the plaque or /and the carious dentin under restorations. Thus, in all the past years, most scientists and clinical dentists focused on adding anticaries substance into restorative materials.

It has been well-known such restorative materials can release copper, Ag–Cu alloy, zinc, calcium, aluminum and fluoride, which are able to inhibit bacteria growth or decrease colonization and acidogenicity of oral plaque, play antibacterial activities and reduce the rate of restoration replacement. The followings are several basic fillings used and researched by clinical dentists and scientists throughout the world: amalgam restorations, zinc oxide eugenol cement; common composite resin (CR); common glass ionomer cement (GIC); and different ion-released restorative materials containing fluoride-containing materials.

Clemens Boeckh et al. investigated the antimicrobial effects of five restorative materials and showed that the most remarkable inhibitory activity was observed with ZOE [Boeckh et al., 2002]. The antimicrobial effects of zinc oxide and ZOE are well recognized [Podbielski et al., 2000; Yap et al., 1999]. Unfortunately, ZOE cannot be widely used except for temporary filling due to its high solubility and insufficient mechanical properties. Different types of amalgam may have different effects on S. mutans growth and bacterial penetration [Fayyad and Ball, 1987]. For instance, a low-copper amalgam can decrease the lesion size significantly [Grossman and Matejka, 1995], non-gamma-2 amalgam can inhibit the metabolic activity of microorganisms due to the release of copper [Wallman-Björklund et al., 1987].

It has been widely shown in long term studies that CR have higher rate of restorations replacement than GIC and amalgam [Leinfelder,et al., 1987; Collins et al., 1998]. An in situ study showed that the percentage of streptococci in plaque on different materials was to be 13.7% on composite, 4.3% on amalgam and 1.1% on glass ionomer cement [Svanberg et al., 1990]. Another study showed up to eight times more microbes beneath composite restorations compared to amalgam and suggested the type of restorative material may have influence on the composition of the microflora [Splieth et al., 2003]. The high rate replacement of CR occurred might be due to its shrinkage and non-fluoride release [Savarino et al., 2004]. Thus, scientists have been making great efforts to improve CR, such as reducing the polymerization shrinkage of composite, increasing the adhesion stress. Remarkably, a modified ion-releasing resin composite (IRCR) has been invented, which can release hydroxyl, calcium, and fluoride ions at low pH [Boeckh et al., 2002]. The rationales of anticaries effect of IRCR include: OH⁻ ions can neutralize the organic acids produced by the plaque bacteria [Heintze, 1999], and the calcium and fluoride ions released from IRCR can prevent demineralization and promote remineralization [ten Cate, 1990; ten Cate and van Duinen, 1995; Featherstone, 1994; Forss and Seppä, 1990; Kraft and Hoyer, 1999]. Thus, the restoration can perform anticaries activities. Studies have shown the release of hydroxyl and calcium can exist for a long period [Heintze, 1999]. Persson and his colleagues showed that IRCR could counter the plaque pH fall and maintain it at levels where less enamel and dentin demineralization can occur [Persson et al., 2004], however, the precious research did not consider IRCR could present significant antibacterial effects [Boeckh et al., 2002].

The inhibition of fluoride at acidic pH is due to the effect of hydrogen fluoride, which can penetrate into the bacteria cell membrane [Nakajo et al., 2009]. The HF can dissociate into hydrogen ion and fluoride ion. Some researchers confirmed that the fluoride can reduce the activities of enolase and proton-extruding ATPase, which are very important for metabolism of bacteria [Hayacibara et al., 2003]. Besides, the hydrogen ion can promote cytoplasmic acidification, which is critical for enzymes of the glycolytic pathway [Hüther et al., 1990]. So the combination effects of hydrogen ion and fluoride can have negative influence on the glycolytic acid production and the metabolism of caries-related bacteria. As a result, fluoride-containing restorative material can inhibit bacteria growth and decrease the demineralization of tooth tissue and the occurrence of secondary caries around restorations. However, these antimicrobial effects in caries prevention are often regarded as little or of no importance as compared to the direct interactions of fluoride with the hard tissue during caries development and progression [Wiegand et al., 2007]. Recent observations have found fluoride in the aqueous phase surrounding the carbonated apatite crystals is much more effective in inhibiting demineralization than fluoride incorporated into the crystal [Rølla and Ekstand, 1996]. Fluoride may precipitate onto tooth surfaces as calcium fluoride-like layer, which serves as a reservoir for fluoride when the pH drops [Rølla et al., 1993]. While amount of in vitro studies showed the inhibitive effect of fluoride on the demineralization of both enamel and dentin around the restoration in primary and permanent teeth[Attar and Önen, 2002; Donly and Gomez, 1994; Francci et al., 1999; Hicks et al., 2002; Tam et al., 1997; Yaman, 2004], the results from some in situ studies are not consistent with that in vitro, which have not confirmed the preventive ability of fluoride to secondary caries[Kielbassa et al., 1999, 2003; Papagiannouslis et al., 2002]. And this conflict is also showed among varieties of clinical studies. In a six-year follow-up assessment, class I restorations in permanent molars exhibited significantly less secondary caries for glass-ionomers(2%) compared to amalgam(10%) [Mandari et al., 2003]. Another five-year evaluation showed the glass-ionomer had a lower survival time and greater loss of anatomic form and marginal integrity, but less secondary caries compared to amalgam [Welbury et al., 1991]. Instead, Van Dijken found no difference in secondary caries development of class III cavities restored with two fluoride-containing materials and one composite in a three-year observation period [van Dijken, 1996]. Moreover, there is no clear evidence for inhibition of secondary caries by glass-ionomer cements as shown in a recent review summarizing extensive literature research [Randall and Wilson, 1999].

The above conflicts might be explained by the following factors: 1) the intrinsic formulation of fluoride-containing materials, the duration of fluoride releasing may influence its effect. The antibacterial effect of dentin is obtained only when the fluoride release is very large

[Kawai et al., 1998]. 2) The ability of fluoride uptake by different dental hard tissue. Due to differences in micro-structure and porosities, the amount of fluoride uptake from restorations and the depth of fluoride penetration are higher for both dentin and cementum than for enamel [Souganidis et al., 1981; Retief et al., 1984]. 3) Other environmental conditions. A decrease in pH increases the dissolution of the material leading to a higher fluoride level and the highest fluoride release is found in acidic and demineralizing-remineralizing regimes and lowest in saliva [Karantakis et al., 2000]. A pellicle forming by the components from saliva on the surface of the restorative material and various bleaching agents can impede fluoride ion release [Behrend and Geurtsen, 2001; Bell at al., 1999; Levallois et al., 1998]. 4) Extra application of fluoride. In a recent research, Cenci et al. found that the fluoride provided either by GI or fluoride dentifrice might be important to decrease demineralization adjacent to fillings, and by using fluoride dentifrice, demineralization adjacent to the restorations were similar [Cenci et al., 2008], which was testified by the previous study [Hara et al., 2006]. 5) In some cases, cavity type may play a significant role in the development of secondary caries [da Rosa Rodolpho et al., 2006], for example class II restorations involve the marginal ridges and significantly reduce the tooth resistance to fracture [Mondelli et al., 1980], and is susceptible to the biodegradation of saliva esterase activity [Finer and Santerre, 2004].

Since the final formation of caries is influenced by multiple factors, the prevention of secondary caries beginning at the time of restoration replacement contains a variety of aspects including the excavation of carious tissue; wise choice of restorative materials; fluoride regimen implementation(rinses, gels, fluoridated toothpastes); salivary flow rate assessment; healthy dietary; oral health or medical education and so on. Therefore, the prevention of secondary cares not only depends on the clinical operation by dentists, but also is influenced by other significant aspects from patients themselves.

4.2 Treatment of secondary caries

Restoration replacement has been invariably deemed as the sequela of clinically diagnosed secondary caries. Although practitioners are suggested should pay attention to the differentiation between secondary caries and discoloration, defective margin and residual caries, generally, a localized surface defect adjacent to restoration features clinically diagnosed secondary carious lesion [Mjör, 2005]. However, Some dental teaching programs related to localized defects on restorations including secondary caries , indicate that repair, rather than replacement, of the restoration is adopted frequently as an alternative to total replacement [Mjör and Gordan, 2002; Blum et al., 2002; Blum et al., 2003; Gordan et al., 2003]. Moreover, the modern conservative dentistry and minimal intervention dentistry call for repairing and refurbishing any localized defects at restoration margins, clinically diagnosed secondary caries rather than total replacement of restoration [Ericson et al., 2003]. Despite of the difficulties of detection and diagnosis of secondary caries, dentists should be trained and should be deliberate in making the decision of total replacement of restoration.

5. Conclusion

Secondary caries has been considered to account for majority of restoration failures and result in restoration replacement. It plays a significant role in human oral health and the longevity of restorations. Until now, there is no standardized criterion for diagnosis of secondary caries, although it is possible to detect the tiny carious lesions using advanced techniques such as QLF and LF. Further experiments and clinical studies are needed to clarify those specific problems. Regardless of those difficulties and conflicts related to secondary caries, the key point is that more care need to be taken to prevent secondary caries and dentists should be cautious when they decide to replace the restoration completely. Besides, patients should be educated to protect the restoration through good oral hygiene and caries-preventive approaches.

6. Acknowledgement

This work was supported by Science and Technology Commission of Shanghai (08DZ2271100) and Shanghai Leading Academic Discipline Project (Project Number: S30206).

7. References

Ando, M., González-Cabezas, C., Isaacs, R. L., Eckert, G. J., & Stookey, G.K. (2004). Evaluation of Several Techniques for the Detection of Secondary Caries Adjacent to Amalgam Restorations. *Caries Research,* Vol. 38(4), pp. 350-356.

Arends, J., Dijkman, T., & Christoffersen, J. (1987). Average mineral loss in dental enamel during demineralization. *Caries Research,* Vol. 21(3), pp. 249-254.

Attar, N., & Önen, A. (2002). Artificial formed caries-like lesions around esthetic restorative materials. *Journal of Clinical Pediatric Dentistry,* Vol. 26(3), pp. 289-296.

Behrend, B., & Geurtsen, W. (2001). Long-term effects of four extraction media on the fluoride release from four polyacid-modified composite resins (compomers) and one resin-modified glass-ionomer cement. *Journal of Biomedical Materials Research,* Vol. 58(6), pp. 631-637.

Beighton, David. (2005). The complex oral microflora of high-risk individuals and groups and its role in the caries process. *Community Dentistry and Oral Epidemiology,* Vol. 33(4), pp. 248-255.

Bell, A., Creanor, S. L., Foye, R. H., & Saunders, W. P. (1999). The effect of saliva on fluoride release by a glass-ionomer filling material. *Journal of Oral Rehabilitation,* Vol. 26(5), pp. 407-412.

Bergman, G., & Lindén, L. A. (1969). The action of the explorer on incipient caries. Svensk Tandläkare Tidskrift. *Swedish Dental Journal,* Vol. 62(10), pp. 629-634.

Bernardo, M., Luis, H., Martin, M. D., Leroux, B. G., Rue, T., Leitão, J., & DeRouen, T. A. (2007). Survival and reasons for failure of amalgam versus composite posterior restorations placed in a randomized clinical trial. *Journal of the American Dental Association,* Vol. 138(6), pp. 775-783.

Black GV. *A work on operative dentistry.* Chicago: Medico-Dental Publishing; 1908. The technical procedures in filling teeth; Vol. 2.

Blum, I R, Schriever, A, Heidemann, D, Mjör, I A, & Wilson, N H F. (2003). The repair of direct composite restorations: an international survey of the teaching of operative techniques and materials. *European Journal of Dental Education,* 7(1), pp. 41-48.

Blum, Igor R, Schriever, Anette, Heidemann, Detlef, Mjör, Ivar A, & Wilson, Nairn H F. (2002). Repair versus replacement of defective direct composite restorations in teaching programmes in United Kingdom and Irish Dental Schools. *The European Journal of Prosthodontics and Restorative Dentistry,* Vol. 10(4), pp. 151-155.

Boeckh, Clemens, Schumacher, E., Podbielski, Andreas, & Haller, Bernd. (2002). Antibacterial Activity of Restorative Dental Biomaterials in vitro. *Caries Research,* Vol. 36(2), pp. 101-107.

Boyd, M. A., & Richardson, A. S. (1985). Frequency of amalgam replacement in general dental practice. *Journal Canadian Dental Association,* Vol. 51(10), pp. 763-766.

Burke, F. J., Cheung, S. W., Mjör, I A, & Wilson, N. H. (1999a). Reasons for the placement and replacement of restorations in vocational training practices. Primary Dental Care: *Journal of the Faculty of General Dental Practitioners,* Vol. 6(1), pp. 17-20.

Burke, F. J., Cheung, S. W., Mjör, I A, & Wilson, N. H. (1999b). Restoration longevity and analysis of reasons for the placement and replacement of restorations provided by vocational dental practitioners and their trainers in the United Kingdom. *Quintessence International,* Vol. 30(4), pp. 234-242.

ten Cate, J. M. (1990). In vitro studies on the effects of fluoride on de- and remineralization. *Journal of Dental Research,* Vol. 69 Spec No, 614-619; discussion pp. 634-636.

ten Cate, J. M., & van Duinen, R. N. (1995). Hypermineralization of dentinal lesions adjacent to glass-ionomer cement restorations. *Journal of Dental Research,* Vol. 74(6), pp. 1266-1271.

Cenci, M S, Pereira-Cenci, T., Cury, J. A., & Ten Cate, J. M. (2009). Relationship between gap size and dentine secondary caries formation assessed in a microcosm biofilm model. *Caries Research,* Vol. 43(2), pp. 97-102.

Cenci, M.S., Tenuta, L. M. A., Pereira-Cenci, T., Del Bel Cury, A. A., ten Cate, J. M., & Cury, J. A. (2008). Effect of Microleakage and Fluoride on Enamel-Dentine Demineralization around Restorations. *Caries Research,* Vol. 42(5), pp. 369-379.

Collins, C. J., Bryant, R. W., & Hodge, K. L. (1998). A clinical evaluation of posterior composite resin restorations: 8-year findings. *Journal of Dentistry,* Vol. 26(4), 311-317.

Dahl, J. E., & Eriksen, H. M. (1978). Reasons for replacement of amalgam dental restorations. *European Journal of Oral Sciences,* Vol. 86(5), pp. 404-407.

Deligeorgi, V., Mjör, I A, & Wilson, N. H. (2001). An overview of reasons for the placement and replacement of restorations. Primary Dental Care: *Journal of the Faculty of General Dental Practitioners,* Vol. 8(1), pp. 5-11.

Dérand, T., Birkhed, D., & Edwardsson, S. (1991). Secondary caries related to various marginal gaps around amalgam restorations in vitro. *Swedish Dental Journal,* Vol. 15(3), pp. 133-138.

Diercke, K., Lussi, A., Kersten, T., & Seemann, R. (2009). Isolated development of inner (wall) caries like lesions in a bacterial-based in vitro model. *Clinical Oral Investigations,* Vol. 13(4), pp. 439-444.

van Dijken, J. W. (1996). 3-year clinical evaluation of a compomer, a resin-modified glass ionomer and a resin composite in Class III restorations. *American Journal of Dentistry,* Vol. 9(5), pp. 195-198.

Donly, K., & Gomez, C. (1994). In vitro demineralization-remineralization of enamel caries at restoration margins utilizing fluoride-releasing composite resin. *Quintessence International,* Vol. 25(5), pp. 355-358.

Ekstrand, K., Qvist, V., & Thylstrup, A. (1987). Light microscope study of the effect of probing in occlusal surfaces. *Caries Research,* Vol. 21(4), pp. 368-374.

Ericson, D., Kidd, E., McComb, D., Mjör, I., & Noack, M. J. (2003). Minimally Invasive Dentistry--concepts and techniques in cariology. *Oral Health & Preventive Dentistry*, Vol. 1(1), pp. 59-72.

Fayyad, M. A., & Ball, P. C. (1987). Bacterial penetration around amalgam restorations. The *Journal of Prosthetic Dentistry*, Vol. 57(5), pp. 571-574.

Featherstone, J. D. (1994). Fluoride, remineralization and root caries. *American Journal of Dentistry*, Vol. 7(5), pp. 271-274.

Featherstone, J. D. B. (2004). The Continuum of Dental Caries--Evidence for a Dynamic Disease Process. *Journal of Dental Research*, Vol. 83(suppl 1), pp. C39-C42.

Finer, Y., & Santerre, J. P. (2004). Salivary Esterase Activity and Its Association with the Biodegradation of Dental Composites. *Journal of Dental Research*, Vol. 83(1), pp. 22 - 26.

Fédération Dentaire Internationale. (1962). Special commission on oral and dental statistics: General principles concerning the international standardization of dental caries statistics. *International Dental Journal*, Vol. 12 pp. 15.

Fontana, M., Li, Y, Dunipace, A. J., Noblitt, T. W., Fischer, G., Katz, B. P., & Stookey, G K. (1996). Measurement of enamel demineralization using microradiography and confocal microscopy. A correlation study. *Caries Research*, Vol. 30(5), pp. 317-325.

Fontana, M., & González-Cabezas, C. (2000). Secondary caries and restoration replacement: An unresolved problem. *Compendium of continuing education in dentistry*, Vol. 21(1), pp. 15.

Forss, H, & Seppä, L. (1990). Prevention of enamel demineralization adjacent to glass ionomer filling materials. *Scandinavian Journal of Dental Research*, Vol. 98(2), pp. 173-178.

Forss, Helena, & Widström, E. (2004). Reasons for restorative therapy and the longevity of restorations in adults. *Acta Odontologica Scandinavica*, Vol. 62(2), pp. 82-86.

Francci, C., Deaton, T. G., Arnold, R. R., Swift, E. J., Perdigao, J., & Bawden, J. W. (1999). Fluoride Release from Restorative Materials and Its Effects on Dentin Demineralization. *Journal of Dental Research*, Vol. 78(10), pp. 1647 -1654.

Friedl, K. H., Hiller, K. A., & Schmalz, G. (1995). Placement and replacement of composite restorations in Germany. *Operative Dentistry*, Vol. 20(1), pp. 34-38.

Fusayama, T. (1988). Clinical guide for removing caries using a caries-detecting solution. *Quintessence International*, Vol. 19(6), pp. 397-401.

Goldberg, J., Tanzer, J., Munster, E., Amara, J., Thal, F., & Birkhed, D. (1981). Cross-sectional clinical evaluation of recurrent enamel caries, restoration of marginal integrity, and oral hygiene status. *Journal of the American Dental Association*, Vol. 102(5), pp. 635-641.

González-Cabezas, C, Li, Y, Gregory, R L, & Stookey, G K. (1999). Distribution of three cariogenic bacteria in secondary carious lesions around amalgam restorations. *Caries Research*, Vol. 33(5), pp. 357-365.

González-Cabezas, Carlos, Li, Yiming, Gregory, Richard L, & Stookey, George K. (2002). Distribution of cariogenic bacteria in carious lesions around tooth-colored restorations. *American Journal of Dentistry*, Vol. 15(4), pp. 248-251.

Gordan, V V, Mjör, I A, Blum I R, & Wilson, N. (2003). Teaching students the repair of resin-based composite restorations: A survey of North American dental schools. The *Journal of the American Dental Association*, Vol. 134(3), pp. 317 -323.

Grossman, E. S., & Matejka, J. M. (1995). Amalgam restoration and in vitro caries formation. *The Journal of Prosthetic Dentistry*, Vol. 73(2), pp. 199-209.

Hals, E. (1975a). Histology of natural secondary caries associated with silicate cement restorations in human teeth. *Archives of Oral Biology*, Vol. 20(4), pp. 291-296.

Hals, E. (1975b). The structure of experimental in vitro lesions around silicate fillings in human teeth. *Archives of Oral Biology*, Vol. 20(4), pp. 283-289.

Hals, E., Andreassen, B. H., & Bie, T. (1974). Histopathology of natural caries around silver amalgam fillings. *Caries Research*, Vol. 8(4), pp. 343-358.

Hals, E., & Nernaes, å. (1971). Histopathology of in vitro Caries Developing around Silver Amalgam Fillings. *Caries Research*, Vol. 5(1), pp. 58-77.

Hals, E., & Norderval, I. T. (1973). Histopathology of experimental in vivo caries around silicate fillings. Acta Odontologica Scandinavica, Vol. 31(6), pp. 357-367.

Hals, E., & Simonsen, L. T. (1972). Histopathology of experimental in vivo caries around silver amalgam fillings. *Caries Research*, Vol. 6(1), pp. 16-33

Hara, A. T., Turssi, C. P., Ando, M., González-Cabezas, C, Zero, D. T., Rodrigues, A. L., Jr, Serra, M. C., et al. (2006). Influence of fluoride-releasing restorative material on root dentine secondary caries in situ. *Caries Research*, Vol. 40(5), pp. 435-439.

Hayacibara, M. F., Rosa, O. P. S., Koo, H., Torres, S. A., Costa, B., & Cury, J. A. (2003). Effects of fluoride and aluminum from ionomeric materials on S. mutans biofilm. *Journal of Dental Research*, Vol. 82(4), pp. 267-271.

Heintze, S. D. (1999). A new material concept for inhibiting the formation of secondary caries. *American Journal of Dentistry*, Vol. 12 Spec No, pp. S4-7.

Hewlett, E. R., Atchison, K. A., White, S. C., & Flack, V. (1993). Radiographic Secondary Caries Prevalence in Teeth with Clinically Defective Restorations. *Journal of Dental Research*, Vol. 72(12), pp. 1604 -1608.

Hicks, J., Garcia-Godoy, F., Donly, K., & Flaitz, C. (2003). Fluoride-releasing restorative materials and secondary caries. *Journal of the California Dental Association*, Vol. 31(3), pp. 229–245.

Hicks, John, Milano, M., Seybold, S., García-Godoy, Franklin, & Flaitz, Catherine. (2002). Fluoride-releasing resin bonding of amalgam restorations in primary teeth: in vitro secondary caries effect. *American Journal of Dentistry*, Vol. 15(6), pp. 361-364.

Huang, C., Tay, F. R., Cheung, G. S. P., Kei, L. H., Wei, S. H. Y., & Pashley, D. H. (2002). Hygroscopic expansion of a compomer and a composite on artificial gap reduction. *Journal of Dentistry*, Vol. 30(1), pp. 11-19.

Hüther, F. J., Psarros, N., & Duschner, H. (1990). Isolation, characterization, and inhibition kinetics of enolase from Streptococcus rattus FA-1. *Infection and Immunity*, Vol. 58(4), pp. 1043-1047.

Irie, M., & Suzuki, K. (1999). Marginal gap formation of light-activated base/liner materials: effect of setting shrinkage and bond strength. *Dental Materials*, Vol. 15(6), pp. 403-407.

Irie, M., Suzuki, K., & Watts, D. C. (2002). Marginal gap formation of light-activated restorative materials: effects of immediate setting shrinkage and bond strength. *Dental Materials*, Vol. 18(3), pp. 203-210.

Iwami, Y., Shimizu, A., Hayashi, M., Takeshige, F., & Ebisu, S. (2005). Three-dimensional evaluation of gap formation of cervical restorations. *Journal of Dentistry*, Vol. 33(4), pp. 325-333.

Jørgensen K. D., & Wakumoto, S. (1968). Occlusal amalgam fillings: marginal defects and secondary caries. *Odontologisk Tidskrift*, Vol. 76(1), pp. 43-54.

Karantakis, P., Helvatjoglou-Antoniades, M., Theodoridou-Pahini, S., & Papadogiannis, Y. (2000). Fluoride release from three glass ionomers, a compomer, and a composite resin in water, artificial saliva, and lactic acid. *Operative Dentistry*, Vol. 25(1), pp. 20-25.

Kawai, K., Tantbirojn, D., Kamalawat, A. S., Hasegawa, T., & Retief, D. H. (1998). In vitro enamel and cementum fluoride uptake from three fluoride-containing composites. *Caries Research*, Vol. 32(6), pp. 463-469.

Kelsey, W. P., 3rd, France, S. J., Blankenau, R. J., Cavel, W. T., & Barkmeier, W. W. (1981). Caries as a cause of restoration replacement: a clinical survey. *Quintessence International*, Vol. 12(9), pp. 971-974.

Kidd, E. A. (1976). Microleakage: a review. *Journal of Dentistry*, Vol. 4(5), pp. 199-206.

Kidd, E. A. (1984). The diagnosis and management of the "early" carious lesion in permanent teeth. *Dental Update*, Vol. 11(2), pp. 69-70, 72-74, 76-78 passim.

Kidd, E. A. (1990). Caries diagnosis within restored teeth. *Adv Dent Res*, Vol. 4, 10-13.

Kidd, E. A. (2001). Diagnosis of secondary caries. *Journal of Dental Education*, 65(10), pp. 997-1000.

Kidd, E. A. (2010). Clinical threshold for carious tissue removal. *Dental Clinics of North America*, Vol. 54(3), pp. 541-549.

Kidd, E. A., & Beighton, D. (1996). Prediction of Secondary Caries around Tooth-colored Restorations: A Clinical and Microbiological Study. *Journal of Dental Research*, Vol. 75(12), pp. 1942 -1946.

Kidd, E. A., & O'Hara, J. W. (1990). The caries status of occlusal amalgam restorations with marginal defects. *Journal of Dental Research*, Vol. 69(6), pp. 1275-1277.

Kidd, E. A., Joyston-Bechal, S., & Beighton, D. (1993). Microbiological validation of assessments of caries activity during cavity preparation. *Caries Research*, Vol. 27(5), pp. 402-408.

Kidd, E. A., Joyston-Bechal, S., & Beighton, D. (1995). Marginal Ditching and Staining as a Predictor of Secondary Caries Around Amalgam Restorations: A Clinical and Microbiological Study. *Journal of Dental Research*, Vol. 74(5), pp. 1206 -1211.

Kielbassa, A. M., Müller, U., & García-Godoy, F. (1999). In situ study on the caries-preventive effects of fluoride-releasing materials. *American Journal of Dentistry*, Vol. 12 Spec No, pp. S13-14.

Kielbassa, A. M., Schulte-Monting, J., Garcia-Godoy, F., & Meyer-Lueckel, H. (2003). Initial in situ secondary caries formation: effect of various fluoride-containing restorative materials. *Operative Dentistry*, Vol. 28(6), pp. 765-772.

Klinke, T., Kneist, S., de Soet, J. J., Kuhlisch, E., Mauersberger, S., Forster, A., & Klimm, W. (2009). Acid production by oral strains of Candida albicans and lactobacilli. *Caries Research*, Vol. 43(2), pp. 83-91.

Kraft U, Hoyer MI(1999): Effect of fluoride released from filling materials on the formation of artificial enamel and dentine lesions (abstract No 75). *Caries Res*, Vol. 33, pp. 306.

Leinfelder, K. F. (1987). Evaluation of criteria used for assessing the clinical performance of composite resins in posterior teeth. *Quintessence International*, Vol. 18(8), pp. 531-536.

Letzel, H., van't Hof, M. A., Vrijhoef, M. M., Marshall, G. W., Jr, & Marshall, S. J. (1989). A controlled clinical study of amalgam restorations: survival, failures, and causes of failure. *Dental Materials*, Vol. 5(2), pp. 115-121.

Levallois, B., Fovet, Y., Lapeyre, L., & Gal, J. Y. (1998). In vitro fluoride release from restorative materials in water versus artificial saliva medium (SAGF). *Dental Materials*, Vol. 14(6), pp. 441-447.

Loesche, W. J. (1986). Role of Streptococcus mutans in human dental decay. *Microbiological Reviews*, Vol. 50(4), pp. 353-380.

Mandari, G. J., Frencken, J. E., & van't Hof, M. A. (2003). Six-year success rates of occlusal amalgam and glass-ionomer restorations placed using three minimal intervention approaches. *Caries Research*, Vol. 37(4), pp. 246-253.

Marsh, P. D. (2006). Dental plaque as a biofilm and a microbial community – implications for health and disease. *BMC Oral Health*, Vol. 6(Suppl 1), pp. S14-S14.

Massler, M. (1967). Pulpal reactions to dental caries. *International Dental Journal*, Vol. 17(2), pp. 441-460.

Mejàre, B., Mejàre, I., & Edwardsson, S. (1979). Bacteria beneath composite restorations--a culturing and histobacteriological study. *Acta Odontologica Scandinavica*, Vol. 37(5), pp. 267-275.

Mjör, I A. (1985). Frequency of secondary caries at various anatomical locations. *Operative Dentistry*, Vol. 10(3), pp. 88-92.

Mjör, I A. (1996). Glass-ionomer cement restorations and secondary caries: a preliminary report. *Quintessence International*, Vol. 27(3), pp. 171-174.

Mjör, I A. (1997). The reasons for replacement and the age of failed restorations in general dental practice. *Acta Odontologica Scandinavica*, Vol. 55(1), pp. 58-63.

Mjör, I A. (1998). The location of clinically diagnosed secondary caries. *Quintessence International*, Vol. 29(5), pp. 313-317.

Mjör, I A. (2005). Clinical diagnosis of recurrent caries. *The Journal of the American Dental Association*, Vol. 136(10), pp. 1426 -1433.

Mjör, I A, & Gordan, V V. (2002). Failure, repair, refurbishing and longevity of restorations. *Operative Dentistry*, Vol. 27(5), pp. 528-534.

Mjör, I A, & Jokstad, A. (1993). Five-year study of Class II restorations in permanent teeth using amalgam, glass polyalkenoate (ionomer) cerment and resin-based composite materials. *Journal of Dentistry*, Vol. 21(6), pp. 338-343.

Mjör, I A, & Qvist, V. (1997). Marginal failures of amalgam and composite restorations. *Journal of Dentistry*, Vol. 25(1), pp. 25-30.

Mjör, I A, & Toffenetti, F. (2000). Secondary caries: a literature review with case reports. *Quintessence International*, Vol. 31(3), pp. 165-179.

Mondelli, J., Steagall, L., Ishikiriama, A., de Lima Navarro, M. F., & Soares, F. B. (1980). Fracture strength of human teeth with cavity preparations. *The Journal of Prosthetic Dentistry*, Vol. 43(4), pp. 419-422.

Mousavinenasab SM, Jafary M (2004): Microleakage of Composite Restorations Following Chemo-mechanical and Conventional Caries Removal. *Journal of Dentistry (TUMS)*, Vol. 1, pp. 12-17.

Nakajo, K., Imazato, S., Takahashi, Y., Kiba, W., Ebisu, S., & Takahashi, N. (2009). Fluoride released from glass-ionomer cement is responsible to inhibit the acid production of caries-related oral streptococci. *Dental Materials*, Vol. 25(6), pp. 703-708.

Nikawa, H., Yamashiro, H., Makihira, S., Nishimura, M., Egusa, H., Furukawa, M., Setijanto, D., et al. (2003). In vitro cariogenic potential of Candida albicans. *Mycoses*, Vol. 46(11-12), pp. 471-478.

Ozer, L., & Thylstrup, A. (1995). What is Known About Caries in Relation to Restorations as a Reason for Replacement? a Review. *Advances in Dental Research*, Vol. 9(4), pp. 394 -402.

Papagiannoulis, L., Kakaboura, A., & Eliades, G. (2002). In vivo vs in vitro anticariogenic behavior of glass-ionomer and resin composite restorative materials. *Dental Materials*, Vol. 18(8), pp. 561-569.

Persson, A., Lingström, P., Bäcklund, T., & Dijken, J. W. V. (2004). Evaluation of a skin reference electrode used for intraoral pH measurements in combination with a microtouch electrode. *Clinical Oral Investigations*, Vol. 8(3), pp. 172-175.

Pimenta, L. A., Navarro, M. F., & Consolaro, A. (1995). Secondary caries around amalgam restorations. *The Journal of Prosthetic Dentistry*, Vol. 74(3), pp. 219-222.

Piwowarczyk, A., Lauer, H., & Sorensen, J. (2005). Microleakage of various cementing agents for full cast crowns. *The Journal of Prosthetic Dentistry*, Vol. 94(6), pp. 548-548.

Podbielski, A, Boeckh, C, & Haller, B. (2000). Growth inhibitory activity of gutta-percha points containing root canal medications on common endodontic bacterial pathogens as determined by an optimized quantitative in vitro assay. *Journal of Endodontics*, Vol. 26(7), pp. 398-403.

Qvist, V., Qvist, J., & Mjör, I A. (1990). Placement and longevity of tooth-colored restorations in Denmark. *Acta Odontologica Scandinavica*, Vol. 48(5), pp. 305-311.

Qvist, V., Thylstrup, A., & Mjör, I A. (1986). Restorative treatment pattern and longevity of amalgam restorations in Denmark. *Acta Odontologica Scandinavica*, Vol. 44(6), pp. 343-349.

Randall, R. C., & Wilson, N.H.F. (1999). Glass-ionomer Restoratives: A Systematic Review of a Secondary Caries Treatment Effect. *Journal of Dental Research*, Vol. 78(2), pp. 628 - 637.

Retief, D. H., Bradley, E. L., Denton, J. C., & Switzer, P. (1984). Enamel and Cementum Fluoride Uptake from a Glass Ionomer Cement. *Caries Research*, Vol. 18(3), pp. 250-257.

Rølla G., Ekstrand J. (1996). *Fluoride in oral fluids and dental plaque*. In: Fluoride in dentistry. 2nd ed. Fejerskov 0, Ekstrand J, Burt J, editors. Copenhagen: Munksgaard, pp. 215-229.

Rølla, G., Ogaard, B., & Cruz, R. de A. (1993). Topical application of fluorides on teeth. New concepts of mechanisms of interaction. *Journal of Clinical Periodontology*, Vol. 20(2), pp. 105-108.

da Rosa Rodolpho, P. A., Cenci, Maximiliano Sérgio, Donassollo, T. A., Loguércio, A. D., & Demarco, F. F. (2006). A clinical evaluation of posterior composite restorations: 17-year findings. *Journal of Dentistry*, Vol. 34(7), pp. 427-435.

Rudolphy, M. P., van Amerongen, J. P., Penning, C., & ten Cate, J. M. (1995). Grey discolouration and marginal fracture for the diagnosis of secondary caries in molars with occlusal amalgam restorations: an in vitro study. *Caries Research*, Vol. 29(5), pp. 371-376.

Savarino, L., Breschi, L., Tedaldi, M., Ciapetti, G., Tarabusi, C., Greco, M., Giunti, A., et al. (2004). Ability of restorative and fluoride releasing materials to prevent marginal dentine demineralization. *Biomaterials*, Vol. 25(6), pp. 1011-1017.

Söderholm, K.-J.; Antonson, D.E.; and Fischlschweiger, W. (1989): *Correlation Between Marginal Discrepancies at the Amalgam-Tooth Interface and Recurrent Caries*. In: Quality Evaluation of Dental Restorations. Criteria for Placement and Replacement. K.J. Anusavice, Ed., Chicago: Quintessence, pp. 95-108.

Souganidis, D. J., Athanassouli, T. M. N., & Papastathopoulos, D. S. (1981). A Study of in vivo Fluoride Uptake by Dental Tissues from Fluoride-containing Silver Amalgams. *Journal of Dental Research*, Vol. 60(2), pp. 105 -108.

Splieth, C., Bernhardt, O., Heinrich, A., Bernhardt, H., & Meyer, G. (2003). Anaerobic microflora under Class I and Class II composite and amalgam restorations. *Quintessence International*, Vol. 34(7), pp. 497-503.

Svanberg, M., Mjör, I.A., & Ørstavik, D. (1990). Mutans Streptococci in Plaque from Margins of Amalgam, Composite, and Glass-ionomer Restorations. *Journal of Dental Research*, Vol. 69(3), pp. 861 -864.

Tam, L. E., Chan, G. P., & Yim, D. (1997). In vitro caries inhibition effects by conventional and resin-modified glass-ionomer restorations. *Operative Dentistry*, Vol. 22(1), pp. 4-14.

Thomas, R. Z., van der Mei, H. C., van der Veen, M. H., de Soet, J. J., & Huysmans, M. C. D. N. J. M. (2008). Bacterial composition and red fluorescence of plaque in relation to primary and secondary caries next to composite: an in situ study. *Oral Microbiology and Immunology*, Vol. 23(1), pp. 7-13.

Thomas, R. Z., Ruben, J. L., ten Bosch, J. J., Fidler, V., & Huysmans, M. C. D. N. J. M. (2007). Approximal secondary caries lesion progression, a 20-week in situ study. *Caries Research*, Vol. 41(5), pp. 399-405.

Totiam, P., González-Cabezas, C., Fontana, M. R., & Zero, D. T. (2007). A New in vitro Model to Study the Relationship of Gap Size and Secondary Caries. *Caries Research*, Vol. 41(6), pp. 467-473.

Wallman-Björklund, C., Svanberg, M., & Emilson, C. G. (1987). Streptococcus mutans in plaque from conventional and from non-gamma-2 amalgam restorations. *Scandinavian Journal of Dental Research*, Vol. 95(3), pp. 266-269.

Welbury, R. R., Walls, A. W., Murray, J. J., & McCabe, J. F. (1991). The 5-year results of a clinical trial comparing a glass polyalkenoate (ionomer) cement restoration with an amalgam restoration. *British Dental Journal*, Vol. 170(5), pp. 177-181.

Wiegand, A., Buchalla, W., & Attin, T. (2007). Review on fluoride-releasing restorative materials—Fluoride release and uptake characteristics, antibacterial activity and influence on caries formation. *Dental Materials*, Vol. 23(3), pp. 343-362.

Wilson, N. H., Burke, F. J., & Mjör, I A. (1997). Reasons for placement and replacement of restorations of direct restorative materials by a selected group of practitioners in the United Kingdom. *Quintessence International*, Vol. 28(4), pp. 245-248.

Yaman, S. D., Er, O., Yetmez, M., & Karabay, G. A. (2004). In vitro inhibition of caries-like lesions with fluoride-releasing materials. *Journal of Oral Science*, Vol. 46(1), pp. 45-50.

Yap, A. U., Khor, E., & Foo, S. H. (1999). Fluoride release and antibacterial properties of new-generation tooth-colored restoratives. *Operative Dentistry*, Vol. 24(5), pp. 297-305.

13

Caries and Periodontal Disease in Rice-Cultivating Yayoi People of Ancient Japan

Tomoko Hamasaki and Tadamichi Takehara
Kyushu Women's University,
Kyushu Dental College,
Japan

1. Introduction

The people of the Yayoi period were the first wet-rice agriculturalists in Japan, and the people of modern Japan are the direct descendents of the Yayoi people. They dominated the Japanese archipelago from the 5th C B.C. to 3rd C A.D. The remains of the Yayoi people have been excavated from several sites in western Japan. It has been proposed that the Yayoi originated in East Asia, based on the morphologic characteristics of the skull and teeth (Hanihara, 1993), as well as genetic evidence(Omoto & Saitou, 1997) . Agriculture practices during the Yayoi period in Japan closely resembled those in southern China and Korea. Based on these findings, the Yayoi people are believed to have been migrants from the Asian continent who introduced wet-rice agriculture to the Japanese islands (Temple, 2010).

Previous studies of ancient populations have revealed a close relationship between oral disease and subsistence patterns (Eshed *et al.*, 2006). In Japan, the incidence of carious teeth among Yayoi period agriculturalists was found to be higher than that among hunter-gatherers from the preceding Jomon period (Temple & Larsen, 2007). Temple and Larsen (Temple & Larsen, 2007) reported that dietary and behavioral variations among the people of the Yayoi period during the transition to an agriculture-based society precipitated an increase in the frequency of carious teeth, as well as variations in carious tooth frequency, based on geographic location and sex.

Most of the carious lesions in ancient populations occurred at or near the cemento-enamel junction–alveolar crest (CEJ–AC). (Hildebolt *et al.*, 1988, Kerr *et al.*, 1988, Lunt, 1974, Moore & Corbett, 1971, Moore & Corbett, 1975, Varrela, 1991, Vodanovic *et al.*, 2005) These lesions appear to be associated with an exposed root surface caused by alveolar bone recession, although a definitive conclusion has not been reached. Exposure of the root surface is a prerequisite for carious lesions of the root, and alveolar bone loss is a major cause of such exposure. Therefore, root caries may occur as a result of alveolar bone loss.

Using multiple sets of remains from the Yayoi period, we investigated carious disease(Haraga, 2006) and alveolar bone loss(Uekubo, 2006) among the Yayoi people. Moreover, we identify the factors associated with root caries, and examine the relationship between root caries and alveolar bone loss(Otani *et al.*, 2009). Our findings may be useful for investigating the pathology of root caries in relation to the Yayoi diet.

2. Relationship between root caries and alveolar bone loss Yayoi people of ancient Japan

2.1.1 Material

We studied 5,010 teeth and the surrounding alveolar bones in 263 ancient human skeletal remains excavated at 49 archeological sites, and which are preserved at the Kyushu University Faculty of Medicine. The distribution of each site are shown in Figure 1. The remains, which were classified as belonging to the Yayoi period, included 152 males, 100 females, and 11 unknowns. The remains were further categorized by age as follows: young adults (estimated age 20–39 years, $n = 126$), and elderly (estimated age 40–59 years, $n = 137$). Gender and age were assigned in accordance with the standard procedures of the Department of Anatomy, Faculty of Medicine, Kyushu University. Only remains with teeth and alveolar bone were selected.

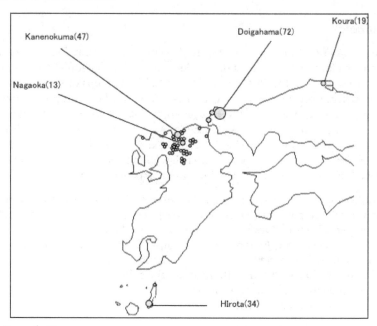

Fig. 1. Location of sites

2.1.2 Methods

Only those teeth with obvious cavities were recorded as being carious (Figure 2). Color changes to the enamel that lacked well-defined cavity edges, possibly as a result of erosion, were not considered to be evidence of caries. Caries was detected on nine different tooth surfaces: the occlusal surface; the distal, buccal, mesial, and lingual (palatal) surfaces of the crown; and the distal, buccal, mesial, and lingual (palatal) surfaces of the root.

Gingivitis leaves no trace in alveolar bone, whereas periodontitis causes alveolar bone loss. Accordingly, periodontitis can be evaluated using bone loss as an index. We measured the CEJ–AC distances only in jawbone specimens with alveolar bone remaining around the teeth using a periodontal probe. Up to four tooth surfaces (distal, buccal, mesial, and lingual/palatal) were examined, and the measurements are expressed in millimeters. For tilted teeth, we measured the vertical distance. Teeth with a fractured alveolar crest or that were missing were excluded from the analysis. Teeth were also excluded if the alveolar bone on the buccal side was lost due to physiologic fenestration or a lesion in the root apex.

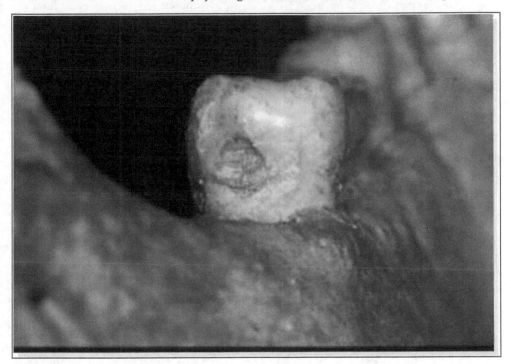

Fig. 2. Caries in Yayoi people

2.2 Distribution of dental caries in Yayoi people

The distribution and site characteristics of dental caries previously identified in a Yayoi population using the aforementioned procedure. We examined 5010 teeth, 941 teeth were classified as antemortem teeth, and 998 teeth were classified as postmortal loss (Otani *et al.*, 2009) (Table 1). The number of teeth in each individual ranged from a minimum of 2 to a maximum of 32, with an average of 19.5. The total number of carious teeth was 883, for a cares ratio of 17.6%. The percent of individuals with caries was 79.1%, and the percent of individuals with root caries was 65.8%

Our analyses indicated that among the Yayoi people, most caries occurred in the root area, particularly on the approximal surface of the tooth root (Haraga, 2006). Moreover, Figure 3 shows the distribution of caries by tooth surface. When categorized into 3 groups, namely occlusal, , the occlusal surface percentage was 10.4%, the crown and root were compared, the crown ratio was 37.4% and the root ratio was 52.2%. When Caries location was classified into 9 tooth surfaces as follows: occlusal surface, crown buccal surface, crown lingual surface, crown approximal surface, root buccal surface, root lingual surface, and root approximal surface. The caries frequency was highest in the root approximal surface area, followed in order by the crown approximal surface and root buccal surface, while it was lowest in the buccal and lingual surfaces of both the crown and root.

Number of teeth present	Mean number of teeth present per person(SD)	Number of antemort em teeth	Numbe r of postmo rtem teeth	Number of teeth lost at unknown timing	Number of carious teeth	Rate of caries (%)a	Caries prevale nce (%)b	Root caries prevale nce (%)c
5010	19.5(7.1)	941	998	999	883	17.6	79.1	65.8

a Rate of caries: Number of carious teeth / Number of teeth present × 100
b Caries prevalence (%): Number of individuals with caries/ Number of individuals× 100
c Root caries prevalence (%)c: Number of individuals with root caries/ Number of individuals× 100

Table 1. Number of teeth present, deciduous teeth, and teeth with caries, and rate and prevalence of caries.

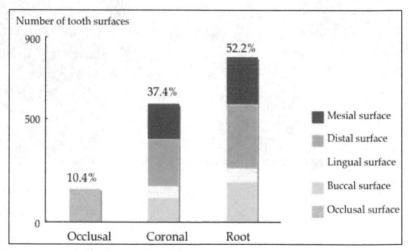

Fig. 3. Distribution of caries by tooth surface

In contrast, we analyzed caries in the Yayoi people and determined the first caries attack site (Haraga, 2006). For determining where caries began in Yayoi people, only caries observed independently on the occlusal surface, crown and root were counted by tooth surface (Figure 4). Large cavities (e.g., spreading in both the tooth crown and root) were excluded from this analysis, and the carious surfaces that were located in only a limited area, such as pits and fissures, crowns, and root surfaces, were determined with certainty as cases. As for the third molar, caries beginning in the occlusal surface accounted for 33.3% in the maxilla and 44.4% in the mandible. Caries beginning in the occlusal surface area were not observed in the upper first premolars and the first molars, the lower first and second premolars, or the first molars. Caries that began in the molars most often originated in the root (70.5% to 86.3%). The percentage of caries beginning in the occlusal surface, crown, and root was

6.9%, 26.9%, and 66.3%, respectively. Thus, most of the molar surfaces affected during the first caries attack were located in the root area. Therefore, these carious lesions may have been initiated in the root area in the Yayoi people. These observations indicate a different pathology from that seen in modern people. Thus, the mechanisms underlying the development of root and coronal caries in the people of the Yayoi period may be different from those in modern people.

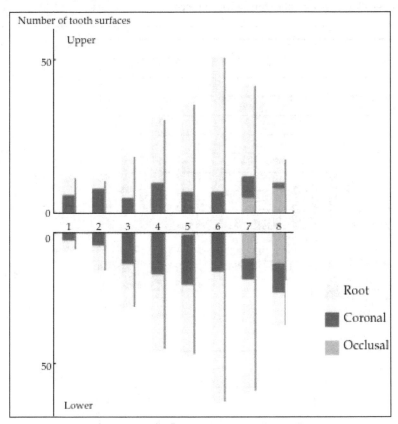

Fig. 4. Distribution of "primary caries" by tooth surfaces in Yayoi people

We have presented here the frequencies of carious lesions in younger and elderly people according to tooth type in Yayoi people (Fig. 5). It is clear that the frequncy of carious lesions was higher in the elderly (Haraga, 2006). In the modern Japanese, the caries ratios in the first molars of younger and elderly people are very similar (Fig 6). These findings also support the suggestion that most of the caries was found in the root area in Yayoi people, likely following the establishment of periodontal disease.

The location of dental caries in the people of the Yayoi period differs from that seen in modern Japanese people. In the skeletal remains of the Yayoi, most carious lesions were located in the root area, while in modern populations, most of these lesions are in the crown. This difference is considered to be associated with dietary variation, particularly the consumption of cariogenic foodstuffs. During the digestion of staple foods, such as rice, acid production causes tooth decalcification (Tayles *et al.*, 2000). Moreover, cooked starch is more easily degraded and fermented by bacteria (Lingstrom *et al.*, 1989). The Yayoi people engaged mainly in agriculture, in contrast to their forebears, the Jomon. Indeed, the Yayoi utilized an advanced system of wet-rice agriculture, which supported an increase in population density in western Japan during the Yayoi period. The increase in whole dental caries was associated to a great extent with the increase in root caries.

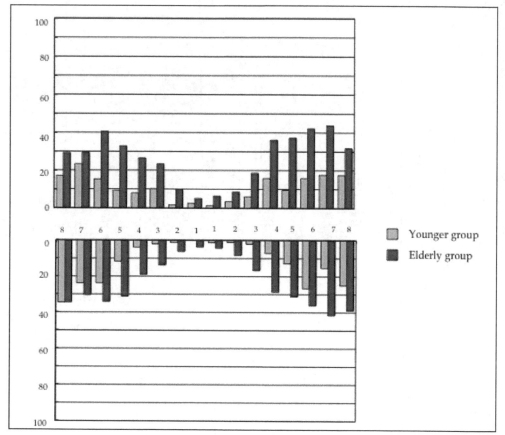

Fig. 5. Number of carious teeth, treated and untreated, by age group and teeth type, in Yayoi people.

However, starch is less cariogenic than sucrose (Lingstrom *et al.*, 1989), and sucrose is a better substrate for *Mutans streptococci* than any other dietary carbohydrate. The high prevalence of root caries yields the most information in this regard. The substrate of the caries in the Yayoi people was most likely a cooked starch, which became a substrate for acid production by oral acid-producing bacteria (not necessarily *Mutans streptococci*), while modern caries are generally induced by *Mutans streptococci* which use sugar as a substrate (Kamp *et al.*, 1983). O'Sullivan (O'Sullivan *et al.*, 1993) compared the skeletal remains of children from an 18th century British population with those of older remains. The results indicated an alteration in pathologic conditions during the 18th century that changed the site of most primary tooth caries from the contact points to the CEJ–AC. In the UK, the average intake of sucrose has consistently increased since the early 1700s (Yudkin, 1972). Yudkin (Yudkin, 1972) reported a positive correlation between the degree of dental caries and the amount of sugar (i.e., sucrose) ingested. Furthermore, the prevalence and distribution of dental decay have changed since the 17th century in Britain (Vodanovic *et al.*, 2005), and these changes may be associated with the importation of sugars.

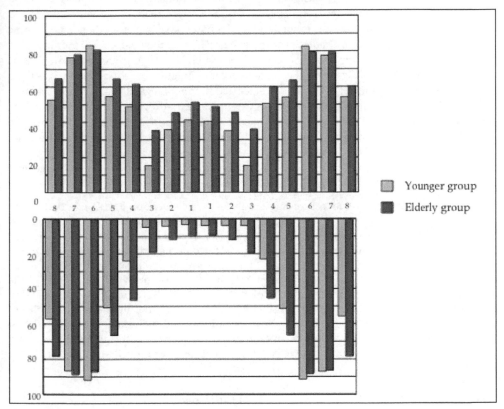

Fig. 6. Number of carious teeth, treated and untreated, by age group and teeth type, in modern Japanese. [From Dental Health Division of Health Policy Bureau, Ministry of Health and Welfare Japan, 1999]

2.3 Alveolar bone loss in Yayoi people

We attempted to clarify the prevalence of periodontal disease in the Yayoi people. Although periodontal disease is characterized by alveolar bone loss, ascertaining the prevalences of periodontal disease in ancient populations is difficult. Although gingivitis does not leave any trace in ancient bones, periodontal disease causes alveolar bone loss, thus periodontal disease can be evaluated by using the degree of alveolar bone loss as a parameter (Stoner, 1972). Therefore, the establishment of an internationally accepted method for quantifying alveolar bone loss would be helpful. There have been few reports regarding periodontal disease in ancient skeletal remains. Notable exceptions include the studies of Clarke et al. (Clarke *et al.*, 1986), Sakashita et al., (Sakashita *et al.*, 1997) and Kerr, (Kerr, 1998) which assessed the prevalence of periodontal disease in ancient populations. Clark et al. (Clarke *et al.*, 1986) investigated ancient human bones stored in 20 museums in 10 countries and reported that the prevalence of periodontal disease was 10% in ancient people. Further, Sakashita et al. (Sakashita *et al.*, 1997) examined bones from the Yin-Shang period in China and reported that periodontal disease prevalence ranged from 20% to 30%. Kerr (Kerr, 1998) reported the prevalence to range from 70% to 100%, however, the investigation method used in that study was detection of lesions while viewing specimens with a stereoscopic microscope. Therefore, it is difficult to compare the results, as they varied depending on the cut-off point employed for alveolar bone loss when evaluating periodontal disease prevalence. A distance of 2 mm in the cementoenamel junction-alveolar crest (CEJ-AC) is generally regarded as normal, while that greater than 2 mm is regarded as a lesion (Lennon & Davies, 1974)., Using that parameter, data can be compared even when not reported by the same researcher. Whittaker et al. (Whittaker *et al.*, 1982) measured the CEJ-AC distance in skulls excavated from human remains of the Roman Empire in England and reported that alveolar bone loss was more remarkable in the elderly group than the adolescent group, as the distance reached 6 mm or more in some of the elderly individuals, which indicated that disease severity was dependent on the CEJ–AC distance.

We investigated alveolar bone loss among the Yayoi people(Uekubo T, 2006). In that study, we measured the CEJ-AC distance in Yayoi specimens to clarify the prevalence of periodontal disease. The minimum CEJ-AC distance was 0 mm and the maximum 17 mm. In most of the site, the elderly group had significantly larger distance values than the adolescent group. As for tooth type, in the adolescent group, the first molar of the maxilla showed the most largest CEJ-AC distance value, followed in order by the first molar of the mandible, canine of the mandible, second molar of the maxilla. In the elderly group, the first molar of the maxilla showed the highest severity, followed in order by the second molar of the maxilla, first molar of the mandible, second molar of the mandible. We reported that alveolar bone loss increased with age among the Yayoi people, with this tendency being most evident in the first molars, and we concluded that alveolar bone loss among the Yayoi was more severe than in other ancient populations.

2.4 Relationship between root caries and alveolar bone loss in Yayoi people

Above mentioned, the people of the Yayoi had carious lesions that were most frequently located on the root surfaces of their teeth. Root surface exposure is a prerequisite for this type of decay, and alveolar bone loss is the main cause of such exposure. Therefore, we identify the factors associated with root caries, and examine the relationship between root caries and alveolar bone loss in the people of the Yayoi period.

As shown in Table 2, the prevalence of root caries was significantly higher (78.7%) among those with a mean CEJ–AC distance ≥3.4 mm than among those with a distance ≤3.3 mm (54.1%). In addition, significant differences in the mean number of teeth with root caries were observed according to age, presence of coronal caries, and the mean CEJ–AC distanceper person. The prevalence of root caries and the mean number of teeth with root caries per person were significantly associated with the mean CEJ–AC distance per person.

		Root caries prevalence (n) (%)	p-value[1]	Mean number of teeth with root caries per person	p-value[2]
Mean CEJ-AC distance per person	<3.3 mm(133)	54.1(72)	< 0.001	1.3±1.7	< 0.001
	>3.4 mm (127)	78.7(100)		2.4±2.6	

[1]χ^2 –test, [2]M-W test

Table 2. Root caries prevalence and mean number of teeth with root caries per person by CEJ-AC distance per person.

Figure 6 shows the percentage of root caries surfaces per tooth surface according to the mean CEJ–AC distance per tooth surface. We calculated the percentage of each root surface (distal, buccal, mesial, and lingual/palatal) affected by caries. Those subjects with a greater mean CEJ–AC distance per tooth surface had a significantly higher percentage of surface root caries for all surfaces compared to those with shorter mean distances.

For the upper and lower molars, the mean CEJ–AC distance per tooth surface was based on the presence of root caries (Table 3). In the upper jaw, root caries on the distal surface of the premolars or on the distal, mesial, and palatal surfaces of the molars, were significantly associated with a greater mean CEJ–AC distance value per tooth surface. In the lower jaw, significantly greater distance values were associated with root caries on the distal, buccal, and mesial surfaces of the molars or on the distal and buccal surfaces of the premolars.

Our results confirm the relationship between root caries and the CEJ–AC distance, which is used as an index of alveolar bone loss, in the bones of the Yayoi people. In ancient agrarian populations, the amount of starchy mass on the tooth surface was probably a key factor in the development of root caries. In addition, alveolar bone loss, which is a major cause of root exposure, tends to precede the development of root caries. Several reports have suggested an association between the occurrence of caries and periodontal disease in ancient populations, although no previous studies have examined this correlation. Thus, the findings of the present study are valuable because they clarify for the first time the relationship between root caries and alveolar bone loss in an ancient population (the Yayoi people). To our knowledge, this is the first study to evaluate the relationship between root caries and CEJ–AC distance using skeletal remains.

Previous reports regarding caries (Haraga, 2006) and alveolar bone loss (Uekubo T, 2006,) among the Yayoi people indicated that carious lesions on the approximal surface were common. The present study, which reveals a CEJ–AC distance-dependent increase in the percentage of surface root caries, confirms these findings (Figure 7). We believe that the close relationship between root caries and alveolar bone loss on the approximal surface is suggestive of the involvement of this bone loss in the manifestation of root caries. Although the mechanism of alveolar bone loss in the Yayoi people has not been elucidated, root caries may be a consequence of alveolar bone loss.

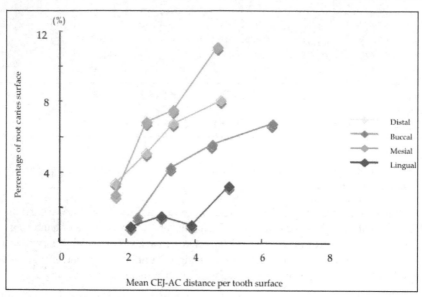

Fig. 7. Relation with percentage of root caries surfaces per tooth surface and mean CEJ-AC distance per tooth surface.

Tooth type	Mean CEJ-AC distance per tooth surface mm±SD (number of tooth surfaces)		p-value [1]
	Without root caries	With root caries	
Upper premolar			
Distal	2.9±1.3(423)	3.6±1.9(23)	0.045
Buccal	3.5±2.0(404)	4.3±3.1(3)	0.490
Mesial	3.0±1.3(405)	3.4±1.4(9)	0.224
Palatal	3.6±1.3(477)	4.00(1)	--------
Upper molar			
Distal	3.3±1.7(311)	3.9±1.2(27)	0.010
Buccal	3.8±2.0(359)	4.3±2.1(16)	0.367
Mesial	3.0±1.4(367)	4.3±1.6(24)	< 0.001
Palatal	4.4±2.1(397)	5.4±1.8(17)	0.011
Lower premolar			
Distal	2.7±1.5(617)	3.6±1.5(32)	0.001
Buccal	4.0±2.1(569)	6.0±2.8(10)	0.013
Mesial	2.6±1.4(618)	3.9±2.8(10)	0.126
Lingual	3.0±1.4(511)	-------- (0)	--------
Lower molar			
Distal	3.1±1.8(453)	4.0±2.0(36)	0.002
Buccal	4.1±2.3(453)	5.7±2.4(39)	< 0.001
Mesial	2.9±1.6(471)	4.6±1.9(27)	< 0.001
Lingual	3.7±1.6(504)	4.3±1.1(16)	0.192

[1] Mann-Whitney test

Table 3. Mean CEJ-AC distance per tooth surface by the presence of root caries.

3. Conclusion

We investigated the relationship between caries and periodontal disease in the people of the Yayoi period. The Yayoi, who dominated the Japanese archipelago around the 5th C B.C., are the direct ancestors of the modern Japanese and were the first people to engage in rice cultivation in Japan.

The people in the Yayoi period had a high prevalence of root caries, and the rate of dental caries, is suggested to be due to changes in dietary habits that occurred concomitant with the development of agriculture. On the other hand, tooth wear and compensatory physiologic growth of the abraded tooth are reduced with a rice diet, and alveolar bone loss occurs due to periodontitis. This results in increased exposure of the root surface, which is thought to result in root caries.

4. Acknowledgment

We thank Dr. Yoshiyuki Tanaka of the Graduate School of Social Science and Cultural Studies, Kyushu University.

5. References

Clarke, N. G., Carey, S. E., Srikandi, W., Hirsch, R. S. & Leppard, P. I. (1986) Periodontal disease in ancient populations. *Am J Phys Anthropol*, 71(2), 173-83.

Eshed, V., Gopher, A. & Hershkovitz, I. (2006) Tooth wear and dental pathology at the advent of agriculture: New evidence from the levant. *Am J Phys Anthropol*, 130(2), 145-59.

Hanihara, K. (1993) [the population history of the japanese]. *Nihon Ronen Igakkai Zasshi*, 30(11), 923-31.

Haraga, S., Hamasaki, T, Ansai, T., Kakuta, S., Akifusa, S., Yoshida, A., Hanada, N., Miyazaki, H. And Takehara, T (2006) Distribution and site characteristics of dental caries in paddy rice-cultivating yayoi people of ancient japan. *Journal of dental health*, 56(558–561.

Hildebolt, C. F., Molnar, S., Elvin-Lewis, M. & Mckee, J. K. (1988) The effect of geochemical factors on prevalences of dental diseases for prehistoric inhabitants of the state of missouri. *Am J Phys Anthropol*, 75(1), 1-14.

Kamp, E. M., Drost, J., Huis in 'T Veld, J. H., Van Palenstein Helderman, W. H. & Dirks, O. B. (1983) Reproducibility of dental caries in balb/c mice induced by the bacterium streptococcus mutans. *Arch Oral Biol*, 28(2), 153-8.

Kerr, N. W. (1998) The prevalence and natural history of periodontal disease in britain from prehistoric to modern times. *Br Dent J*, 185(10), 527-35.

Kerr, N. W., Bruce, M. F. & Cross, J. F. (1988) Caries experience in the permanent dentition of late mediaeval scots (1300-1600 a.D.). *Arch Oral Biol*, 33(3), 143-8.

Lennon, M. A. & Davies, R. M. (1974) Prevalence and distribution of alveolar bone loss in a population of 15-year-old schoolchildren. *J Clin Periodontol*, 1(3), 175-82.

Lingstrom, P., Holm, J., Birkhed, D. & Bjorck, I. (1989) Effects of variously processed starch on ph of human dental plaque. *Scand J Dent Res*, 97(5), 392-400.

Lunt, D. A. (1974) The prevalence of dental caries in the permanent dentition of scottish prehistoric and mediaeval populations. *Arch Oral Biol*, 19(6), 431-7.

Moore, W. J. & Corbett, M. E. (1971) The distribution of dental caries in ancient british populations. 1. Anglo-saxon period. *Caries Res,* 5(2), 151-68.

Moore, W. J. & Corbett, M. E. (1975) Distribution of dental caries in ancient british populations. Iii. The 17th century. *Caries Res,* 9(2), 163-75.

O'sullivan, E. A., Williams, S. A., Wakefield, R. C., Cape, J. E. & Curzon, M. E. (1993) Prevalence and site characteristics of dental caries in primary molar teeth from prehistoric times to the 18th century in england. *Caries Res,* 27(2), 147-53.

Omoto, K. & Saitou, N. (1997) Genetic origins of the japanese: A partial support for the dual structure hypothesis. *Am J Phys Anthropol,* 102(4), 437-46.

Otani, N., Hamasaki, T., Soh, I., Yoshida, A., Awano, S., Ansai, T., Hanada, N., Miyazaki, H. & Takehara, T. (2009) Relationship between root caries and alveolar bone loss in the first wet-rice agriculturalists of the yayoi period in japan. *Arch Oral Biol,* 54(2), 192-200.

Sakashita, R., Inoue, M., Inoue, N., Pan, Q. & Zhu, H. (1997) Dental disease in the chinese yin-shang period with respect to relationships between citizens and slaves. *Am J Phys Anthropol,* 103(3), 401-8.

Stoner, J. E. (1972) An investigation into the accuracy of measurements made on radiographs of the alveolar crests of dried mandibles. *J Periodontol,* 43(11), 699-701.

Tayles, N., Domett, K. & Nelsen, K. (2000) Agriculture and dental caries? The case of rice in prehistoric southeast asia. *World Archaeol,* 32(1), 68-83.

Temple, D. H. (2010) Patterns of systemic stress during the agricultural transition in prehistoric japan. *Am J Phys Anthropol,* 142(1), 112-24.

Temple, D. H. & Larsen, C. S. (2007) Dental caries prevalence as evidence for agriculture and subsistence variation during the yayoi period in prehistoric japan: Biocultural interpretations of an economy in transition. *Am J Phys Anthropol,* 134(4), 501-12.

Uekubo T, H. T., Kakuta, S, Sogame, K., Awano, S., Hanada, N., Miyazaki, H., Ansai, T. And Takehara, T (2006) Alveolar bone loss in rice-cultivating yayoi people of ancient japan. *Journal of dental health,* 56(171-177.

Varrela, T. M. (1991) Prevalence and distribution of dental caries in a late medieval population in finland. *Arch Oral Biol,* 36(8), 553-9.

Vodanovic, M., Brkic, H., Slaus, M. & Demo, Z. (2005) The frequency and distribution of caries in the mediaeval population of bijelo brdo in croatia (10th-11th century). *Arch Oral Biol,* 50(7), 669-80.

Whittaker, D. K., Parker, J. H. & Jenkins, C. (1982) Tooth attrition and continuing eruption in a romano-british population. *Arch Oral Biol,* 27(5), 405-9.

Yudkin, J. (1972) Sugar and disease. *Nature,* 239(5369), 197-9.

14

Molar Incisor Hypomineralization: Morphological, Aetiological, Epidemiological and Clinical Considerations

Márcia Pereira Alves dos Santos[1,2] and Lucianne Cople Maia[2]
1School of Dentistry, Fluminense Federal University,
2School of Dentistry, Federal University of Rio de Janeiro,
Brazil

1. Introduction

The prevalence of dental caries has been reduced over the years due to increased access of fluorides, such as fluoride tooth paste, to dental services and to oral health education on the great part of the population. However, a significant portion of the same population still remains undertreated and show dental cavities as after-effects of this oral disease. In spite of dental caries is strongly influenced by social, economic, cultural, religious and environmental factors, its severity may be increased by structural changes of enamel/dentin such those observed in cases of molar incisor hypomineralization (MIH). In a Brazilian survey, children with MIH showed higher caries experience in the permanent dentition than the general population of similar age. (da Costa-Silva et al., 2010) The MIH increases the dental caries risk as consequence of affected teeth because they are not only soft and porous enamel teeth but also very sensitive to stimuli making effective oral hygiene difficult. (Kilpatrick, 2009) Several aetiological factors are mentioned as the cause of MIH (Alaluusua, 2010, Lygidakis et al., 2010, Crombie et al., 2009, Brook, 2009) and they are frequently associated with childhood diseases or nutritional conditions during the first three years of life. (Fagrell et al., 2011)

Clinically, MIH can create serious drawbacks for the dentist as well as for the child affected. For dentists, the problems are related to unexpectedly rapid caries development in the erupting first permanent molar and unpredictable behaviour of apparently intact opacities. Moreover, these teeth are very sensitive and often require extensive treatment since rapid breakdown of tooth structure may occur, giving rise to acute symptoms and complicated treatments. Defected enamel teeth require complex treatment solutions and the different treatment options will depend on the extension of the defect, the degree of tooth eruption, the oral hygiene and diet habits of the patient. According to the severity of the case, the treatment ranges from topical fluoride varnish, to the use of adhesive materials for restorative procedures, or even the extraction of the teeth associated with orthodontic therapy. (Lygidakis et al., 2010, Lygidakis, 2010) The child, on the other hand, will experience pain and sensitivity, even when the enamel is intact, suffering from toothache during teeth brushing. Often, there is more difficulty to anaesthetize the MIH molars when treatment is indicated. Furthermore, children may also complain about the appearance and stainment of their affected incisor. (William et al., 2006a) In such circumstance, the esthetic complaint may also be considerable. Apart from the restorative difficulties faced by clinicians, children with MIH have dental fear and anxiety and these behaviour problems can be related to pain experienced by the patients during multiple treatment appointments, as many of them were either inadequately anesthetized or even had treatment without local analgesia (Jalevik & Klingberg, 2002). It has been shown that children with MIH receive much more dental treatment that unaffected children. (Jalevik & Klingberg, 2002, Kotsanos et al., 2005) Thus, treatment planning should also consider the long-term prognosis of teeth suffering from this condition.

Children during the period of eruption of their first permanent molars and/or incisors should be monitored very carefully in order to obtain an early diagnosis and immediate treatment for MIH. Considering all aspects mentioned above, MIH is one of the biggest challenges to great challenger of great clinical interest for dental practice because MIH has a great impact on the oral health as consequently, on the quality of life of children and adolescents. Thus, the objective of this chapter is to describe some epidemiological, morphological and treatment management considerations about MIH.

1.1 Definition

Developmental defects of enamel were commonly defined as hypoplasia, but according to the FDI Commission on Oral Health, Research and Epidemiology (1992), these defects are best classified into two distinct categories: a) hypomineralized enamel or enamel opacities (Figures 1A and 1B) and enamel hypoplasia (Figures 1C and 1D). While opacity is defined as a qualitative defect of the enamel, hypoplasia is defined as a quantitative defect of the enamel. (Suckling, 1989) There are others differences between developmental defects of enamel that can be seen in Table 1.

In the dental literature a wide variety of terminology or definitions were used for developmental defects of enamel in molars, with or without association with post eruptive breakdown of enamel as non-fluoride enamel opacities, internal enamel hypoplasia, non-endemic mottling of enamel, opaque spots, idiopathic enamel opacities, enamel opacities or cheese molars. (Koch et al., 1987, van Amerongen & Kreulen, 1995) However, to better understand the occurrence of molar incisor hypomineralisation and its impact on the oral health, the use of a uniform terminology is strongly recommended. (Weerheijm, 2004, Weerheijm et al., 2003)

The term molar incisor hypomineralisation (MIH) was firstly cited by WEERHEIJM ET AL., 2001. (Weerheijm et al., 2001) and further, this terminology was definitively adopted by the international dental scientific community as a result of a consensus after innumerous discussions in relation to developmental defects of enamel (Weerheijm et al., 2003). Then, MIH was defined as the clinical appearance of morphological enamel defects involving the occlusal and/or incisal third of one or more permanent molars or incisors as result as "hypomineralisation of systemic origin." (Weerheijm, 2004) The first permanent molar enamel is affected to an extent ranging from mild to severe; in many cases the incisor enamel is affected, but often, minimally not necessarily involving a macroscopic defect of tooth. Furthermore, this specific form of developmental defects of enamel (Baroni & Marchionni, 2011) show opacities asymmetrically often distributed, with marked variation in severity within an individual and ranges from small demarcated white, yellow or brown opacities (Figures 2A to 2F) to those covering much or the entire crown affecting cuspal areas and sparing the cervical areas. (Brook, 2009) CHAWLA ET AL. 2008 (Chawla et al., 2008) suggested that yellow–brown enamel defects are more severe than white-opaque ones it means that the stained degree of MIH enamel, may be used clinically to reflect the severity of the defect. (Farah et al., 2010a) In severe cases, the defective enamel is lost shortly after molar eruption, exposing underlying dentine favoring the tooth sensitivity and the dental carious lesion. (Kilpatrick, 2009)

Developmental defects of enamel		
Characteristics	Hypomineralised enamel or enamel opacities	Enamel hypoplasia
Enamel defect	Qualitative	quantitative
Clinical aspects	Normal thickness of the enamel Demarcated opacities of white to yellow-brown coloration Enamel is soft, porous and poorly delineated from normal tooth tissue Post eruptive breakdown in molars Assymmetrical opacities	Partial or total absence of enamel White colored lesions Deep fissures, horizontal or vertical grooves Edges with adjacent normal enamel are smooth Symmetrical or isolated lesions
Clinical appearance	Fig. 1. A – Assymmetrical opacities in incisors Fig. 1. B – Assymmetrical opacities in upper first permanent molars	Fig. 1. C – Symmetrical opacities in incisors Fig. 1. D – Isolated opacity in left upper incisor
Aetiological factors	Remains obscure	Identifiable systemic or local insult (trauma or local infection in primary teeth)

Table 1. Differences between two developmental defects of enamel according to FDI Commission on Oral Health, Research and Epidemiology (FDI, 1982)

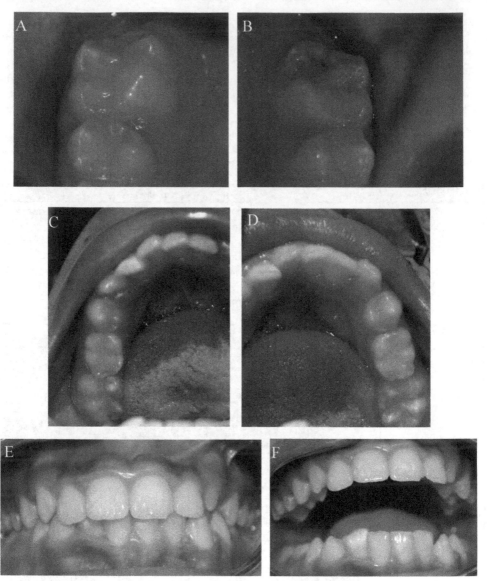

Fig. 2. A to F – In the same patient, note the presence of asymmetry and the different levels severity of lesions associated to the color opacities in molars and incisors.

Lately, MIH is understood as a hypocalcified subtype of enamel defect with reduced mineral content, low residual content of amelogenins and the presence of more than 16 types of proteins in affected teeth, thirteen of which are found in saliva and crevicular fluid (Kojima et al., 2000, Denny et al., 2008) and the three others (hemoglobin, albumin, complement C3) are major components of blood. Moreover, protein composition of MIH enamel varies with severity of enamel defect. (Mangum et al., 2010a)

2. Morphological considerations about MIH

2.1 Amelogenesis and developmental defects of enamel

Tooth development is strictly genetically controlled but sensitive to environmental disturbances (Suckling et al., 1988) since teeth have been formed they do not undergo remodeling. (Brook, 2009) During dental development, a single layer of inner enamel epithelial cells undergoes a remarkable change in cell shape in preparation for the secretion of enamel extracellular matrix. These cells develop into tall ameloblasts with cellular extensions called Tomes' processes, which function during enamel matrix secretion. Following generation of the enamel layer, the ameloblasts shorten and reorganize during the transition stage; they then enter maturation, where they change histologically from ruffle-ended to smooth-ended at the location where Tomes' processes have retracted. These cells reduce the enamel protein content and increase the mineral content so that the enamel layer can develop into the hardest tissue in the body. Finally, the cells shorten further and adhere to the enamel surface until just before eruption of the tooth into the oral cavity (Smith , 1979). In other words, enamel formation occurs in three stages:

1. matrix formation during which proteins involved in amelogenesis are produced;
2. calcification during which mineral content is acquired and the proteins are removed;
3. maturation during which the enamel is calcified and the remaining proteins are removed.

The mineralization of the enamel matrix is described as a two-step process. Firstly, the ameloblasts secrete an organic matrix that is immediately mineralized to about 30% by weight. Secondly, when the full thickness of enamel has been secreted by an ameloblast, a progressive increases in mineral content begin. Smooth-ended ameloblasts remove of water and proteins from the enamel matrix, whereas ruffle-ended ameloblasts participate in the active transport of calcium and phosphate into the matrix. The principal proteins acted in the enamel matrix are:

a. amelogenins (the major protein ~90% secreted into the enamel matrix) is a group of heterogeneous proteins (20-30 kDa) that are hydrophobic and rich in proline, histidine and glutamine and they are thought to play a role in the organization and regulation of crystal growth;
b. ameloblastins (Amelin, Sheathelin) constitutes 5-10% of the enamel matrix. It is thought to promote mineralization and crystal elongation; and
c. enamelins (60-80 kDa) are a heterogeneous group of proteins that may be involved in crystal nucleation. They are responsible for the progressive proteolytic cleavage of amelogenins. The processing of amelogenins to smaller peptides is necessary for the regulation of crystal organization and growth of enamel.

According to BROOK, 2009 (Brook, 2009) in the secretory stage the enamel protein matrix deposited by the ameloblasts is predominantly formed of amelogenin (85%). At the mid-secretory stage for appositional crystal growth and structural maintenance amelogenin is essential. However, while enamelin contributes less than 5% of the matrix it plays a major role in controlling the initiation of hydroxyapatite formation in early amelogenesis, being necessary for creating and maintaining enamel crystallite elongation at the mineralization front immediately adjacent to ameloblasts. The further enamel protein ameloblastin is a cell-adhesion molecule that maintains the differentiation stage of secreting ameloblasts and controls their secretion. The subsequent breakdown and removal of matrix proteins by means of proteolytic processing is essential for further development and mineralisation. Enamelysin (Mmp20), a matrix metalloproteinase, and the enamel serine protease kallikrein 4 (Klk4) are two major molecules involved in this process. (Wright et al., 2009, Bartlett et al., 2011) Mmp20 is expressed in secretory stage ameloblasts and also has effects on them maturation stage as well as on the mineralisation of mantle dentine. Klk4, present in both ameloblasts and odontoblasts, is expressed at the enamel transition and maturation phase. KLK4 which is secreted into the enamel by ameloblasts during the transition and maturation stages of amelogenesis. Klk4 degrades the organic matrix remaining from the secretion stage. This facilitates the continued deposition of minerals into enamel required for full mineralisation of hard enamel. Amelogenin is cleaved by Mmp20 and later degraded during maturation by Klk4. Within the ameloblasts Dlx3 and Dlx6 are expressed throughout the presecretory, secretory and maturation stages. During secretion Dlx2 is switched off and Dlx1 expression is upregulated. The Dlx homeobox genes may influence enamel formation by the regulation of amelogenin expression. Normal enamel thickness may be achieved by Runx2 suppressing enamel protein expression at the end of the secretory stage to give normal enamel thickness. In the maturation phase Runx2 induces Klk4 and upregulates basal membrane protein expression to induce ameloblast attachment to the enamel matrix. (Brook, 2009, Wrightet al., 2009, Bartlett et al., 2011)

In general, systemic factors that disturb the ameloblasts during the secretory stage cause restrictions of crystal elongation and result in pathologically thin, or hypoplastic enamel. On the other hand, disturbances during the transitional and/or maturation stage of amelogenesis result in pathologically soft (hypomaturated, hypomineralised) enamel of normal thicknesses. (Suga, 1989) According to REID AND DEAN, 2006 (Reid & Dean, 2006), enamel formation as a whole takes approximately one thousand days. Two thirds of this time is devoted to the maturation stage of amelogenesis. Considering this, the most critical period for enamel defects of first permanent molars and incisors is the first year of life coinciding with their early maturation (Alaluusua, 2010). In this period ameloblasts are highly sensitive to environmental disturbances. (Suckling, 1989) Hypomineralisation may also develop later because enamel maturation in the first permanent molars takes several years (later maturation stage). (Alaluusua, 2010)

2.2 Amelogenesis and MIH

As mentioned previously, there are no hypoplastic defects in MIH affected teeth because there is not any discernable reduction in enamel thickness teeth. (Farah et al., 2010a, Fearne et al., 2004) It suggests that any reduction in enamel thickness seen clinically is indicative of post-eruption disintegration of enamel. Furthermore, this clarify that whatever insult affects the developing tooth it happens after the enamel secretion is completed and affects the maturation phase of the mineralization process in a localized area of enamel. (Farah et al., 2010a)

2.3 Characteristics of MIH affected teeth

MIH is a qualitative defective enamel classified as hypomineralised type that follows the natural incremental lines of enamel formation, from cuspal to cement-enamel junction. (Farah et al., 2010a, Fearne et al., 1994) In the most cervical section, the enamel is sound with no evidence of defective structure. At a more occlusal level, the defect is confined to the inner enamel while the outer enamel does not appear to be affected. As move occlusally, the hypomineralisation becomes more evident, eventually spreading to span the entire thickness of the enamel. The defects usually did not involve the cusp tips; but if a marginal ridge was involved, its maximum height was affected. (Farah et al., 2010a)

Microstructural analysis of sound and hypomineralised enamel showed two marked changes in microstructure in the MIH affected enamel region; less dense prism structure with loosely packed apatite crystals and wider sheath regions. (Xie et al., 2008) These changes appear to occur during enamel maturation and may be responsible for the marked reduction in hardness and elastic modulus of the affected enamel. (Fagrell et al., 2010) In addition, the enamel in the transitional region adjacent to the demarcated defects in MIH has also notable alterations in their prism sheaths. Despite the translucent, normal appearance, the transitional region between the affected and unaffected regions in MIH teeth had weakened prism sheaths which compromised its overall mechanical properties. (Chan et al., 2010) The reason for this is unclear but may be also related to the lack of organization of the enamel crystals due poorly demarcated prism boundaries in the affected regions (Mahoney et al., 2004) and the packing of the crystals seemed to be less tight and less well organized in the porous parts. The borders of the enamel rods were indistinct and the interrods zones hardly visible, or the rods were very thin with wide interrod zones. (Jalevik et al., 2005)

Semi-quantitative analysis by energy dispersive X-ray spectrometry in extracted MIH affected teeth showed that the mineral composition of this type of enamel is low (Javelik & Norén, 2001), on average the mineral density is about 19 % lower than sound enamel (Baroni & Marchionni, 2011, Farah et al., 2010a, Jalevik & Noren, 2000, Schulze et al., 2004), there is a decrease in Ca:P ratio in the enamel (Rodd et al., 2007a, Jalevik, 2001) related to an increase in C content. (Fearne et al., 2004)

Also, MIH enamel has substantially higher protein content than normal enamel, but a near-normal level of residual amelogenins. This characteristic distinguishes MIH from hypomaturation defects that contain high residual amelogenins such as *Amelogenesis Imperfecta* or Fluorosis (Mangum et al., 2010a, Wright et al., 1996, Wright et al., 1997) and in turn typifies MIH as a hypocalcification defect as mentioned above. Pathogenically, it points to a pre-eruptive disturbance of mineralization involving albumin probably due to an over-abundance of albumin that interferes with the mineralisation process. It justifies the porosities exhibited in the subsurface (Jalevik & Noren, 2000) because albumin degradation may be a prerequisite for maximal crystal growth in the maturation stage of enamel. (Farah et al., 2010b, Farah et al., 2010c, Mangum et al., 2010b) The presence of excessive albumin seemed to be promote KLK4 inactivity resulting in enamel with elevated protein content and reduced mineral content. In cases of MIH with post-eruptive breakdown, on the exposed surface there is a subsequent protein adsorption on the exposed hydroxyapatite matrix. An indicator of the severity of MIH affected teeth is the actual organic content of its enamel (Farah et al., 2010a) Brown enamel, the most severe MIH lesion, has the highest protein content (15–21-fold greater), whilst the protein content of white/opaque and yellow enamel are both markedly higher (8-fold greater) than sound enamel. (Farah et al., 2010a) For sound enamel, when subjected to mechanical forces the controlling deformation mechanism was distributed shearing within nanometer thick protein layer between its constituent mineral crystals; whereas for hypomineralised enamel micro cracking and subsequent crack growth were more evident in its less densely packed microstructure. (Xie et al., 2009) Thereafter, the ability of dental enamel to absorb energy and sustain deformation without catastrophic failure is attributed to its viscoelastic protein layers. Thus, the change in the protein content in teeth with MIH induces the enamel fracture when subjected to the masticatory efforts.

In relation to the dentin of MIH affected teeth it was observed that the Ca/P ratios for dentin below hypomineralized enamel were in principle identical to those of normal enamel; but when the Ca/C ratio was analyzed, dentin below hypomineralized enamel had the lowest values and the level of C was highest for dentin below hypomineralized enamel. In addition, O and P levels in dentin below normal enamel were higher compared with values in dentin below hypomineralized and N values for dentin below hypomineralized enamel are the highest. (Heijs et al., 2007)

This enhanced knowledge concerning the microstructural changes in hypomineralised enamel improves the understanding of some of the problems associated with the clinical management of these teeth. In particular, the frequent occurrence of enamel fractures and inadequate retention of adhesive materials both of which are recognized as significant clinical challenges preventing successful restoration of these compromised teeth. It is known that organic matter such as proteins have poor acid solubility. The presence of increased amounts of organic matter in the hypomineralised enamel, specifically within both prism structure and sheath regions may inhibit the creation of an adequate etch profile which in turn compromises the adhesion between resin based restorative materials and the defective enamel. (William et al., 2006b) Improved clinical outcomes are likely to depend, at least in part, on the successful treatment of these proteins prior to any enamel etching or adhesive strategies. (Baroni & Marchionni, 2011, Xie et al., 2008)

3. Aetiological considerations

Etiological factors of causing changes in organic/inorganic composition of MIH affected teeth are still unknown as showed by two systematic reviews. (Alaluusua, 2010, Crombie et al., 2009) As far, MIH may have a multifactor aetiology (Figure 3) acting additionally or even synergistically (Alaluusua, 2010, Crombie et al., 2009, Fagrell et al., 2011), with a genetic predisposition associated with one or more of a range of systemic insults occurring at a susceptible stage in the development of specific teeth. (Figure 3) It explains why in a seeming random manner several teeth are severely affected while their antimeres are unaffected. (Brook, 2009)

Notwithstanding, FAGRELL et al., 2011 (Fagrell et al., 2011) evaluated the etiological factors for severe demarcated enamel opacities in the first permanent molars from a database that contained approximately 4,000 variables with the purpose to prospectively investigate risk factors for immune mediate diseases in All Babies in Southeast Sweden project. Approximately, 17,000 children take part in the study. Medical data, information from interviews, questionnaires were collected at delivery, at 1, 2.5 years, of age with follow up at 5, at 8-9 and at 12 years. All information collected, about 4,000 variables for each child covering somatic growth: in pre-, peri-, and neonatal data from the child and its mother; diseases during first 3 years of child life; medication and vaccinations during the same period, socioeconomic factors and nutrition during first 3 years of child life were entered into databank. Besides, in this study, randomly, there were two-age and sex-matched children to each MIH child. After a regression logistic analyses, the results showed a positive association between severe demarcated opacities in permanent first molars with breastfeeding for more than 6 months, late introduction of gruel and late introduction of infant formula. Moreover, a combination of these variables increased the risk to develop severe demarcated opacities by more five times. According these results, the authors concluded that nutritional conditions during first 6 months of life may influence the risk to develop severe demarcated opacities in first permanent molars. (Fagrell et al., 2011)

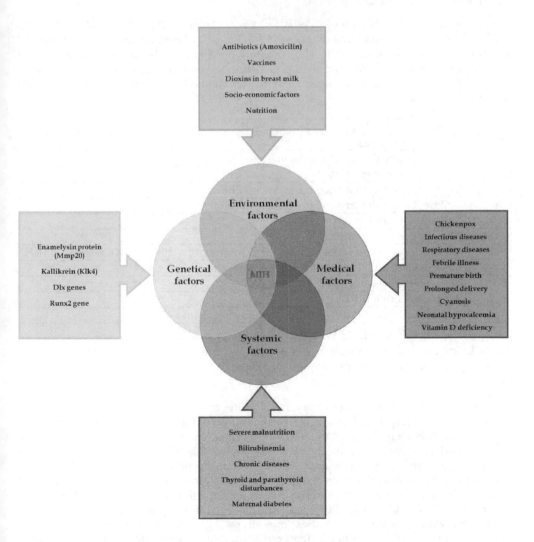

Fig. 3. Multifactorial aetiology of MIH

4. Epidemiological considerations about MIH

4.1 Diagnose of MIH

Traditionally, a wide variety of terms and definitions have been used to describe various developmental defects of enamel (DDE). However, this original index turned out to be too complicated to use in practice and a modified DDE index (mDDE) was presented by FDI (1992). The modified development dental enamel (DDE) index was considered to be too time consuming and not adequate for MIH prevalence studies because the post-eruptive breakdown is a pathognomonic feature in MIH but the mDDE index does not clearly distingue PEB from enamel hypoplasia.

According to European Academy of Pediatric Dentistry seminar (EAPD) placed in Athens in 2003. (Weerheijmet al., 2003) The diagnose of MIH must be based on scores range from 0 to 10 (Table 2). (Ghanim et al., 2011) The screening of MIH must be done in children eight years of age; examination for MIH should be performed on wet teeth after removing debris with cotton roll; first permanent molars and incisors should be examined, each tooth as seen in Table 2.

Code	Criteria
0	Enamel defect free
1	White/creamy demarcated opacities, no PEB
1a	White/creamy demarcated opacities, with PEB
2	Yellow/brown demarcated opacities, no PEB
2a	Yellow/brown demarcated opacities, with PEB
3	Atypical restoration
4	Missing because of MIH
5	Partially erupted (i.e., less than one-third of the crown high) with evidence of MIH
6	Unerupted/partially erupted with no evidence of MIH
7	Diffuse opacities (not MIH)
8	Hypoplasia (not MIH)
9	Combined lesion (diffuse opacities/hypoplasia with MIH)
10	Demarcated opacities in incisors only

Table 2. Criteria for scoring molar incisor hypomineralisation (MIH) according to European Academy of Paediatric Dentistry recommendations cited by GHANIM et al., 2011 (Ghanim et al., 2011).

Clinically, the enamel defects can vary from white, cream, yellow to brownish, but they always show a sharp demarcation between the affected and sound enamel. The tooth surface enamel initially develops to a normal thickness, but can chip off under masticatory forces called post eruption breakdown (PEB) (Figure 2B) PEB is characterized by poor aesthetic appearance and sensitivity to thermal and mechanical stimuli. After such PEB, the clinical pictures can resemble enamel hypoplasia. However, the margins of the disintegrated areas are irregular, whereas those in hypoplasia are smooth and rounded. The demarcated lesions in MIH should also be distinguished from the diffuse opacities typical of fluorosis. Dentitions with generalized opacities present on all teeth such as in Amelogenesis *Imperfecta*, rather than limited to the first permanent molars and incisors, are not considered to have MIH. Nowadays, to simplify the use of MIH scores, the severity of MIH can be determined by dividing the affected teeth in only two groups: mild defect (demarcated opacities) (Figures 4A, B) and moderate/severe defect (enamel breakdown and atypical restorations) (Lygidakis et al., 2008) (Figures 4B, C).

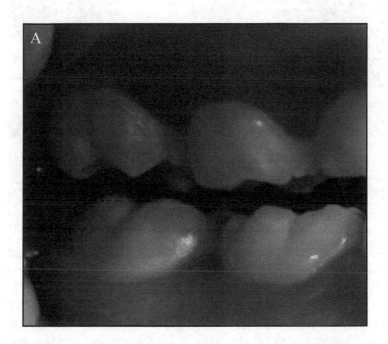

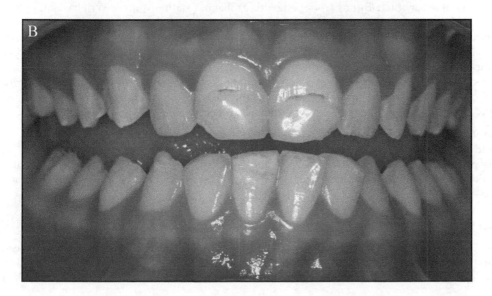

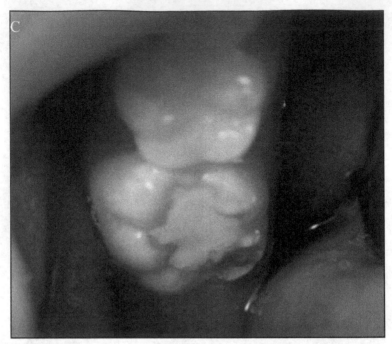

Fig. 4. A to C – Mild defect opacities in right FPM (A). Atypical restorations in upper incisors (B) and in left lower FPM (C). Note the opacities in the vestibular surface of the right lower incisor (B), left upper FPM (B). Post restoration enamel fracture in lower right FPM (C).

Dental diseases have a detrimental effect on quality of life both in childhood and older age. (Moynihan & Petersen, 2004) Several authors have discussed whether developmental defects of enamel (DDE) are a public health problem. (Mathu-Muju & Wright, 2006) For a condition to be considered of public health significance, several criteria need to be reviewed, particularly the prevalence its impact on an individual in terms of symptoms, functioning, psychological and social should be considerate. (Marshman et al., 2009) Besides its clinical implications in the field of public health, MIH have taken on importance as strong predictors of dental caries. This result highlights the importance of establishing priority programs of prevention and early treatment for these groups of children both for aesthetic and functional reasons, as well as to minimize the increased risk of dental caries.

In view of MIH having a potentially large impact on treatment needs in child populations and a cost-effectiveness treatment from public or private health insurance, it is relevant to identify the prevalence of MIH in epidemiological studies, with the concern only studies using the MIH index as epidemiological criteria. (Weerheijm et al., 2003, Weerheijm et al., 2001, Weerheijm, 2003)

4.2 Prevalence of MIH

A first epidemiological study was carried out in Swedish children in the late 1970s, whose first permanent molars (FPM) called "cheese" molars, were described as creamy-white to yellow-brown enamel opacities; or with disintegration in severe cases (Koch et al., 1987)

After that, epidemiological data comes from studies conducted in European countries and reported the prevalence of MIH had varied from 3.6 to 25%.(Weerheijm & Mejare, 2003) Lately, a systematic review showed a wide variation in the prevalence of MIH (2.4 - 40.2 %) and stated that the cross comparison of the results of the various studies were difficult because of use of different indices and criteria, examination variability, methods of recording and different age groups. (Jalevik, 2010)

Based on this, we performed a nonsystematic hand-searching screening in the PUBMED data base using the terms: EAPD; MIH; limited to: at least 100 subjects and the data of study - after 2003 and the results could be found (Table 3). According to results, it was possible observed that at least one country in each continent already demonstrates concern for the impact of MIH regarding the condition of oral health of the population, which makes it a public health problem. Taking searching results of the more recent studies into account, the prevalence of MIH varies from 3.5% to 40.2%. This could be explained by methodological variability, by different socio-demographic-ethnical characteristics of samples and by the access to health services (favorable x unfavorable). It worthwhile mentions that only one population-based well designed study could be found and it highlights the prevalence of 3.5% for MIH in Southeast Sweden. (Fagrell et al., 2011) These results are also found in China and Bulgaria epidemiological surveys.

Country	Prevalence	Subjects (n)	Years age (mean ± SD)	Authors
Argentina	15.9%	1,098	11.3 years (11.08-11.39)	Biondi et al, 2011 (Biondi et al., 2011)
Boznia and Herzegovina	12.3%	560	12 years	Muratbegovic et al., 2008 (Muratbegovic et al., 2008)
Brazil	19.8%	918	6-12 years	da Costa-Silva et al., 2010 (da Costa-Silva et al., 2010)
Brazil	40.2%	249	7-13 years	Soviero et al., 2009 (Soviero et al., 2009)
Bulgaria	3.58%	2,960	7-14 years	Kukleva et al., 2008 (Kukleva et al., 2008)
China	2.8%	2,635	11.0-14.0 years (12 years ±0.6)	Cho et al., 2008 (Cho et al., 2008)
Germany	14.3%	442	9 years	Jasulaityte et al., 2008 (Jasulaityte et al., 2008)
Greece	10.2%	3,518	5.5-12 years (8.17±1.38)	Lygidakis et al., 2008 (Lygidakis et al., 2008)
Instanbul	14.9%	147	7-9 years	Kusku et al., 2008 (Kusku et al., 2008)
Iraq	21.5%	823	7-9 years	Ghanim et al., 2011 (Ghanim et al., 2011)
Jordan	17.6%	3,666	7-9 years	Zawaideh et al., 2011 (Zawaideh et al., 2011)

Country	Prevalence	Subjects (n)	Years age (mean ± SD)	Authors
Libya	9%	378	7-8.9 years	Fteita et al., 2006 (Fteita et al., 2006)
Lithuania	14.9%	1,277	7-9 years	Jasulaityte et al.,2007 (Jasulaityte et al., 2007)
Norhern England	15.9%	3,233	12 years	Balmer et al., 2011 (Balmer et al., 2011)
Southeast Sweden	3.5%	17,055	Children born from1,October-1997 to 1, 1999	Fagell et al., 2011 (Fagrell et al., 2011)
Spain	17.8%	505	6-14 years	Martinez Gomez et al., 2011 (Martinez Gomez et al., 2011)

Table 3. Distribution of MIH in some countries in the world. Selected studies were conducted using only MIH index criteria as suggested by EAPD.

In spite of having still need of further investigation considering population-based samples, with standardization of methodology, it is clearly seen that different countries from different regions of the world are performing epidemiological surveys using MIH index. This is essential to ascertain the occurrence of the MIH and may otherwise be systematized not only strategies to MIH diagnosis, but also treatments and monitoring as well as outlining scientific researches considering this topic. Thus, it is essential to do well design clinical studies considering MIH pathology.

5. Clinical considerations and management of MIH

5.1 Dentino-pulpal complex considerations and MIH

Patients with MIH affected teeth suffer from dentine sensitivity once often report exacerbated sensitivity to a variety of normally innocuous thermal, mechanical and osmo-chemical stimuli (Jalevik & Klingberg, 2002) due to the presence of porous enamel and sometimes, the exposed dentine. Based on the immunocytochemical findings in hypomineralised permanent first molars, changes in pulpal innervation, vascularity, and immune cell accumulation were indicative of an inflammatory response.(Rodd et al.,2007a) Besides, the morphological aspects of MIH may favor ingress of bacterial contaminants (Fagrell et al., 2008), thereby resulting in chronic inflammation of the pulp (Rodd et al., 2007b) Following tissue inflammation, a variety of morphological and cytochemical neuronal changes may occur including neuronal branching and altered expression of neuropeptides and ion channels (Rodd et al., 2007b, Rodd & Boissonade, 2002) that seems to be related with an overexpressed dental sensitive.

From a clinical perspective, these findings would support early interventions in order to avoid the development of pulpal inflammation and associated hypersensitivity. Thus, toothpastes and/or chewing gums with mineralizing products, such as Casein

Phosphopeptide-Amorphous Calcium Phosphate (CCP-ACP) (Baroni & Marchionni, 2011) or the application of desensitizers (2 % potassium nitrate plus 2% sodium fluoride) or sealers have been indicated. (Lygidakis et al., 2010, Lygidakis, 2010)

Dental pain and the severity of hypomineralisation or enamel loss in molar-incisor hypomineralisation are major determinants for the choice of treatment. (William et al., 2006a) The most conservative interventional treatment consists of bonding a tooth colored material to the tooth to protect it from further wear or sensitivity although the nature of the enamel prevents formation of an acceptable bond. (William et al., 2006b) Less conservative treatment options, but frequently necessary include use of stainless steel crowns, permanent cast crowns or extraction of affected teeth in association with the orthodontic appliance or teeth replacement with a bridge or implant.

5.2 Clinical management of MIH

In accordance with the European Academy of Pediatric Dentistry until now there are only a limited number of evidence based research papers on MIH affected teeth. (Lygidakis et al., 2010) Because of this, the guidelines diagram according to Scottish Intercollegiate Guidelines Network (SIGN) methodology (SIGN, 1999) is impossible to be made. However, treatment modalities in children with teeth affected by MIH were systematically reviewed by LYGIDAKIS, 2010. (Lygidakis, 2010) Thus, the clinical management of MIH was resumed by the present authors as seen in Figure 5. These clinical guidelines approach were organized considering the type of MIH affected teeth (permanent first molars or incisors) and the severity of defects. Then, it was also considered, the treatment management of the first permanent molars (FPM) without post eruptive breakdown (PEB) or with post-eruptive breakdown; as well as to the incisors with different levels of opacities (Figure 3). It worthwhile be emphasized the necessity of not only randomized controlled clinical trials but also the laboratory studies to support and better understand the specificities of MIH condition.

Therefore, a detailed study under magnification of the unerupted molar and incisor crowns on any available radiographs should be done. (William et al., 2006a) During teeth eruption, when MIH is confirmed, it should be made a diet counseling for dietary modifications to avoid dental caries, dental erosion and dental sensitivity; It should be recommended a toothpaste with a fluoride or, in cases of dental sensitivity, aiming to produce a non-sensitivity and hypermineralized surface layer which provides a super saturated environment of calcium and phosphate on enamel surface, a desensitizing toothpaste with casein phosphopeptide-amorphous calcium phosphate (CPP-ACP) should be indicated. (Baroni & Marchionni, 2011)

Fissure sealants should be applied early after molars eruption and before enamel breakdown. (Kilpatrick, 2009, Lygidakis et al., 2010, Lygidakis, 2010, William et al., 2006a, Crombie et al., 2008) Taking the morphological aspects of MIH affected teeth into account, for first permanent molars, highly viscosity glass ionomer cements can be considered as an alternative material of choice for fissure sealing due to its stable chemical adhesion on the substrate (Welbury et al., 2004) which ensures its clinical longevity even if disappeared macroscopically in the follow-ups. (Frencken &Wolke, 2010)

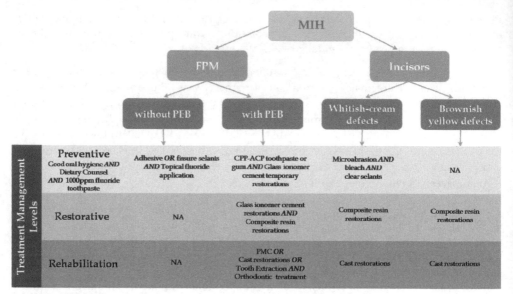

The flow chart (Fig. 5) content:

| MIH |
| FPM | | | Incisors |
| without PEB | with PEB | Whitish-cream defects | Brownish yellow defects |

Treatment Management Levels		without PEB	with PEB	Whitish-cream defects	Brownish yellow defects
	Preventive	Adhesive *OR* fissure selants *AND* Topical fluoride application	CPP-ACP toothpaste or gum *AND* Glass ionomer cement temporary restorations	Microabrasion *AND* bleach *AND* clear selants	NA
	Restorative	NA	Glass ionomer cement restorations *AND* Composite resin restorations	Composite resin restorations	Composite resin restorations
	Rehabilitation	NA	PMC *OR* Cast restorations *OR* Tooth Extraction *AND* Orthodontic treatment	Cast restorations	Cast restorations

NA – Not applicable

Fig. 5. Flow chart illustrated by the authors of clinical management of MIH Children with a history of putative aetiological factors in the first 3 years should be screening at risk for MIH (Alaluusua, 2010, Crombie et al., 2009, Fagrell et al., 2011)

As suggested by LIGYDIKIS ET AL., 2010 (Lygidakis et al., 2010), when children express their concern on mild discolorations, at late mixed dentition, incisors with whitish-creamy opacities may occasionally respond to bleaching with carbamide peroxide. (Fayle, 2003) Another conservative approach is microabrasion with either 18% hydrochloric acid or 37% phosphoric acid and pumice for 60s. (Lygidakis et al., 2010, Wright, 2002, Gotler & Ratson, 2010, Willmott et al., 2008) More pronounced enamel defects might be dealt with by combining the two methods (Sundfeld et al., 2007a), bleaching and microabrasion. However, bleaching for young children may induce hypersensitivity, mucosal irritation and enamel surface alterations (Joiner, 2006), whilst microabrasion may result in loss of enamel. (Sundfeld et al., 2007b) An etch-bleach-seal technique by involving:

a.   60 seconds etch with 37% phosphoric acid;
b.   bleach with 5% sodium hypochlodite for 5-10 min.
c.   re-etch and application of fissure sealant over the surface to occlude the porosities appears as another management treatment possibility. (Wright, 2002)

On the other hand, the replacement of micro-abrasion by local enamel thickness reduction, using high-speed headpiece, should be also evaluated by the professional.

The others clinical problems for patients with MIH are attrition, exposed dentin, atypical cavities or complete coronal destruction. (Kilpatrick, 2009, Jalevik & Noren, 2000) Moreover, pain experience during dental treatment has led some MIH children to be significantly less compliant and more dentally anxious than their peers.(Jalevik & Klingberg, 2002) In this case, the adjunctive use of nitrous oxide-oxygen analgesia may alleviate anxiety and reduce dental pain. In last case, general anesthesia may be required for restorative treatment. (William et al., 2006a) The maintenance of existing tooth structure and pain relief can be achieved with temporary restorations, often in sub-optimal clinical conditions, through the use of glass ionomer cements. In mild and moderate MIH cases composite restorations using self-etching primer adhesive bonding systems is the treatment of choice (William et al., 2006b) and may last for many years until indirect restorations would be placed. (Lygidakis et al., 2010, Lygidakis, 2010) For cavities involving large areas of dentine, glass ionomer cement has been proposed to be used as a sub-layer under the composite restoration (Mathu-Muju & Wright, 2006). A more definitive restorative approach, albeit still temporary solution, is the preformed metal crown (PMC) which placed on first permanent molars provide an excellent medium term restorative solution. (Kilpatrick, 2009) For that, it requires an excellent analgesia and patient cooperation which may not be forthcoming. In severe cases, transitional treatment for function and aesthetics can be provided until adolescence when permanent prosthetic approach with crowns in molars and veneers or crowns in incisors can be indicated. Cast restorations (full coverage crown, tooth-colored crown, porcelains or veneers) have been used. (Lygidakis et al., 2010, Lygidakis, 2010) However, they are not recommended for teeth in early post-eruptive stage because of the continuous eruption exposing the crown margins, the large pulp size, short crown height, and difficulties in obtaining a good impression for subgingival crown margins. (Koch & Garcia-Godoy, 2000) At last case, any extraction of first permanent molars should only be carried out with consideration of the possible orthodontic implications.

6. Conclusion

Despite a fall in the prevalence and in the speed of progression of dental caries disease, often, the clinicians and the pedodontics can find first permanent molars and incisors with hypomineralised enamel defected. MIH must be regarded as a public health problem which brings painful consequences, aesthetic and a negative impact on the quality of life of individuals suffering from MIH. A difficult and complex problem resolution, therefore all effort should converge towards the sense of real knowledge of the MIH aetiology to allow more accurate diagnosis and more appropriate treatment. People seized with MIH pathology have made sure that their expectations in relation to intervention proposal is based on high efficiency and effectiveness scientific evidences by ensuring the quality of life not only these people but also of their families. The etiology of MIH as a result of synergistic action of environmental factors and, suddenly genetic expressions leaving disturbances in enamel formation of molars and incisors in the first year of life, is the challenge to be overcome. Ultimately, the discovery of new genes and novel proteins such as amelotin and apin (Nishio, 2008) that they are also produced by ameloblasts, but during the stage of maturation, with important enamel mineralization function in relation to obtaining final hardness of enamel point to a promissory future in relation to knowledge of dental development. Well-being, understanding the genetic sequential and signaling pathways of developmental normal of enamel will provide us with an invaluable tool for understanding the pathways and mechanisms of tissue maintenance, repair and regeneration. It will enable us to manipulate genetic and environmental factors and ultimately, aid in the development of dental develpomental defects of enamel therapy.

7. Acknowledgment

We would like to thank Ms. Maja Bozicevic for giving us the opportunity to write this chapter, Andre Caula for illustrations and Andre Alves for technical support.

8. References

(1992). A review of the developmental defects of enamel index (DDE Index). Commission on Oral Health, Research & Epidemiology. Report of an FDI Working Group. Int Dent J. Vol. 42, No. 6, (Dec, 1992), pp. 411-426. 0020-6539 (Print) 0020-6539 (Linking) 0164-1263 (Linking)

Alaluusua, S. (2010). Aetiology of Molar-Incisor Hypomineralisation: A systematic review. Eur Arch Paediatr Dent. Vol. 11, No. 2, (Apr, 2010), pp. 53-58. 1818-6300 (Print) 1818-6300 (Linking)

Balmer, R. et al. (2011). The prevalence of molar incisor hypomineralisation in Northern England and its relationship to socioeconomic status and water fluoridation. Int J Paediatr Dent, No., (Oct 20, 2011), 1365-263X (Electronic) 0960-7439 (Linking)

Baroni, C. & Marchionni, S. (2011). MIH supplementation strategies: prospective clinical and laboratory trial. J Dent Res. Vol. 90, No. 3, (Mar, 2011), pp. 371-376. 1544-0591 (Electronic) 0022-0345 (Linking)

Bartlett, J. D. et al. (2011). MMP20 cleaves E-cadherin and influences ameloblast development. Cells Tissues Organs. Vol. 194, No. 2-4, 2011), pp. 222-226. 1422-6421 (Electronic) 1422-6405 (Linking)

Biondi, A. M. et al. (2011). Prevalence of molar incisor hypomineralization in the city of Buenos Aires. Acta Odontol Latinoam. Vol. 24, No. 1, 2011), pp. 81-85. 0326-4815 (Print) 0326-4815 (Linking)

Brook, A. H. (2009). Multilevel complex interactions between genetic, epigenetic and environmental factors in the aetiology of anomalies of dental development. Arch Oral Biol. Vol. 54 Suppl 1, No., (Dec, 2009), pp. S3-17. 1879-1506 (Electronic) 0003-9969 (Linking)

Chan, Y. L. et al. (2010). Degraded prism sheaths in the transition region of hypomineralized teeth. J Dent. Vol. 38, No. 3, (Mar, 2010), pp. 237-244. 1879-176X (Electronic) 0300-5712 (Linking)

Chawla, N. et al. (2008). Clinical studies on molar-incisor-hypomineralisation part 1: distribution and putative associations. Eur Arch Paediatr Dent. Vol. 9, No. 4, (Dec, 2008), pp. 180-190. 1818-6300 (Print) 1818-6300 (Linking)

Cho, S. Y. et al. (2008). Molar incisor hypomineralization in Hong Kong Chinese children. Int J Paediatr Dent. Vol. 18, No. 5, (Sep, 2008), pp. 348-352. 1365-263X (Electronic) 0960-7439 (Linking)

Crombie, F. A. et al. (2008). Molar incisor hypomineralization: a survey of members of the Australian and New Zealand Society of Paediatric Dentistry. Aust Dent J. Vol. 53, No. 2, (Jun, 2008), pp. 160-166. 0045-0421 (Print) 0045-0421 (Linking)

Crombie, F. et al. (2009). Aetiology of molar-incisor hypomineralization: a critical review. Int J Paediatr Dent. Vol. 19, No. 2, (Mar, 2009), pp. 73-83. 1365-263X (Electronic) 0960-7439 (Linking) da Costa-Silva, C. M. et al. (2010). Molar incisor hypomineralization: prevalence, severity and clinical consequences in Brazilian children. Int J Paediatr Dent. Vol. 20, No. 6, (Nov, 2010), pp. 426-434. 1365-263X (Electronic) 0960-7439 (Linking)

Denny, P. et al. (2008). The proteomes of human parotid and submandibular/sublingual gland salivas collected as the ductal secretions. J Proteome Res. Vol. 7, No. 5, (May, 2008), pp. 1994-2006. 1535-3893 (Print) 1535-3893 (Linking)

Fagrell, T. G. et al. (2008). Bacterial invasion of dentinal tubules beneath apparently intact but hypomineralized enamel in molar teeth with molar incisor hypomineralization. Int J Paediatr Dent. Vol. 18, No. 5, (Sep, 2008), pp. 333-340. 1365-263X (Electronic) 0960-7439 (Linking)

Fagrell, T. G. et al. (2010). Chemical, mechanical and morphological properties of hypomineralized enamel of permanent first molars. Acta Odontol Scand. Vol. 68, No. 4, (Jul, 2010), pp. 215-222. 1502-3850 (Electronic) 0001-6357 (Linking)

Fagrell, T. G. et al. (2011). Aetiology of severe demarcated enamel opacities--an evaluation based on prospective medical and social data from 17,000 children. Swed Dent J. Vol. 35, No. 2, 2011), pp. 57-67. 0347-9994 (Print) 0347-9994 (Linking)

Farah, R. A. et al. (2010b). Protein content of molar-incisor hypomineralisation enamel. J Dent. Vol. 38, No. 7, (Jul, 2010b), pp. 591-596. 1879-176X (Electronic) 0300-5712 (Linking)

Farah, R. A. et al. (2010c). Mineral density of hypomineralised enamel. J Dent. Vol. 38, No. 1, (Jan, 2010c), pp. 50-58. 1879-176X (Electronic) 0300-5712 (Linking)

Farah, R. et al. (2010a). Linking the clinical presentation of molar-incisor hypomineralisation to its mineral density. Int J Paediatr Dent. Vol. 20, No. 5, (Sep 1, 2010a), pp. 353-360. 1365-263X (Electronic) 0960-7439 (Linking)

Fayle, S. A. (2003). Molar incisor hypomineralisation: restorative management. Eur J Paediatr Dent. Vol. 4, No. 3, (Sep, 2003), pp. 121-126. 1591-996X (Print) 1591-996X (Linking)

Fearne, J. et al. (2004). 3D X-ray microscopic study of the extent of variations in enamel density in first permanent molars with idiopathic enamel hypomineralisation. Br Dent J. Vol. 196, No. 10, (May 22, 2004), pp. 634-638; discussion 625. 0007-0610 (Print) 0007-0610 (Linking)

Fearne, J. M. et al. (1994). Deciduous enamel defects in low-birth-weight children: correlated X-ray microtomographic and backscattered electron imaging study of hypoplasia and hypomineralization. Anat Embryol (Berl). Vol. 189, No. 5, (May, 1994), pp. 375-381. 0340-2061 (Print) 0340-2061 (Linking)

Frencken, J. E. & Wolke, J. (2010). Clinical and SEM assessment of ART high-viscosity glass-ionomer sealants after 8-13 years in 4 teeth. J Dent. Vol. 38, No. 1, (Jan, 2010), pp. 59-64. 1879-176X (Electronic) 0300-5712 (Linking)

Fteita, D. et al. (2006). Molar-incisor hypomineralization (MIH) in a group of school-aged children in Benghazi, Libya. Eur Arch Paediatr Dent. Vol. 7, No. 2, (Jun, 2006), pp. 92-95. 1818-6300 (Print) 1818-6300 (Linking)

Ghanim, A. et al. (2011). Molar-incisor hypomineralisation: prevalence and defect characteristics in Iraqi children. Int J Paediatr Dent. Vol. 21, No. 6, (Nov, 2011), pp. 413-421. 1365-263X (Electronic) 0960-7439 (Linking)

Gotler, M. & Ratson, T. (2010). Molar incisor hypomineralization (MIH)--a literature review. Refuat Hapeh Vehashinayim. Vol. 27, No. 2, (Apr, 2010), pp. 10-18, 60. 0792-9935 (Print) 0792-9935 (Linking)

Heijs, S. C. et al. (2007). Morphology and chemical composition of dentin in permanent first molars with the diagnose MIH. Swed Dent J. Vol. 31, No. 4, 2007), pp. 155-164. 0347-9994 (Print) 0347-9994 (Linking)

Jalevik, B. (2001). Enamel hypomineralization in permanent first molars. A clinical, histo-morphological and biochemical study. Swed Dent J Suppl, No. 149, 2001), pp. 1-86. 0348-6672 (Print) 0348-6672 (Linking)

Jalevik, B. (2010). Prevalence and Diagnosis of Molar-Incisor- Hypomineralisation (MIH): A systematic review. Eur Arch Paediatr Dent. Vol. 11, No. 2, (Apr, 2010), pp. 59-64. 1818-6300 (Print) 1818-6300 (Linking)

Jalevik, B. et al. (2005). Scanning electron micrograph analysis of hypomineralized enamel in permanent first molars. Int J Paediatr Dent. Vol. 15, No. 4, (Jul, 2005), pp. 233-240. 0960-7439 (Print) 0960-7439 (Linking)

Jalevik, B. & Klingberg, G. A. (2002). Dental treatment, dental fear and behaviour management problems in children with severe enamel hypomineralization of their permanent first molars. Int J Paediatr Dent. Vol. 12, No. 1, (Jan, 2002), pp. 24-32. 0960-7439 (Print) 0960-7439 (Linking)

Jalevik, B. & Noren, J. G. (2000). Enamel hypomineralization of permanent first molars: a morphological study and survey of possible aetiological factors. Int J Paediatr Dent. Vol. 10, No. 4, (Dec, 2000), pp. 278-289. 0960-7439 (Print) 0960-7439 (Linking)

Jasulaityte, L. et al. (2007). Molar incisor hypomineralization: review and prevalence data from the study of primary school children in Kaunas/Lithuania. Eur Arch Paediatr Dent. Vol. 8, No. 2, (Jun, 2007), pp. 87-94. 1818-6300 (Print) 1818-6300 (Linking)

Jasulaityte, L. et al. (2008). Prevalence of molar-incisor-hypomineralisation among children participating in the Dutch National Epidemiological Survey (2003). Eur Arch Paediatr Dent. Vol. 9, No. 4, (Dec, 2008), pp. 218-223. 1818-6300 (Print) 1818-6300 (Linking)

Joiner, A. (2006). The bleaching of teeth: a review of the literature. J Dent. Vol. 34, No. 7, (Aug, 2006), pp. 412-419. 0300-5712 (Print) 0300-5712 (Linking)

Kilpatrick, N. (2009). New developments in understanding development defects of enamel: optimizing clinical outcomes. J Orthod. Vol. 36, No. 4, (Dec, 2009), pp. 277-282. 1465-3133 (Electronic) 1465-3125 (Linking)

Koch, G. et al. (1987). Epidemiologic study of idiopathic enamel hypomineralization in permanent teeth of Swedish children. Community Dent Oral Epidemiol. Vol. 15, No. 5, (Oct, 1987), pp. 279-285. 0301-5661 (Print) 0301-5661 (Linking)

Koch, M. J. & Garcia-Godoy, F. (2000). The clinical performance of laboratory-fabricated crowns placed on first permanent molars with developmental defects. J Am Dent Assoc. Vol. 131, No. 9, (Sep, 2000), pp. 1285-1290. 0002-8177 (Print) 0002-8177 (Linking)

Kojima, T. et al. (2000). Human gingival crevicular fluid contains MRP8 (S100A8) and MRP14 (S100A9), two calcium-binding proteins of the S100 family. J Dent Res. Vol. 79, No. 2, (Feb, 2000), pp. 740-747. 0022-0345 (Print) 0022-0345 (Linking)

Kotsanos, N. et al. (2005). Treatment management of first permanent molars in children with Molar-Incisor Hypomineralisation. Eur J Paediatr Dent. Vol. 6, No. 4, (Dec, 2005), pp. 179-184. 1591-996X (Print) 1591-996X (Linking)

Kukleva, M. P. et al. (2008). Molar incisor hypomineralisation in 7-to-14-year old children in Plovdiv, Bulgaria--an epidemiologic study. Folia Med (Plovdiv). Vol. 50, No. 3, (Jul-Sep, 2008), pp. 71-75. 0204-8043 (Print) 0204-8043 (Linking)

Kusku, O. O. et al. (2008). The prevalence and aetiology of molar-incisor hypomineralisation in a group of children in Istanbul. Eur J Paediatr Dent. Vol. 9, No. 3, (Sep, 2008), pp. 139-144. 1591-996X (Print) 1591-996X (Linking)

Lygidakis, N. A. (2010). Treatment modalities in children with teeth affected by molar-incisor enamel hypomineralisation (MIH): A systematic review. Eur Arch Paediatr Dent. Vol. 11, No. 2, (Apr, 2010), pp. 65-74. 1818-6300 (Print) 1818-6300 (Linking)

Lygidakis, N. A. et al. (2008). Molar-incisor-hypomineralisation (MIH). Retrospective clinical study in Greek children. I. Prevalence and defect characteristics. Eur Arch Paediatr Dent. Vol. 9, No. 4, (Dec, 2008), pp. 200-206. 1818-6300 (Print) 1818-6300 (Linking)

Lygidakis, N. A. et al. (2010). Best Clinical Practice Guidance for clinicians dealing with children presenting with Molar-Incisor-Hypomineralisation (MIH): An EAPD Policy Document. Eur Arch Paediatr Dent. Vol. 11, No. 2, (Apr, 2010), pp. 75-81. 1818-6300 (Print) 1818-6300 (Linking)

Mahoney, E. et al. (2004). Mechanical properties across hypomineralized/hypoplastic enamel of first permanent molar teeth. Eur J Oral Sci. Vol. 112, No. 6, (Dec, 2004), pp. 497-502. 0909-8836 (Print) 0909-8836 (Linking)

Mangum, J. E. et al. (2010a). Surface integrity governs the proteome of hypomineralized enamel. J Dent Res. Vol. 89, No. 10, (Oct, 2010a), pp. 1160-1165. 1544-0591 (Electronic) 0022-0345 (Linking)

Mangum, J. E. et al. (2010b). Proteomic analysis of dental tissue microsamples. Methods Mol Biol. Vol. 666, No., 2010b), pp. 309-325. 1940-6029 (Electronic) 1064-3745 (Linking)

Marshman, Z. et al. (2009). The impact of developmental defects of enamel on young people in the UK. Community Dent Oral Epidemiol. Vol. 37, No. 1, (Feb, 2009), pp. 45-57. 1600-0528 (Electronic) 0301-5661 (Linking)

Martinez Gomez, T. P. et al. (2011). Prevalence of molar-incisor hypomineralisation observed using transillumination in a group of children from Barcelona (Spain). Int J Paediatr Dent, No., (Aug 24, 2011), 1365-263X (Electronic) 0960-7439 (Linking)

Mathu-Muju, K.&Wright, J. T. (2006). Diagnosis and treatment of molar incisor hypomineralization. Compend Contin Educ Dent. Vol. 27, No. 11, (Nov, 2006), pp. 604-610; quiz 611. 1548-8578 (Print) 1548-8578 (Linking)

Moynihan, P. & Petersen, P. E. (2004). Diet, nutrition and the prevention of dental diseases. Public Health Nutr. Vol. 7, No. 1A, (Feb, 2004), pp. 201-226. 1368-9800 (Print) 1368-9800 (Linking)

Muratbegovic, A. et al. (2008). Molar-incisor-hypomineralisation impact on developmental defects of enamel prevalence in a low fluoridated area. Eur Arch Paediatr Dent. Vol. 9, No. 4, (Dec, 2008), pp. 228-231. 1818-6300 (Print) 1818-6300 (Linking)

Nishio C. Formação do esmalte dentário, novas descobertas, novos horizontes. R Dental Press Ortodon Ortop Facial Maringá, v. 13, n. 4, p. 17-18, jul./ago. 2008.

Reid, D. J. & Dean, M. C. (2006). Variation in modern human enamel formation times. J Hum
    Evol. Vol. 50, No. 3, (Mar, 2006), pp. 329-346. 0047-2484 (Print) 0047-2484 (Linking)
Reid, D. J. & Ferrell, R. J. (2006). The relationship between number of striae of Retzius and
    their periodicity in imbricational enamel formation. J Hum Evol. Vol. 50, No. 2,
    (Feb, 2006), pp. 195-202. 0047-2484 (Print) 0047-2484 (Linking)
Rodd, H. D. et al. (2007a). Pulpal status of hypomineralized permanent molars. Pediatr
    Dent. Vol. 29, No. 6, (Nov-Dec, 2007a), pp. 514-520. 0164-1263 (Print) 0164-1263
    (Linking)
Rodd, H. D. et al. (2007b). Pulpal expression of TRPV1 in molar incisor hypomineralisation.
    Eur Arch Paediatr Dent. Vol. 8, No. 4, (Dec, 2007b), pp. 184-188. 1818-6300 (Print)
    1818-6300 (Linking)
Rodd, H. D. & Boissonade, F. M. (2002). Comparative immunohistochemical analysis of the
    peptidergic innervation of human primary and permanent tooth pulp. Arch Oral
    Biol. Vol. 47, No. 5, (May, 2002), pp. 375-385. 0003-9969 (Print) 0003-9969 (Linking)
Schulze, K. A. et al. (2004). Micro-Raman spectroscopic investigation of dental calcified
    tissues. J Biomed Mater Res A. Vol. 69, No. 2, (May 1, 2004), pp. 286-293. 1549-3296
    (Print) 1549-3296 (Linking) Scottish Intercollegiate Guidelines Network. Clinical
    guidelines and SIGN. March,2004, pp:1
    http://cys.bvsalud.org/lildbi/docsonline/9/5/159-sign50section1.pdf   Acessed:
    Nov 2011.
Smith, C. E. (1979). Ameloblasts: secretory and resorptive functions. J Dent Res. Vol. 58, No.
    Spec Issue B, (Mar, 1979), pp. 695-707. 0022-0345 (Print) 0022-0345 (Linking)
Soviero, V. et al. (2009). Prevalence and distribution of demarcated opacities and their
    sequelae in permanent 1st molars and incisors in 7 to 13-year-old Brazilian
    children. Acta Odontol Scand. Vol. 67, No. 3, 2009), pp. 170-175. 1502-3850
    (Electronic) 0001-6357 (Linking)
Suckling, G. et al. (1988). The macroscopic and scanning electron-microscopic appearance
    and microhardness of the enamel, and the related histological changes in the
    enamel organ of erupting sheep incisors resulting from a prolonged low daily dose
    of fluoride. Arch Oral Biol. Vol. 33, No. 5, 1988), pp. 361-373. 0003-9969 (Print) 0003-
    9969 (Linking)
Suckling, G. W. (1989). Developmental defects of enamel--historical and present-day
    perspectives of their pathogenesis. Adv Dent Res. Vol. 3, No. 2, (Sep, 1989), pp. 87-
    94. 0895-9374 (Print) 0895-9374 (Linking)
Suga, S. (1989). Enamel hypomineralization viewed from the pattern of progressive
    mineralization of human and monkey developing enamel. Adv Dent Res. Vol. 3,
    No. 2, (Sep, 1989), pp. 188-198. 0895-9374 (Print) 0895-9374 (Linking)
Sundfeld, R. H. et al. (2007a). Enamel microabrasion followed by dental bleaching for
    patients after orthodontic treatment--case reports. J Esthet Restor Dent. Vol. 19, No.
    2, 2007a), pp. 71-77; discussion 78. 1496-4155 (Print) 1496-4155 (Linking)
Sundfeld, R. H. et al. (2007b). Considerations about enamel microabrasion after 18 years. Am
    J Dent. Vol. 20, No. 2, (Apr, 2007b), pp. 67-72. 0894-8275 (Print) 0894-8275 (Linking)
van Amerongen, W. E. & Kreulen, C. M. (1995). Cheese molars: a pilot study of the etiology
    of hypocalcifications in first permanent molars. ASDC J Dent Child. Vol. 62, No. 4,
    (Jul-Aug, 1995), pp. 266-269. 1945-1954 (Print) 1945-1954 (Linking)

Weerheijm, K. L. (2003). Molar incisor hypomineralisation (MIH). Eur J Paediatr Dent. Vol. 4, No. 3, (Sep, 2003), pp. 114-120. 1591-996X (Print) 1591-996X (Linking)

Weerheijm, K. L. (2004). Molar incisor hypomineralization (MIH): clinical presentation, aetiology and management. Dent Update. Vol. 31, No. 1, (Jan-Feb, 2004), pp. 9-12. 0305-5000 (Print) 0305-5000 (Linking)

Weerheijm, K. L. et al. (2001). Molar-incisor hypomineralisation. Caries Res. Vol. 35, No. 5, (Sep-Oct, 2001), pp. 390-391. 0008-6568 (Print) 0008-6568 (Linking)

Weerheijm, K. L. et al. (2003). Judgement criteria for molar incisor hypomineralisation (MIH) in epidemiologic studies: a summary of the European meeting on MIH held in Athens, 2003. Eur J Paediatr Dent. Vol. 4, No. 3, (Sep, 2003), pp. 110-113. 1591-996X (Print) 1591-996X (Linking)

Weerheijm, K. L. & Mejare, I. (2003). Molar incisor hypomineralization: a questionnaire inventory of its occurrence in member countries of the European Academy of Paediatric Dentistry (EAPD). Int J Paediatr Dent. Vol. 13, No. 6, (Nov, 2003), pp. 411-416. 0960-7439 (Print) 0960-7439 (Linking)

Welbury, R. et al. (2004). EAPD guidelines for the use of pit and fissure sealants. Eur J Paediatr Dent. Vol. 5, No. 3, (Sep, 2004), pp. 179-184. 1591-996X (Print) 1591-996X (Linking)

William, V. et al. (2006a). Molar incisor hypomineralization: review and recommendations for clinical management. Pediatr Dent. Vol. 28, No. 3, (May-Jun, 2006a), pp. 224-232. 0164-1263 (Print) 0164-1263 (Linking)

William, V. et al. (2006b). Microshear bond strength of resin composite to teeth affected by molar hypomineralization using 2 adhesive systems. Pediatr Dent. Vol. 28, No. 3, (May-Jun, 2006b), pp. 233-241. 0164-1263 (Print) 0164-1263 (Linking)

Willmott, N. S. et al. (2008). Molar-incisor-hypomineralisation: a literature review. Eur Arch Paediatr Dent. Vol. 9, No. 4, (Dec, 2008), pp. 172-179. 1818-6300 (Print) 1818-6300 (Linking)

Wright, J. T. (2002). The etch-bleach-seal technique for managing stained enamel defects in young permanent incisors. Pediatr Dent. Vol. 24, No. 3, (May-Jun, 2002), pp. 249-252. 0164-1263 (Print)

Wright, J. T. et al. (1996). Protein characterization of fluorosed human enamel. J Dent Res. Vol. 75, No. 12, (Dec, 1996), pp. 1936-1941. 0022-0345 (Print) 0022-0345 (Linking)

Wright, J. T. et al. (1997). The protein composition of normal and developmentally defective enamel. Ciba Found Symp. Vol. 205, No., 1997), pp. 85-99; discussion 99-106. 0300-5208 (Print) 0300-5208 (Linking)

Wright, J. T. et al. (2009). Human and mouse enamel phenotypes resulting from mutation or altered expression of AMEL, ENAM, MMP20 and KLK4. Cells Tissues Organs. Vol. 189, No. 1-4, 2009), pp. 224-229. 1422-6421 (Electronic) 1422-6405 (Linking)

Xie, Z. et al. (2008). Transmission electron microscope characterisation of molar-incisor-hypomineralisation. J Mater Sci Mater Med. Vol. 19, No. 10, (Oct, 2008), pp. 3187-3192. 0957-4530 (Print) 0957-4530 (Linking)

Xie, Z. et al. (2009). Structural integrity of enamel: experimental and modeling. J Dent Res. Vol. 88, No. 6, (Jun, 2009), pp. 529-533. 1544-0591 (Electronic) 0022-0345 (Linking)

Zawaideh, F. I. et al. (2011). Molar incisor hypomineralisation: prevalence in Jordanian children and clinical characteristics. Eur Arch Paediatr Dent. Vol. 12, No. 1, (Feb, 2011), pp. 31-36. 1818-6300 (Print) 1818-6300 (Linking)

Permissions

The contributors of this book come from diverse backgrounds, making this book a truly international effort. This book will bring forth new frontiers with its revolutionizing research information and detailed analysis of the nascent developments around the world.

We would like to thank LI, Ming-yu, for lending his expertise to make the book truly unique. He has played a crucial role in the development of this book. Without his invaluable contribution this book wouldn't have been possible. He has made vital efforts to compile up to date information on the varied aspects of this subject to make this book a valuable addition to the collection of many professionals and students.

This book was conceptualized with the vision of imparting up-to-date information and advanced data in this field. To ensure the same, a matchless editorial board was set up. Every individual on the board went through rigorous rounds of assessment to prove their worth. After which they invested a large part of their time researching and compiling the most relevant data for our readers. Conferences and sessions were held from time to time between the editorial board and the contributing authors to present the data in the most comprehensible form. The editorial team has worked tirelessly to provide valuable and valid information to help people across the globe.

Every chapter published in this book has been scrutinized by our experts. Their significance has been extensively debated. The topics covered herein carry significant findings which will fuel the growth of the discipline. They may even be implemented as practical applications or may be referred to as a beginning point for another development. Chapters in this book were first published by InTech; hereby published with permission under the Creative Commons Attribution License or equivalent.

The editorial board has been involved in producing this book since its inception. They have spent rigorous hours researching and exploring the diverse topics which have resulted in the successful publishing of this book. They have passed on their knowledge of decades through this book. To expedite this challenging task, the publisher supported the team at every step. A small team of assistant editors was also appointed to further simplify the editing procedure and attain best results for the readers.

Our editorial team has been hand-picked from every corner of the world. Their multi-ethnicity adds dynamic inputs to the discussions which result in innovative outcomes. These outcomes are then further discussed with the researchers and contributors who give their valuable feedback and opinion regarding the same. The feedback is then collaborated with the researches and they are edited in a comprehensive manner to aid the understanding of the subject.

Apart from the editorial board, the designing team has also invested a significant amount of their time in understanding the subject and creating the most relevant covers. They scrutinized every image to scout for the most suitable representation of the subject and create an appropriate cover for the book.

The publishing team has been involved in this book since its early stages. They were actively engaged in every process, be it collecting the data, connecting with the contributors or procuring relevant information. The team has been an ardent support to the editorial, designing and production team. Their endless efforts to recruit the best for this project, has resulted in the accomplishment of this book. They are a veteran in the field of academics and their pool of knowledge is as vast as their experience in printing. Their expertise and guidance has proved useful at every step. Their uncompromising quality standards have made this book an exceptional effort. Their encouragement from time to time has been an inspiration for everyone.

The publisher and the editorial board hope that this book will prove to be a valuable piece of knowledge for researchers, students, practitioners and scholars across the globe.

List of Contributors

Andréa C.B. Silva
Center of Sciences, Technology and Health, Brazil

Daniela C.C. Souza, Gislaine S. Portela and Fábio C. Sampaio
State University of Paraiba, Araruna, Paraiba, Brazil
Health Science Center, Federal University of Paraiba, João Pessoa, Paraiba, Brazil

Demetrius A.M. Araújo
Center of Biotechnology, Federal University of Paraiba, João Pessoa, Paraiba, Brazil

Tsuneyuki Oku, Michiru Hashiguchi and Sadako Nakamura
University of Nagasaki Siebold, Japan

Alexandra Saldarriaga Cadavid
Faculty of Odontology, Pediatric Dentistry and Epidemilogy, Research Department, Colombia

Rubén Darío Manrique Hernández
Department of Epidemiology, Colombia

Clara María Arango Lince
Faculty of Odontology, Pediatric Dentistry Department, CES University, Medellín , Colombia

Elżbieta Jodkowska
Medical University of Warsaw, Poland

Arezoo Tahmourespour
Islamic Azad University, Khorasgan- Isfahan Branch, Iran

Cafer Türkmen
Marmara University, Dentistry Faculty, Depertment of Restorative Dentistry, Istanbul, Turkey

Airton O. Arruda, Scott M. Behnan and Amy Richter
University of Michigan, USA

Adriana Bona Matos, Cynthia Soares de Azevedo, Patrícia Aparecida da Ana, Sergio Brossi Botta and Denise Maria Zezell
University of São Paulo, School of Dentistry and Nuclear and Energetic Research Institute, Brazil

Laura Emma Rodríguez-Vilchis, Rosalía Contreras-Bulnes, Felipe González-Solano, Judith Arjona-Serrano, María del Rocío Soto-Mendieta and Blanca Silvia González-López
Centro de Investigación y Estudios Avanzados en Odontología, Facultad de Odontología de la Universidad Autónoma del Estado de México, México

Hamidreza Poureslami
Associate Professor, Department of Paediatric Dentistry, Dental School, Kerman, University of Medical Sciences, Iran

Tayebeh Malek Mohammadi
Kerman University of Medical Sciences, Iran

Elizabeth Jane Kay
Peninsula Dental School, UK

Guang-yun Lai
Department of Restorative Dentistry and Periodontology, Ludwig-Maximilians-University, Munich, Germany

Ming-yu Li
Shanghai Key Laboratory of Stomatology, Shanghai Research Institute of Stomatology, Ninth People's Hospital, Medical College, Shanghai Jiao Tong University, Shanghai,P.R. China

Tomoko Hamasaki and Tadamichi Takehara
Kyushu Women's University, Kyushu Dental College, Japan

Márcia Pereira Alves dos Santos
School of Dentistry, Fluminense Federal University, Brazil
School of Dentistry, Federal University of Rio de Janeiro, Brazil

Lucianne Cople Maia
School of Dentistry, Federal University of Rio de Janeiro, Brazil

Printed in the USA
CPSIA information can be obtained
at www.ICGtesting.com
JSHW011452221024
72173JS00005B/1046

9 781632 421869